TIPS AND TRICKS IN ENDOVASCULAR SURGERY

Tips and Tricks in Endovascular Surgery is a practical, experience-driven guide to mastering both the fundamentals and the most advanced aspects of endovascular procedures.

From basic interventions to complex cases, this book walks readers through the often-unspoken details that are usually learned through years of practice – or trial and error. Each Tip is designed to stand alone, providing actionable insights that can immediately improve technique, decision-making, and outcomes. Richly illustrated with step-by-step diagrams and supported by real-world clinical experience, this volume bridges the gap between academic learning and the realities of daily vascular surgery.

As new technologies and techniques reshape the field at an unprecedented pace, this is a much-needed "toolbox" for endovascular surgeons, interventional radiologists, and interventional cardiologists who want to stay sharp, safe, and effective in their work. More than just a manual, this is a companion in the operating room – built from observation, mistakes, and small victories, and written for those who believe that the best surgeons never stop learning.

TIPS AND TRICKS IN ENDOVASCULAR SURGERY

A "HOW TO" GUIDE FOR REACHING THE NEXT LEVEL IN ENDOVASCULAR SURGERY

Giovanni Solimeno, MD

Division of Vascular and Endovascular Surgery
Pineta Grande Hospital
Castelvolturno (CE), Italy

CRC Press
Taylor & Francis Group
Boca Raton London New York

CRC Press is an imprint of the
Taylor & Francis Group, an **informa** business

Cover images: Giovanni Solimeno © (Figures 3.11, 4.7, 4.9 and 5.5)

First edition published 2026
by CRC Press
4 Park Square, Milton Park, Abingdon, Oxon, OX14 4RN

and by CRC Press
2385 NW Executive Center Drive, Suite 320, Boca Raton, FL 33431

British Library Cataloguing-in-Publication Data
A catalogue record for this book is available from the British Library

ISBN: 978-1-032-93672-7 (hbk)
ISBN: 978-1-032-93671-0 (pbk)
ISBN: 978-1-003-56708-0 (ebk)

DOI: 10.1201/9781003567080

Typeset in Minion Pro
by Apex CoVantage, LLC

To my wonderful Mihaela and Camilla, who lovingly endure my head-in-the-clouds nature every single day.

To my parents, without whose support and example I could never have become the person I am today.

To Pasquale Valitutti and Matteo Salcuni, without whom you wouldn't be reading most of the Tips & Tricks in this book!

Conflict of Interest Statement

The author declares that no financial support, sponsorship, or funding of any kind was received for the mention of specific devices, brands, or products throughout this book. All references to such devices reflect solely the author's personal clinical experience and opinion, without any commercial influence or endorsement.

CONTENTS

Preface   ix

Section 1 GENERAL PRINCIPLES   1
Toolkit A – Radiation Protection Principles: Repetita Iuvant   2
Toolkit B – Tips & Tricks for Percutaneous Access   4
Toolkit C – Handling Guidewires   20
Toolkit D – Handling Catheters   28
Toolkit E – Tips & Tricks for Managing Hemostasis of Percutaneous Access   37

Section 2 TIPS & TRICKS IN INFRAINGUINAL PATHOLOGY   41
Toolkit A – Tips & Tricks in CTO Recanalization   42
Toolkit B – Tips & Tricks in Complex Recanalization   52
Toolkit C – CTO Crossing Algorithm   65
Toolkit D – Tips & Tricks in Vessel Preparation   68
Toolkit E – Tips & Tricks for the Use of Drug-Coated Balloons   78
Toolkit F – Anastomotic PTA and PTA of Stenotic Patches   80
Toolkit G – Tips & Tricks in the Endovascular Treatment of Acute Arterial Lesions   81
Toolkit H – Tips & Tricks in Popliteal Aneurysms   86

Section 3 TIPS & TRICKS IN AORTOILIAC OBSTRUCTIVE DISEASES   91
Toolkit A – Management of Percutaneous Access in Aortoiliac Pathology   92
Toolkit B – Tips & Tricks for Aortoiliac Stenoses and Occlusions   97
Toolkit C – The CERAB Technique   108
Toolkit D – Hybrid Procedures in the Context of Iliac–Femoral Recanalizations   114

Section 4 TIPS & TRICKS IN ABDOMINAL AORTIC ANEURYSMS   123
Toolkit A – Tips & Tricks in Infrarenal AAAs   124
Toolkit B – Tips & Tricks for Challenging Necks in AAA   141
Toolkit C – Tips & Tricks in the Choice of Infrarenal Endograft   154

Section 5 TIPS & TRICKS IN THE MANAGEMENT OF ILIAC ANEURYSMS   171
Toolkit A – Isolated Aneurysms of the Iliac Arteries   172
Toolkit B – Algorithm for the Treatment of Iliac Aneurysms   178
Toolkit C – Tips & Tricks in the Management of Hypogastric Aneurysms   183

Section 6 ADVANCED TIPS & TRICKS IN THE MANAGEMENT OF
               ENDOLEAKS AND PSEUDOANEURYSMS   187
Toolkit A – Tips & Tricks in Endoleak Treatment   188
Toolkit B – Tips & Tricks in the Percutaneous Treatment of Iatrogenic Femoral
               Pseudoaneurysms   205

Index   215

Note to readers: *The colored circles next to Tips – green, orange, or red (the traffic light system) – reflect the increasing level of technical difficulty required. This simple visual code reflects a progressive technical learning path:*

🟢 Green

🟠 Orange

🔴 Red

Note: *Some Tips, particularly the orange and red, require greater experience and should only be attempted by more experienced clinicians.*

PREFACE

This book does not stem from any particular technical talent of mine – quite the opposite. Rather, it originates from the awareness of certain gaps that, over the years, I came to recognize in myself: gaps that pushed me to search, observe, study, and – above all – take notes.

The notes, observations, and Tips collected over time – accompanied, whenever possible, by the scientific evidence they refer to and which I will cite throughout the text – emerged from multiple sources: from closely watching colleagues at work, from daily practice, from unexpected successes, and – not least – from mistakes.

They form the core of this volume and, because of how they were gathered over the years, they naturally took on an anecdotal tone. Each of them represents a self-contained, independent concept that still helps me today to recall what to do – and more importantly, how to do it. They are an invitation to be methodical and consistent, leaving aside improvisation – something that may be useful in art, but certainly not in science.

The book is organized into thematic sections. Each section addresses a specific area of endovascular practice and is further divided into chapters, each structured around Tips & Tricks, meant to be read and absorbed even in a non-sequential way.

This is not a book to be read from cover to cover, but rather a toolbox to consult as needed, according to your clinical context at any given time.

Next to each Tip, you will find a colored circle – green, orange, or red – based on the logic of a traffic light. These colors reflect the increasing level of technical difficulty required to apply that particular suggestion. I designed this simple visual code to help guide you along a progressive technical learning path: some Tips, particularly the orange and red ones, require greater experience and should only be attempted once you feel truly confident.

We have all learned that our beautiful discipline is based not only on study and evidence, but also – and perhaps most importantly – on the everyday reality of the operating room, with everything it entails.

This book aims to shed light precisely on that reality: the part of our craft that we all experience daily, yet which remains the hardest to learn, as it is rarely formalized and often underrepresented in the literature.

Many of the things we know, we have "stolen" by watching others. Others we have learned the hard way – through mistakes, trial and error, and frustration.

I hope this book can return some of that lived, hidden knowledge. And if even just one of the Tips & Tricks you find here sparks an idea or proves useful to you, then the effort behind its publication will have been worthwhile.

Enjoy the read!

(This book was created to share experiences and encourage practical reflection – it is not intended to provide absolute rules. The application of the suggested techniques always requires the critical judgment of the surgeon and in no way replaces official guidelines or the recommendations of scientific societies.)

Section 1

GENERAL PRINCIPLES

Toolkit A – Radiation Protection Principles: Repetita Iuvant   2
- Tips 1 to 6

Toolkit B – Tips & Tricks for Percutaneous Access   4
- Tips 7 to 13

Toolkit C – Handling Guidewires   20
- Tips 14 to 19

Toolkit D – Handling Catheters   28
- Tips 20 to 30

Toolkit E – Tips & Tricks for Managing Hemostasis of Percutaneous Access   37
- Tips 31 to 36

DOI: 10.1201/9781003567080-1

We will not delve into the theoretical concepts underlying medical physics as applied to radiation protection.

The role of the endovascular operator is to minimize radiation exposure for both themselves and the patient, reducing it to the minimum dose necessary for the procedure being performed.

TIP #1

Our discussion must necessarily begin by emphasizing the importance of properly positioning protective devices, such as the lead apron (which should have a thickness of at least 0.35 mm), the lead collar, and radiation-protective eyewear (the latter with protective lenses of at least 0.75 mm thickness). The correct placement of dosimeters is equally critical, including the wrist dosimeter, eye lens dosimeter, and body dosimeter. These dosimeters should be worn with their sensitive side positioned as closely as possible to the radiation source.

For instance, the wrist dosimeter should be worn with the sensor plate facing the volar surface of the wrist, as operators generally keep their hands oriented downward – toward the radiation source – during the procedure.

The eye lens dosimeter should be attached to the side of the eyewear closest to the radiation source, which is typically the left side for right-handed operators. Additionally, two dosimeters should be positioned on the torso: one outside the lead apron and one underneath it. The difference in absorbed doses between these two dosimeters reveals the level of protection provided by the apron.

TIP #2

To minimize the patient's exposure dose, the operating table should be positioned as close as possible to the detector (Figures 1.1–1.1a; this also improves the quality of intra-procedural imaging). The image field should be reduced as much as possible by using collimation (Figures 1.2–1.2a), which not only decreases the patient's absorbed dose but also improves image quality by reducing scattered radiation.

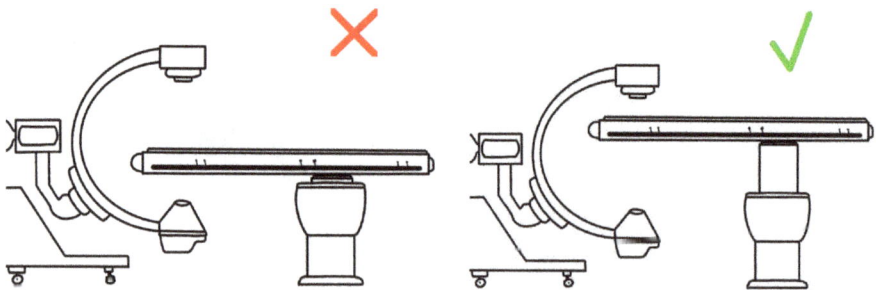

Figures 1.1–1.1a Radiation protection measures – the bed should be positioned as close as possible to the detector.

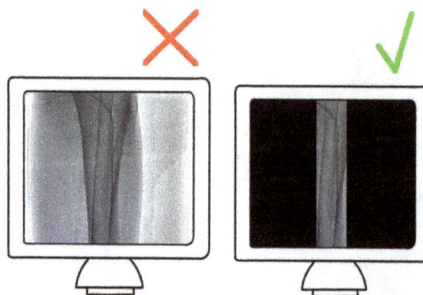

Figures 1.2–1.2a Radiation protection measures – minimize the image field using collimation.

It is important to note that image magnification increases the patient's dose. When magnification is necessary, digital zoom can be used instead, achieving a similar effect with approximately a 30% reduction in the radiation dose.

Set peripheral angiography to 1 FPS and thoracic and abdominal aortic angiography to a maximum of 2–4 FPS. Whenever possible, fluoroscopic imaging should be preferred over angiographic imaging.

To protect both the operator and the patient, the guiding principle to follow is *A.L.A.R.A. (As Low As Reasonably Achievable)*.

TIP #3

Prefer pulsed fluoroscopy over continuous fluoroscopy, setting it to the lowest pulse rate compatible with adequate image quality (the optimal pulse rate recommended by guidelines is 7.5).

TIP #4

Avoid placing hands under the fluoroscopic source. This often occurs unintentionally, such as during arterial puncture when the operator relies solely on fluoroscopy to guide the angiographic needle and localize the puncture site over the femoral head.

This underscores the critical importance of ultrasound-guided arterial puncture, a technique detailed later in this text.

TIP #5

Reserve oblique projections for only those phases when they are strictly necessary, avoiding them whenever possible. In such cases, ensure that the radiation source is not directed toward the operator. Always use radiation-protective shields (Figures 1.3–1.4) and step away from the operating table, retreating to the control room during angiographic phases whenever feasible.

TIP #6

Last but not least: meticulously plan the endovascular procedure in the preoperative phase, down to the smallest possible details. Entering the angiographic suite with a clear plan for the intervention is invaluable for reducing radiation doses during the procedure.

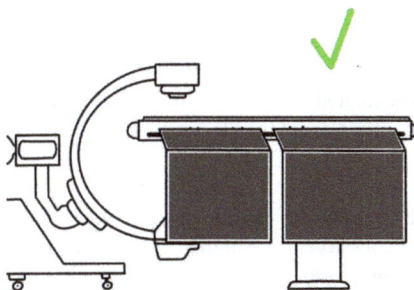

Figure 1.3 Radiation protection measures – Always use protective shields.

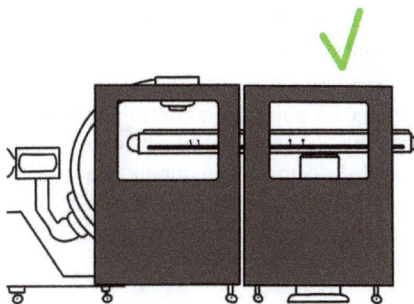

Figure 1.4 Radiation protection measures – Always use protective shields.

It may seem unusual to novices, but performing a proper percutaneous access is the most important part of any procedure. Therefore, always take the time needed before starting an endovascular procedure to plan a safe and effective access strategy, as this represents the best path to a successful outcome.

Planning the access should include the following.

1. A review of preoperative CT angiography images, if available.

2. A preoperative ultrasound mapping of the access sites, preferably performed by the primary operator.

3. A physical examination of the patient and an evaluation of their body habitus. Additionally, assessing the patient's compliance with the procedure is essential: endovascular interventions are often lengthy – and sometimes uncomfortable – and significant intraoperative restlessness can jeopardize the success of the procedure. Coordination with the anesthesiologist is critical – starting in the preoperative phase – to plan the best anesthetic strategy. It is not always necessary to perform the procedure under local anesthesia! In some cases – barring absolute contraindications – subarachnoid anesthesia may be the optimal choice.

   In other scenarios, such as patients with intractable foot pain or when subarachnoid anesthesia is contraindicated, an effective alternative could be a combination of local inguinal anesthesia and plexus anesthesia at the sciatic-popliteal level.

The access strategy should begin with an evaluation of the type of procedure to be performed. If an ultradistal procedure is planned, an antegrade access is mandatory. This approach is feasible in most cases, and its feasibility should be assessed based on the following.

- The patency of the first few centimeters of the superficial femoral artery (SFA).
- The quality of the ipsilateral common femoral artery (CFA).
- The absence of significant disease in the upstream iliac system.

In principle, antegrade access is preferred for infrainguinal pathology. This approach avoids navigating devices through the aortoiliac segment, provides greater pushability (the force the operator must apply to advance the catheter to the desired position), and facilitates the manipulation of wires and catheters. By bypassing the aortoiliac segment, the procedure is faster, and fluoroscopic exposure during aortic bifurcation crossing is avoided.

A retrograde femoral access, on the other hand, is preferable in the following scenarios.

- When iliac disease needs to be treated in conjunction with infrainguinal pathology.
- When treating the first few centimeters of the SFA, as this represents the most convenient and safest option.
- When the ipsilateral CFA is severely diseased or has been previously revascularized via open surgery (due to the presence of patches or prostheses at this level, which I consider near-absolute contraindications to percutaneous access due to the risk of septic complications or challenging hemostasis following arterial puncture).
- In patients with significant obesity, where antegrade access becomes difficult because the patient's abdomen creates a physical obstacle during arterial puncture and the procedure itself. A prominent abdomen can also push the introducer downward, causing an angulation that impedes the smooth and safe advancement of wires and catheters.

(*Note:* Literature reports the experience of some operators performing antegrade access at the origin of the SFA in cases when CFA puncture is contraindicated or challenging [e.g., obese patients or diseased arteries]. This access should be performed under ultrasound guidance and should include the use of a labeled closure system for antegrade accesses distant from the femoral head. The incidence of inguinal hematoma is higher with this approach, and it requires adequate expertise.)

Ultrasound-guided arterial puncture: This is a must for anyone performing percutaneous proce-dures. It is simple, safe, and quick. The most important advice is to standardize your own method in which you feel comfortable and confident: always use the same approach, hold the probe with the same hand, orient the probe in the same direction, and use the same ultrasound preset and settings. There is no room during this phase for improvisation or deviations from the routine.

The steps are as follows.

1. **Pre-puncture scanning:** Perform both longitudinal and transverse scans of the entire femoral tripod, including the origins of the superficial and deep femoral arteries. Evaluate the quality of the arterial wall (especially the superior wall, which will be traversed by the needle), its texture (calci-fied, fibrocalcified, or elastic), and the presence of any stenosis in the common femoral artery or at the origin of the superficial femoral artery. Even a minor stenosis at the origin of the superficial femoral artery can sometimes make guidewire engagement more challenging. In the absence of sterile gel, povidone iodine solution can be used, as it provides excellent ultrasound transparency.

2. **Positioning the probe:** Place the ultrasound probe at the chosen puncture site, ensuring that the femoral head is clearly visualized. The orientation of the probe (longitudinal or transverse) during the puncture depends on personal preference, with no option being inherently superior. Person-ally, after an initial scan in both orientations and confirming the chosen arterial puncture site in the longitudinal projection (Figures 1.5–1.5a), I prefer a transverse orientation for the ultrasound probe during the puncture. This allows precise centering of the vessel and avoids accidental venous puncture.

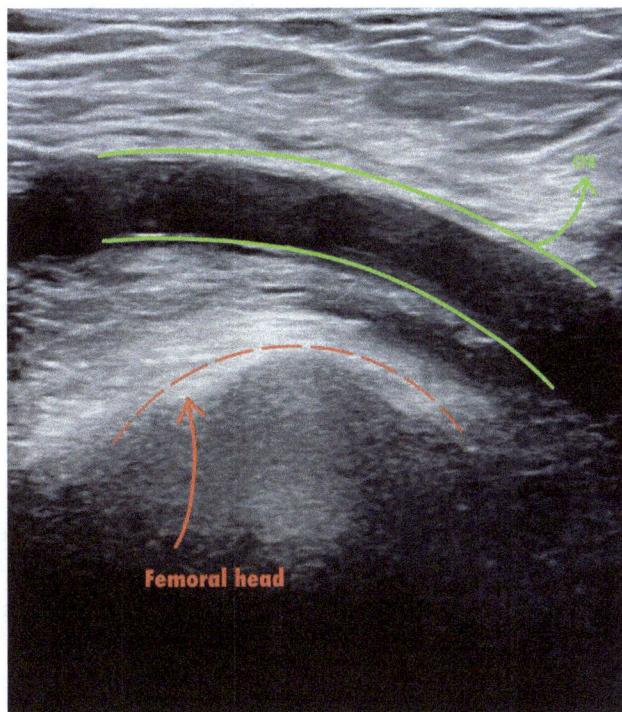

Figure 1.5 Ultrasound-guided puncture: The optimal entry point should be identified in the best-quality arterial segment lying on the femoral head.

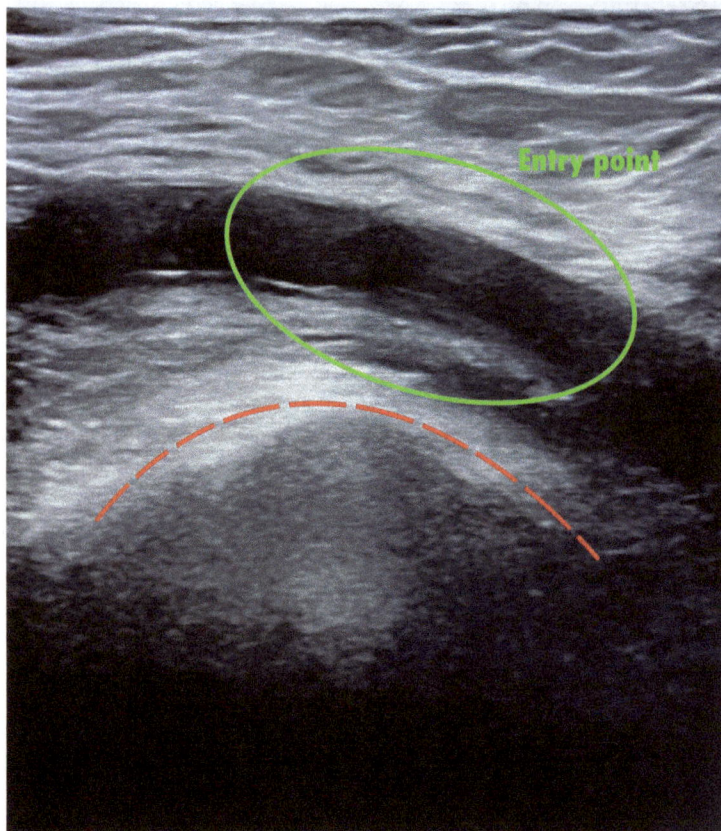

Figure 1.5a (Continued)

3. **Advancing the needle:** Slowly advance the needle through the soft tissues, clearly visualizing the point where it will enter the artery. This step is straightforward, and in most cases, the vessel can be successfully traversed in a single attempt.

4. **Maintaining needle control:** Once the artery is successfully punctured, do not release the needle to grasp the guidewire. Allowing the needle to move freely risks dislodging it from its correct intraluminal position. Instead, continue holding the needle firmly and remain still, asking your assistant to insert the guidewire.

During this phase, for antegrade access, it may be helpful to reorient the ultrasound probe longitudinally. With this perspective, by tilting the probe to visualize the superficial femoral artery in direct continuity with the common femoral artery, it is often possible to advance the guidewire into the superficial femoral artery.

If this approach does not succeed (or if antegrade puncture fails to easily direct the guidewire into the superficial femoral artery), the following steps are necessary.

- Set the ultrasound probe aside and transition to fluoroscopy.
- Switch the hand holding the needle (for right-handed operators, the right hand is typically used for arterial puncture).
- Use one hand to guide the wire into the superficial femoral artery under fluoroscopic guidance, while the other hand holds the needle firmly in position.

ANTEGRADE ACCESS UNDER FLUOROSCOPY

Referring to Figure 1.6, the femoral head can be used as a bony landmark to guide the angiographic needle. By dividing the femoral head into four quadrants, the ideal entry point for the needle to perforate the artery is the inferomedial quadrant. During antegrade access, this result can typically be achieved by puncturing the skin at the superomedial quadrant (green tick in the figure).

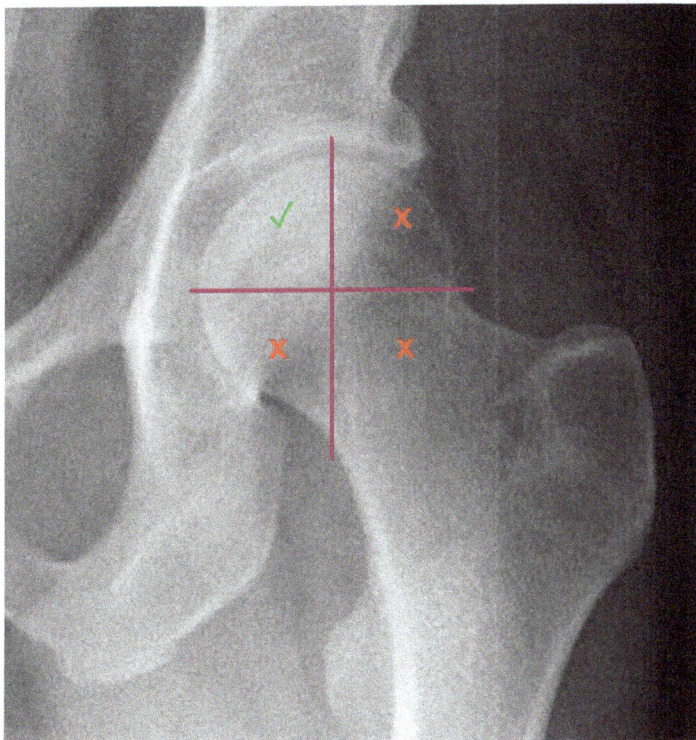

Figure 1.6 Antegrade puncture: under fluoroscopy, for correct introducer placement, the needle pierces the skin at the superomedial quadrant.

When directing the needle toward the artery, it should be held at an angle of approximately 60° to the skin plane. This approach generally ensures that the needle enters the artery at the inferomedial quadrant.

The steps we typically follow for a safe and effective antegrade access using a fully fluoroscopic technique are the following.

- **Puncture the skin and artery:** Use the technique described previously.
- **Inject contrast medium:** Perform this step under fluoroscopic guidance or using road mapping to confirm that the needle is correctly positioned in the common femoral artery. Under fluoroscopic guidance, orient the guidewire until it engages the origin of the superficial femoral artery, into which it is then directed.
- **Insert the introducer:** Once the guidewire is correctly positioned, proceed to insert the introducer.

TIP #8

In cases when, during antegrade access, the guidewire enters the profunda femoral artery and it becomes difficult to access the ostium of the superficial femoral artery, several techniques can be employed.

Wesley Moore, in his book *Endovascular Surgery*, describes the steps illustrated in Figures 1.7–1.7e:

1. Insert a standard hydrophilic guidewire into the profunda femoral artery and advance a Cobra-type catheter over it, then remove the guidewire (Figure 1.7a).

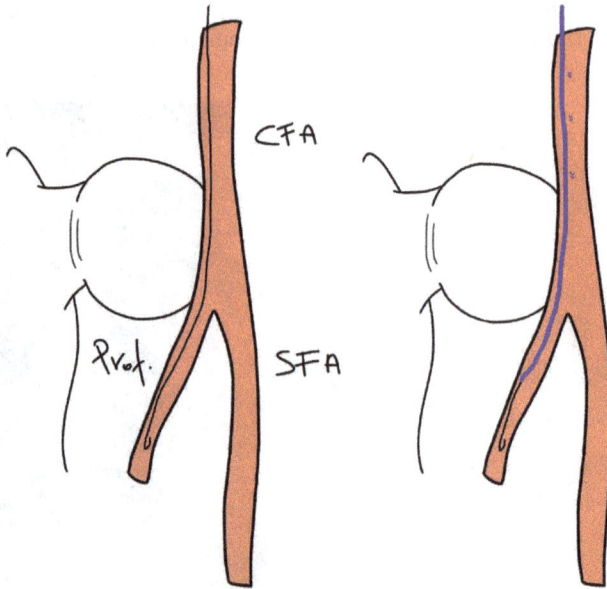

Figures 1.7–1.7a Antegrade puncture: How to redirect the introducer into the superficial femoral artery (Option 1).

2. Gently inject contrast while slowly retracting the catheter until it reaches the common femoral artery (Figures 1.7b–1.7c).

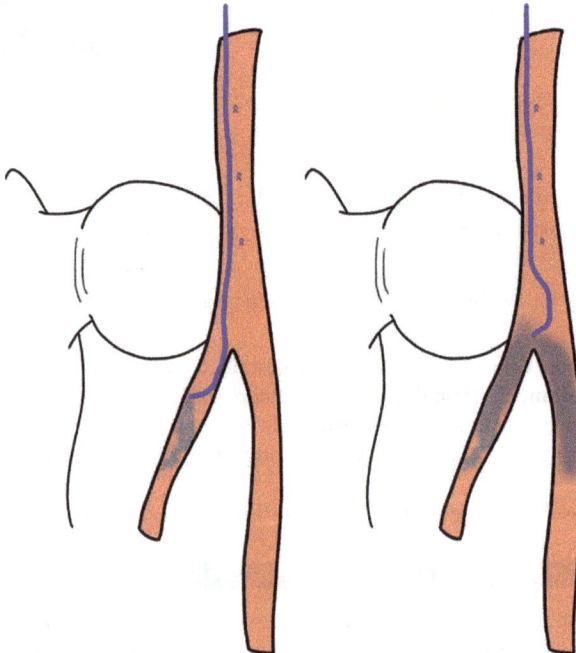

Figures 1.7b–1.7c (Continued)

3. Rotate the tip of the catheter while continuing to inject contrast until the ostium of the superficial femoral artery is visualized (Figure 1.7d).

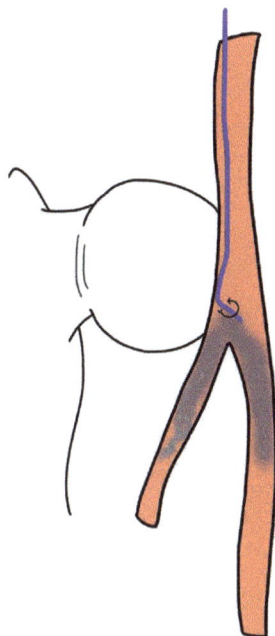

Figure 1.7d (Continued)

4. Reinsert the hydrophilic guidewire and direct it toward the superficial femoral artery. This maneuver is facilitated by the curvature of the catheter (Figure 1.7e).

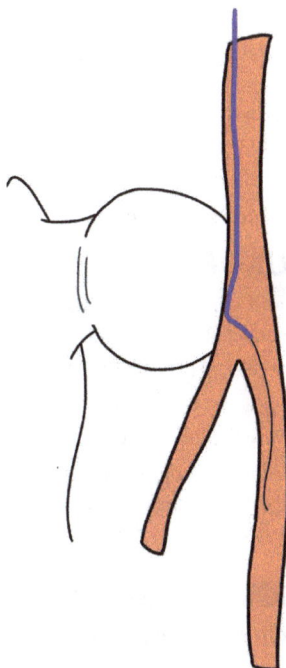

Figure 1.7e (Continued)

5. Remove the catheter and proceed with the standard technique.

An elegant solution is illustrated in Figure 1.8.

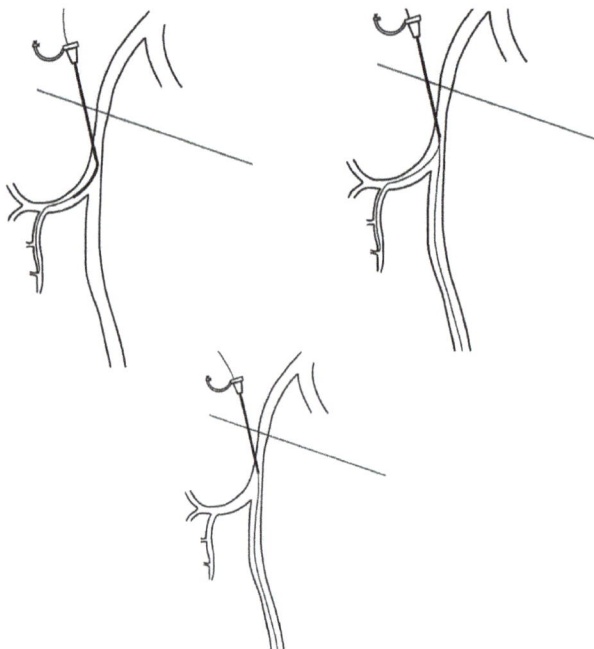

Figure 1.8 Antegrade puncture – How to redirect the introducer into the superficial femoral artery (Option 2).

1. Advance the introducer along the guidewire until it reaches the profunda femoral artery.
2. Remove the guidewire and replace it with a 0.018" wire. With this wire in place, retract the introducer while gently injecting contrast under fluoroscopy until the introducer reaches the common femoral artery.
3. Once the introducer is positioned in the common femoral artery, insert a second standard hydrophilic guidewire and use it to access the ostium of the superficial femoral artery.
4. Once the superficial femoral artery is engaged, remove the 0.018" wire from the profunda femoral artery and continue with the standard technique.

RETROGRADE ACCESS UNDER FLUOROSCOPY

This approach is easier to perform and generally presents fewer challenges compared to antegrade access. Referring to Figure 1.9, the needle, starting from below, should always enter the artery in the inferomedial quadrant. Retrograde access typically allows for greater precision without significant difficulties.

The steps according to our technique are the following.

- Insert the needle into the skin at an angle of approximately 30°, about 2–3 cm below the target zone.
- Once in the subcutaneous tissue, slightly increase the needle's angle to approximately 45°, orienting it toward the selected quadrant (the green tick in Figure 1.9).

TIP #9

FEMORAL-FEMORAL RETROGRADE CROSSOVER ACCESS

In retrograde crossover catheterization of the contralateral femoral artery, various catheters can be used to engage the ostium of the contralateral common iliac artery. The most commonly used include

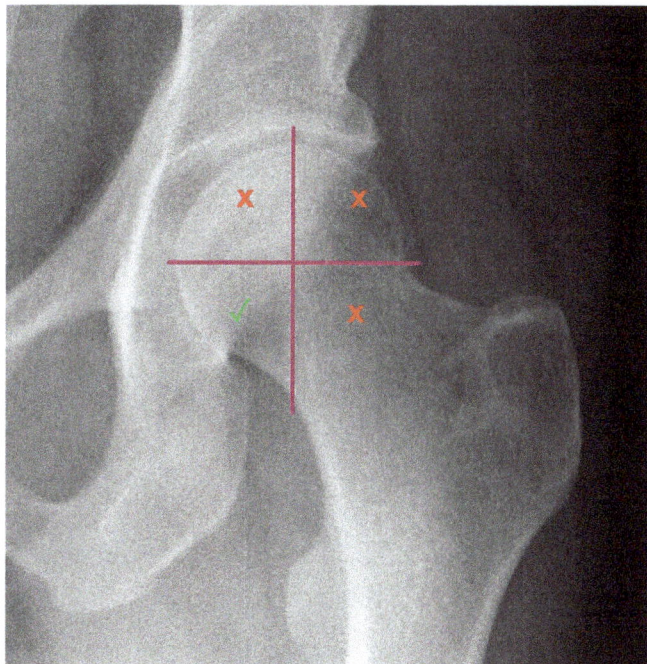

Figure 1.9 Retrograde puncture – Under fluoroscopy, the needle enters the artery at the inferomedial quadrant.

Contra, IM, RIM, UF, and Pigtail catheters. There is no universally superior catheter or technique; each operator must develop their preferred method.

My choice is generally the IM, RIM, or Contra catheter. The technique for the latter is a bit more elaborate and is as follows.

1. Once inserted into the system, advance it up to the thoracic aorta and reconstitute its curvature by withdrawing the guidewire inside the catheter (Figures 1.10–1.10a).

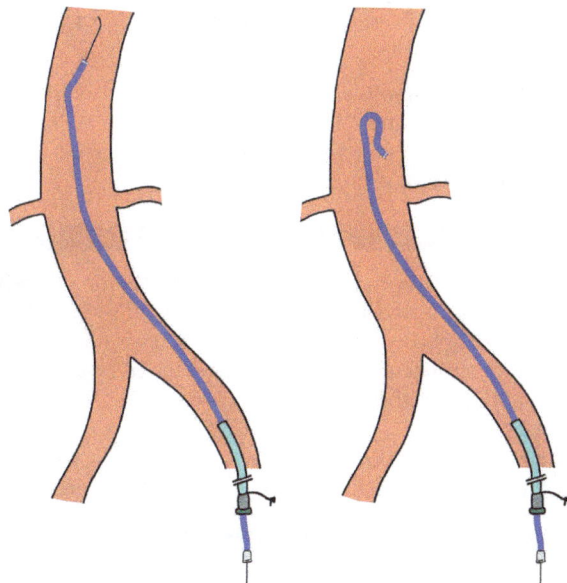

Figures 1.10–1.10a Retrograde puncture – Using the Contra catheter for crossing the aortoiliac bifurcation.

2. From this point, retract the catheter downward until it accesses the contralateral system. During this phase of retraction toward the contralateral iliac axis, extend a few centimeters of the guidewire from the catheter. Additionally, orient the catheter tip toward the right aortic wall; below the renal artery, there are no major branches on this side where the catheter could become trapped (Figures 1.10b–1.10c).

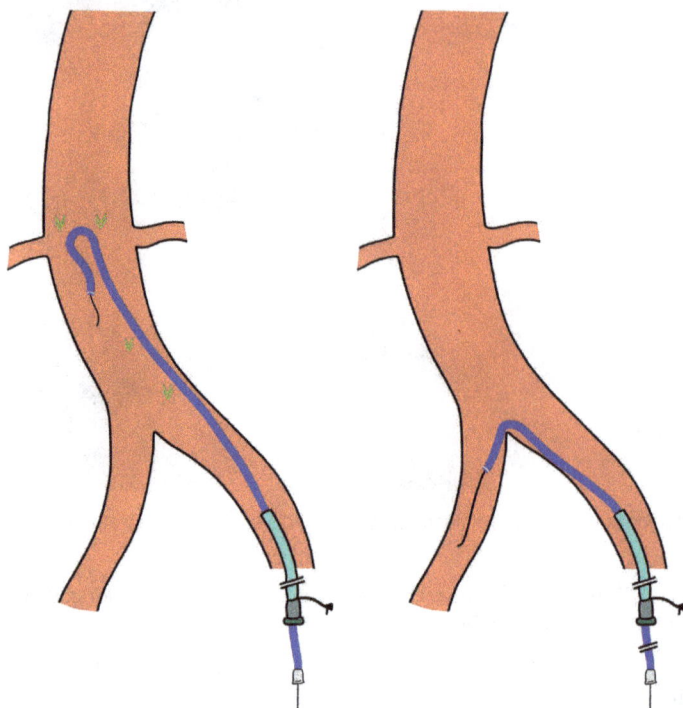

Figures 1.10b–1.10c (Continued)

3. Once near the aortic bifurcation, it becomes straightforward to direct the catheter toward the axis to be engaged.

Advance the hydrophilic guidewire into the common femoral artery and then the catheter over it. Once the catheter reaches the contralateral femoral axis, replace the hydrophilic guidewire with a more supportive one (typically a stiff or super-stiff Teflon-coated guidewire) to facilitate the necessary exchange of the short introducer with one 45 cm long.

TIP #10

Sometimes, after engaging the contralateral iliac axis with a hydrophilic guidewire, the catheter used for the crossover maneuver does not advance. This obstacle is usually caused by a narrow and highly angulated aortoiliac bifurcation or by severe calcification of the vessel wall, which creates resistance to the passage of the catheter. In such cases, the issue can be resolved by using a catheter with greater trackability, like a Bern or a Straight catheter. If these also prove ineffective, an alternative solution is to use a hydrophilic catheter (GlideCath – Terumo), which generally can navigate effectively in most anatomies. However, some anatomies – albeit rare – are truly challenging for crossover access from the contralateral side; therefore, do not overlook the possibility of a left brachial access in these situations.

TIP #11

If difficulties are encountered during the crossover advancement of the long sheath into the contralateral iliac artery, the following strategies can be employed.

- **Advance the introducer over its dilator:** Gradually reposition the dilator into its correct position, then continue advancing the introducer over it (Figures 1.11–1.11d). By proceeding step by step in this manner, the contralateral access is typically achieved without significant issues.
- **Use a stiffer guidewire:** Opt for a guidewire with greater stiffness to facilitate advancement.
- **Replace the introducer:** Switch to a reinforced introducer, such as the Terumo Destination.

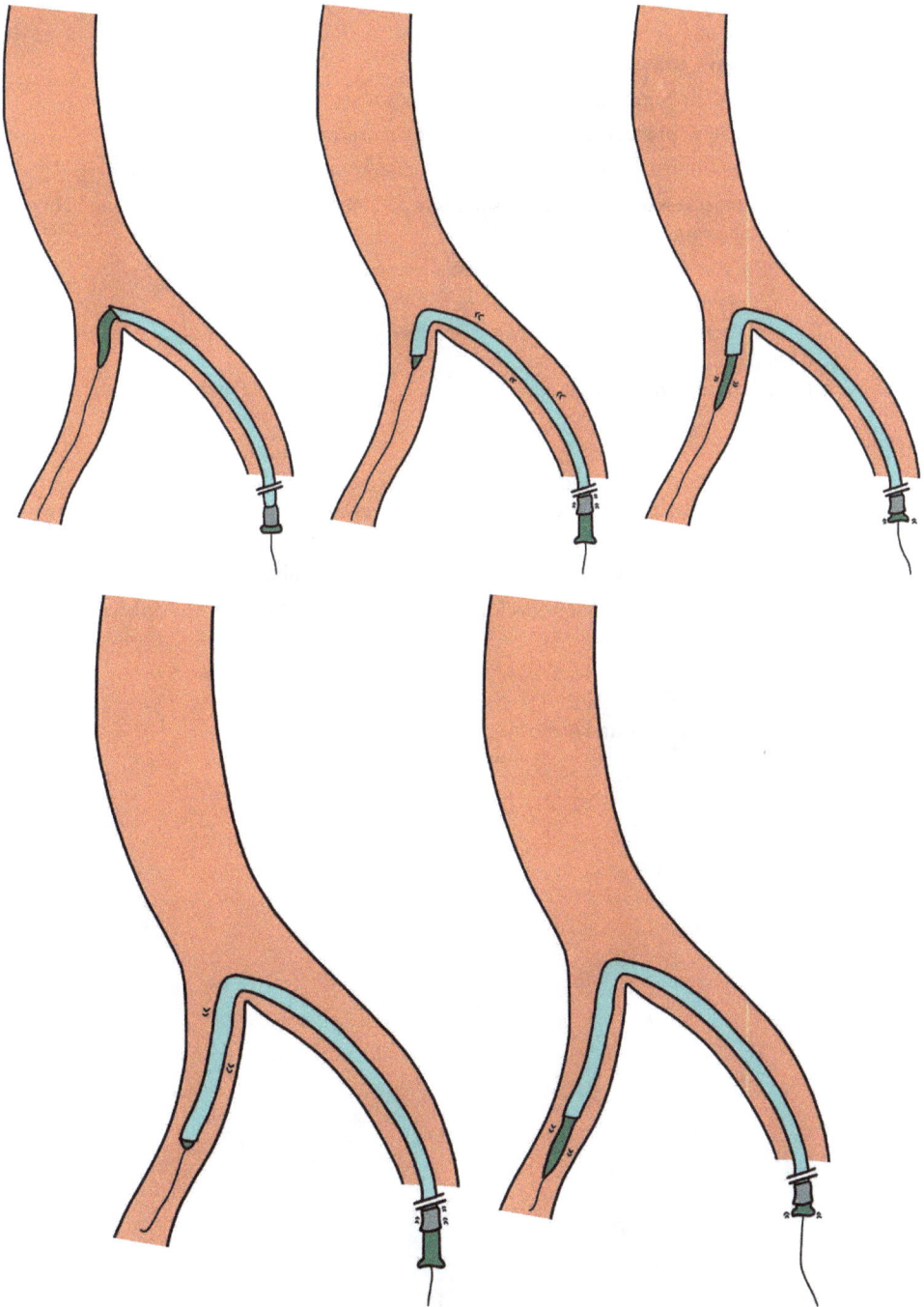

Figures 1.11–1.11d Retrograde puncture – How to navigate difficult bifurcation crossings.

● BRACHIAL ACCESS

The brachial approach is usually a valid alternative to femoral access for aortoiliac procedures. It is rarely used for infrainguinal procedures, except when femoral access is contraindicated (noting that the shaft length of current devices allows brachial access to perform procedures at most up to the superficial femoral artery).

The most frequent indications for brachial access are the following.

1. **Aortoiliac occlusions** when recanalization from below has failed or in conjunction with mono- or bifemoral retrograde access.
2. **Flush occlusion** of the common iliac artery, when contralateral recanalization is not possible.
3. As a **service access** for procedures aimed at repairing thoracoabdominal aneurysms.
4. As a **service access** for performing diagnostic angiography in aortoiliac occlusive disease.
5. When **femoral access is contraindicated**, such as in patients with previous aortobifemoral bypass grafts or infected groins.

Advantages of brachial access for aortoiliac occlusive disease are the following.

*   Excellent pushability for guidewires and catheters.
*   When subintimal recanalization of an iliac occlusion is required, an upper approach reduces the risk of extensive abdominal aortic dissections.
*   Enables advanced recanalization techniques (e.g., dual approach, Railroad Technique, etc.).

Steps for Successful Brachial Access

1. The left brachial artery is preferred because it provides a direct path to the abdominal aorta and iliac axes. Additionally, it avoids manipulating guidewires and catheters in the aortic arch, which may be diseased and prone to embolic complications in patients with occlusive pathology.
2. Always perform a preoperative ultrasound mapping to rule out subclavian artery stenosis.
3. Use an ultrasound-guided access approach as a standard, preferably combined with a micropuncture kit.
4. Puncture the brachial artery under ultrasound guidance, typically 0.5–1 cm above the antecubital crease. The arterial pulse at this level is usually strong, and the humeral head provides effective compression for post-procedural hemostasis (Figure 1.12).

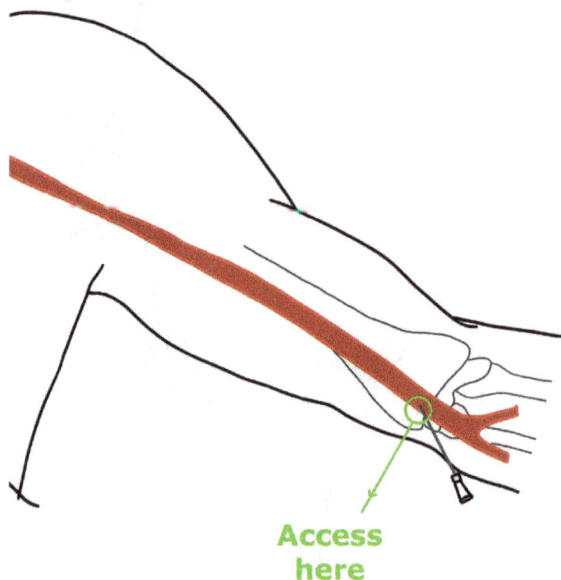

Figure 1.12 Brachial access.

5.   Begin with a short 4 Fr sheath. Bern, Contra 2, or Cobra C2 catheters can be used to easily reach the descending thoracic aorta (Figures 1.12a–1.12d).

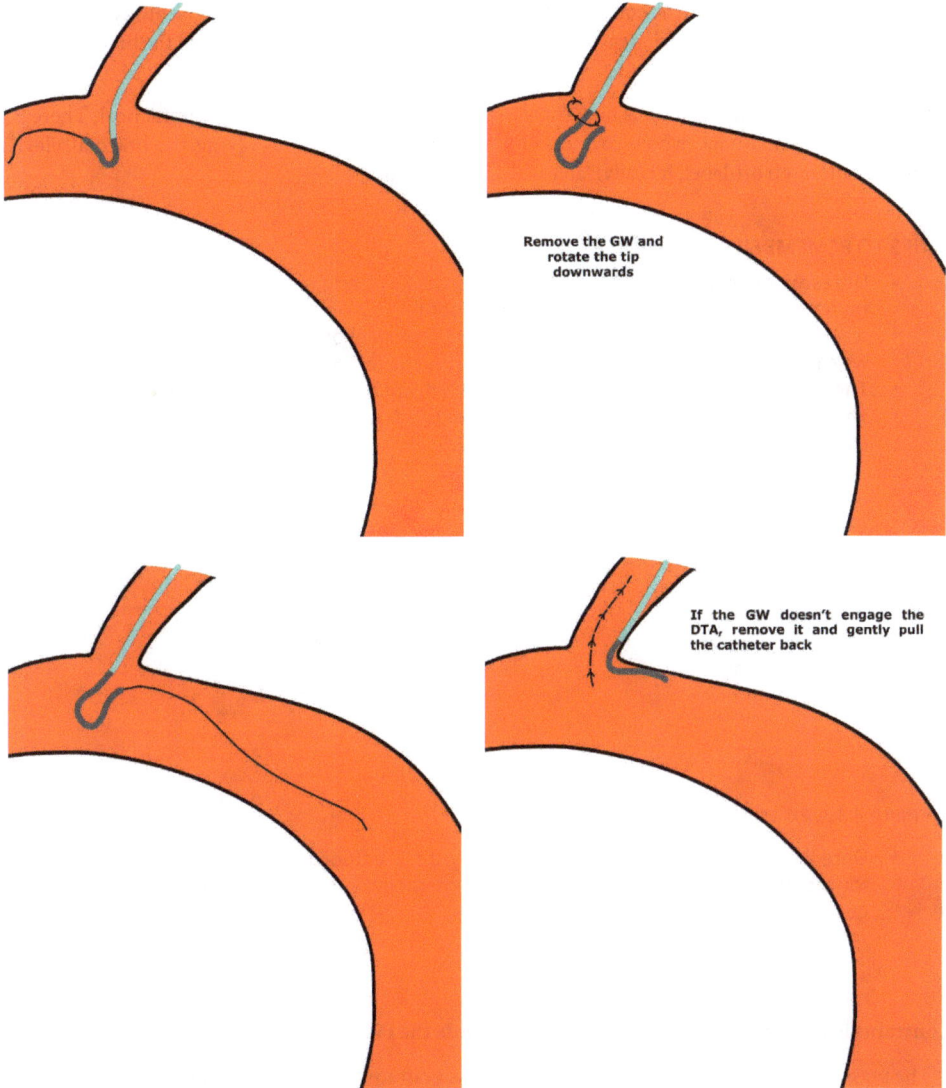

Remove the GW and
rotate the tip
downwards

If the GW doesn't engage the
DTA, remove it and gently pull
the catheter back

Figures 1.12a–1.12d (Continued)

6.   Once the target area is reached, replace the introducer with a 90 cm long sheath (4–6 Fr).

7.   At the end of the procedure, apply manual compression (percutaneous closure devices are off-label in this setting).

If a sheath larger than 6 Fr is required – or if the brachial artery is small or non-palpable – a surgical approach is recommended, according to the French school of thought. In such cases, the complication rate associated with the access tends to increase (the average complication rate for brachial access is approximately 5–6% in international studies). For this reason, brachial access should always be considered a secondary strategy to be used when necessary.

Due to its larger size and the usual absence of atherosclerotic disease at this level, some authors prefer – especially when a service access is required during endovascular procedures for thoracoabdominal aneurysmal disease – an access obtained at the axillary artery. However, this should also be considered an option only for those with adequate expertise and in limited cases. Puncture is always performed under ultrasound guidance, and great care must be taken regarding the branches of the brachial plexus that surround the artery.

Manual compression at this level is not straightforward and can sometimes be impractical. There is a risk of axillary hematoma, which can lead to neurological sequelae involving the brachial plexus. Therefore, although off-label, it is advisable to use a closure device.

TIPS TO REMEMBER

- **Ultrasound-guided percutaneous access** should be performed with the probe oriented transversely to the vessel. Some authors prefer positioning a roll of cotton towels between the scapulae to open the joint, while others prefer hyperextension of the arm. The debate about which segment of the axillary artery to use (usually the first or third segment) remains open.
- **The left axillary artery is generally preferred**, but this is not a strict requirement.
- **The complication rate is significantly reduced** when the axillary artery's diameter (lumen-to-lumen) is at least 5 mm (Figure 1.13).

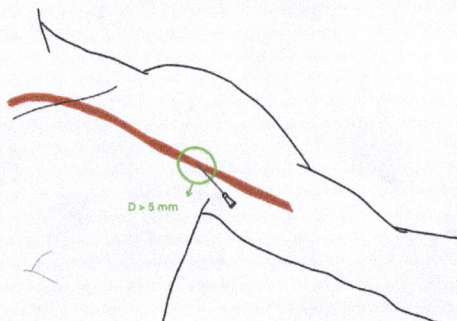

Figure 1.13 Axillary access.

- Once the guidewire is advanced into the artery, a quick **fluoroscopic check** should be performed to confirm its correct position before inserting the introducer. This ensures that the guidewire is not located in the vertebral artery.

Contraindications for the Axillary Approach Include the Following

- The presence of an internal mammary artery bypass graft to the coronary arteries.
- The presence of an arteriovenous fistula (AVF) for hemodialysis.
- The presence of a pacemaker in situ.
- Scars from prior surgical interventions or the presence of an axillobifemoral bypass.

ACCESS STRATEGY: HOW I DO IT

The debate between performing a fully fluoroscopic femoral access versus a fully ultrasound-guided access remains open and is often a source of discussion.

While ultrasound-guided puncture is preferable due to the advantages we will outline shortly, the best technique today likely lies in the middle: a hybrid approach that leverages the benefits of both methods.

Disadvantages of a Fully Fluoroscopic Technique

- The need to position hands and arms under the fluoroscopic beam, sometimes for several minutes in cases of challenging access.
- The inability to precisely define – only approximately estimate – the exact point where the needle (and subsequently the introducer) enters the artery. This can lead, sometimes unknowingly, to puncturing the most diseased portion of the CFA or an area with plaque. This issue becomes particularly concerning if a hemostatic closure device with an intra-arterial plug (such as Terumo FemoSeal or AngioSeal) is planned for use, making ultrasound-guided femoral access effectively mandatory.

Disadvantages of a Fully Ultrasound-Guided Technique

- The technical skill required, as hand coordination during the puncture and guidewire insertion phase must be precise and methodical.
- The use of a probe cover often impairs optimal visualization due to the presence of air inside the cover, which interferes with the ultrasound beam.
- Difficulty, especially in obese patients, in accurately determining the quadrant of the femoral head where the needle enters the artery. A precise puncture aligned with the femur is critical: it ensures accurate manual hemostasis during manual compression and (consequently) prevents complications related to femoral access, which remain the most common. These include complications from a high puncture (retroperitoneal bleeding) or a low puncture (superficial or deep femoral pseudoaneurysms and other vessel complications) (Figure 1.14).

This is the point...

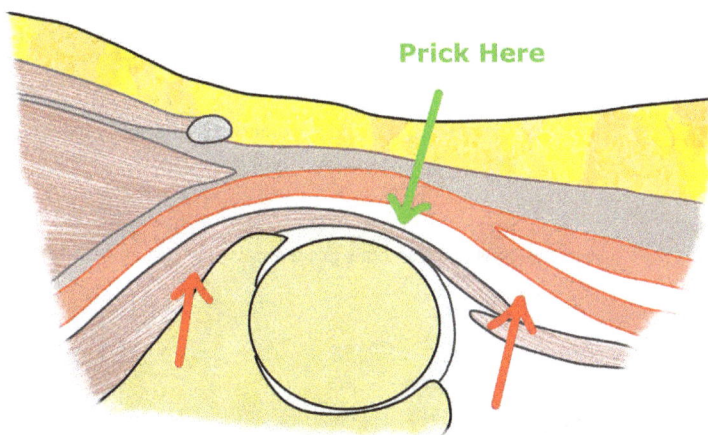

Prick Here

Figure 1.14 Anatomy of the femoral puncture (lateral view).

THE HYBRID APPROACH

This approach, which is preferred by our team and one that has caused minimal issues over thousands of endovascular procedures, is characterized by the following simple steps.

1. **Pre-procedural ultrasound mapping:** Perform an ultrasound mapping of both femoral tripods a few minutes before starting the procedure. This determines the best technique for the specific case (antegrade, retrograde, or retrograde crossover).
2. **Initial fluoroscopic guidance:** Begin by verifying the position of the needle under fluoroscopy to clearly identify its entry point relative to the femoral head, following the topographical indications described in previous tips. At this stage, you can puncture the skin (only the skin) to confirm the correct positioning of the needle.

3. **Continue with ultrasound guidance:** Use ultrasound to guide the needle precisely to the point of arterial entry.

4. **Reverse hybrid approach:** Alternatively, start by puncturing the skin under ultrasound guidance. Once the artery is reached at the area where it will be pierced with the needle, perform a fluoroscopic scan to check if the chosen access point is correctly located relative to the femoral head.

   (*Note:* In a limited number of cases, I personally opt for a fully fluoroscopic access [after preoperative evaluation of the arterial wall quality via ultrasound mapping]. This is typically for very thin patients without significant adipose tissue. In such cases, the artery lies practically under the fingers, making it very easy to puncture, with the only consideration being ensuring the correct position relative to the femoral head.)

TIP #13

It may happen that the introducer does not advance into the artery, or that the guidewire bends or loops under the skin during the insertion maneuver. This typically occurs due to the "step" created by the differing consistency between subcutaneous fat and the muscular fascia – particularly in overweight patients (Figures 1.15–1.15b). Calcification of the arterial wall further complicates the task for the guidewire/introducer system, as it adds additional resistance to the pathway.

In such cases, the following solutions can be employed.

- After arterial puncture and advancing the guidewire into the artery, ask your assistant to press with the fingers of both hands on the skin around the access site. This compresses the thickness of the adipose tissue, equalizing its resistance with that of the underlying muscular fascia.
- Thread the dilator of a 4 Fr introducer onto the guidewire. Gradually dilate the created channel until the desired introducer can be advanced.
- If at least the 4 Fr dilator has been inserted but further sheath escalation is not possible, replace the guidewire with a stiff or super-stiff Teflon-coated wire.
- Make a small skin incision.

With time and experience, you will be able to anticipate potential challenges with arterial access and adjust accordingly. The most common situations where difficulties arise include the following.

- Highly calcified arterial walls.
- Obese patients.
- Groins with scars or sites of previous percutaneous procedures.

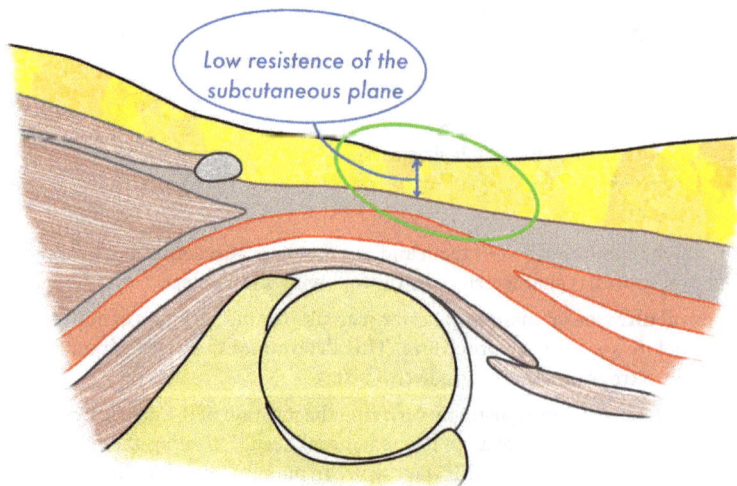

Low resistence of the subcutaneous plane

Figure 1.15 Point of greatest resistance in cases of difficulty advancing the introducer into the artery.

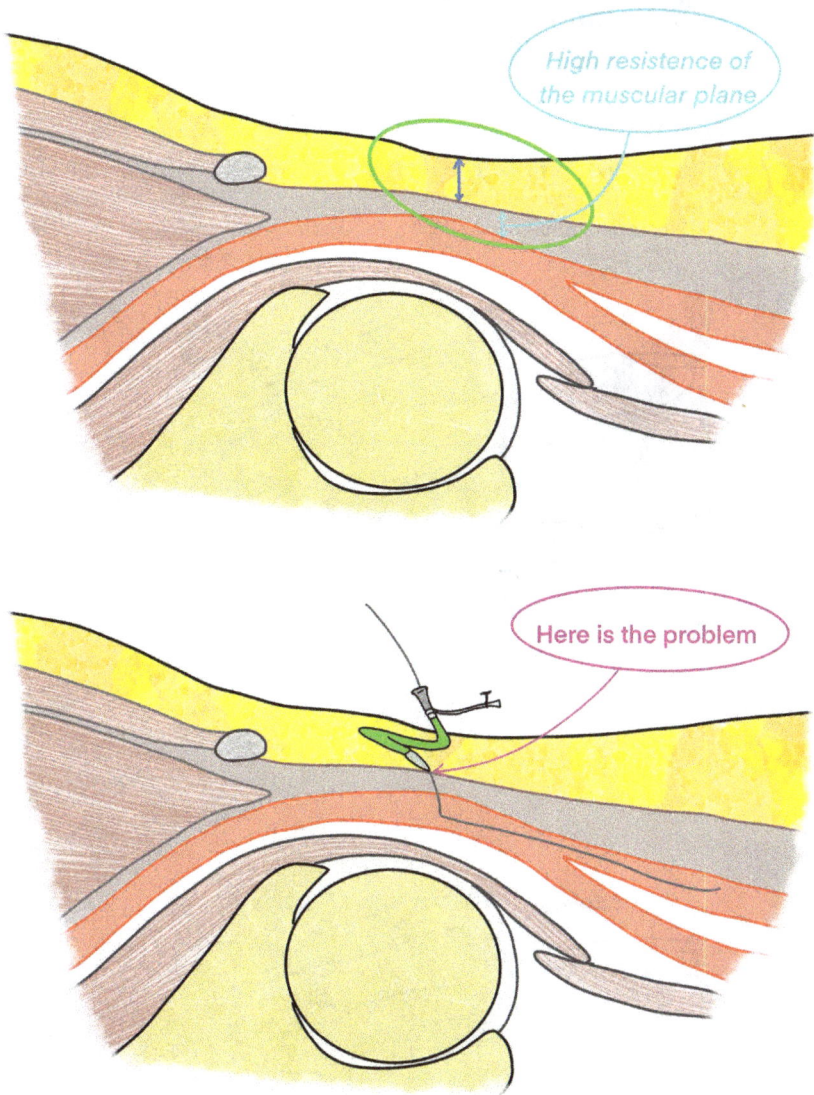

Figures 1.15a–1.15b (Continued)

In these cases, using an **advanced approach** from the outset is always a good idea. The most effective steps are the following.

- Use a stiff or super-stiff guidewire (preferably 70–80 cm in length; longer wires hinder movement at this stage) instead of a standard guidewire.
- Thread the dilator of a 4 or 5 Fr introducer onto this guidewire, then advance the desired introducer.

  (*Note:* One of the advantages of ultrasound-guided access is the ability to assess the condition of the arterial wall and select the most suitable and accommodating puncture site [Figure 1.15a].)

It is also helpful to have various types of introducers available, as some offer greater pushability but may be too rigid in certain situations.

In obese patients, it is very useful to reposition the abdomen upward and contralaterally using adhesive bands secured to the steel side rails of the operating table.

TIP #14

0.035" Hydrophilic guidewires, such as Radifocus (especially the stiff type), should preferably be advanced by gripping them firmly, sometimes even using fingernails (Figure 1.16a). Often, when held only with fingertips, their hydrophilic coating creates the illusion of advancing within the vessel, while

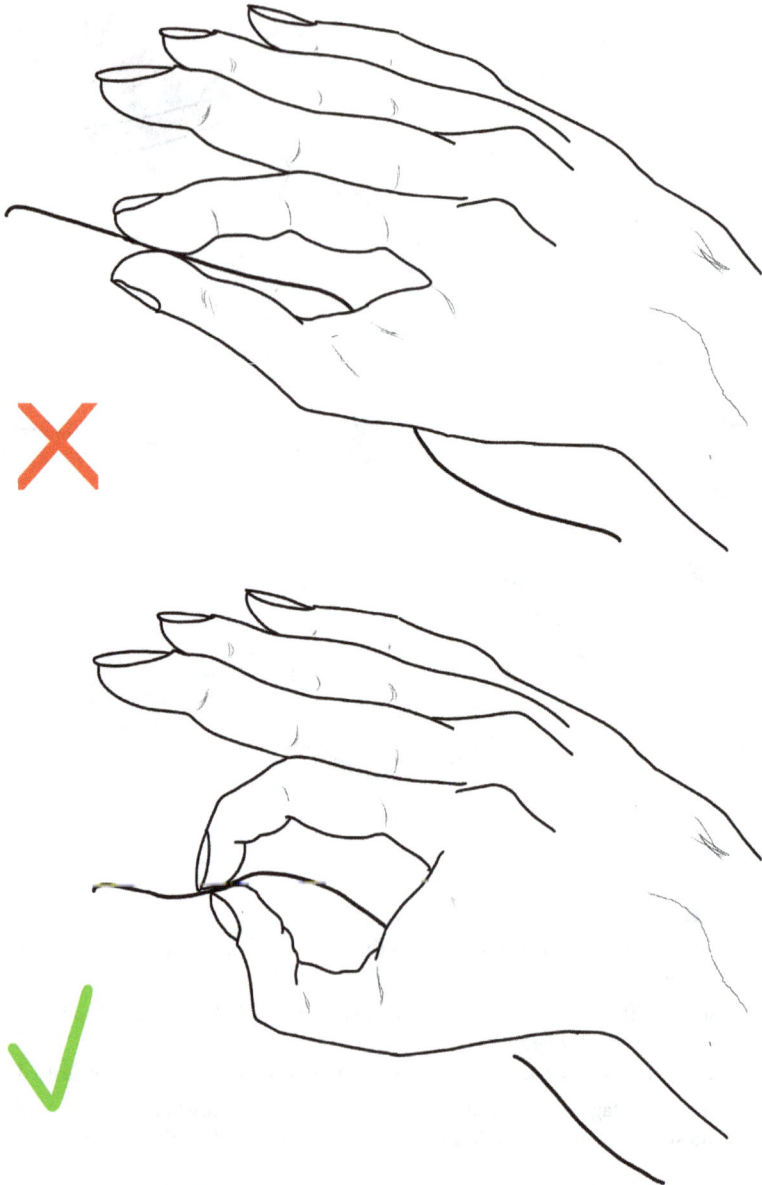

Figures 1.16–1.16a Hydrophilic guidewires often slip between the fingers; to prevent this, firmly grasp them with your fingertips.

they are actually just slipping between the fingers. **Nitrile gloves** can help increase friction, making them easier to handle.

TIP #15

High tip-load guidewires (tip load > 20–25 g) should be used with caution in below-the-knee vessels due to the risk of vessel perforation if they advance non-linearly. These guidewires should not be used as supportive wires during a PTA; once the vessel has been recanalized, they should be replaced with a supportive guidewire. When crossing a chronic total occlusion (CTO), they must progress linearly without deviating toward the vessel wall, as this poses a significant risk of perforation.

TIP #16

When the proximal cap of a CTO is particularly calcified and impenetrable, it can sometimes be helpful – in experienced hands – to perforate it using the posterior (non-floppy) end of a 0.035 hydrophilic guidewire, either standard or stiff. In such cases, extreme caution must be exercised to avoid vessel perforation.

The procedure involves reaching the CTO with a guidewire and catheter using the standard technique and positioning the catheter adjacent to it (Figures 1.17–1.17a). At this point, withdraw the guidewire from the catheter and reinsert it reversed (Figures 1.17b–1.17c). The stiff end of the guidewire should then be used as though it were a needle, advancing it only 1–2 cm beyond the catheter while ensuring it progresses in a straight line along the vessel and into the CTO cap (Figure 1.17d).

To help center the guidewire on the cap and avoid directing it toward the vessel wall, it may be useful to perform this technique with an inflated short balloon in place of a standard catheter.

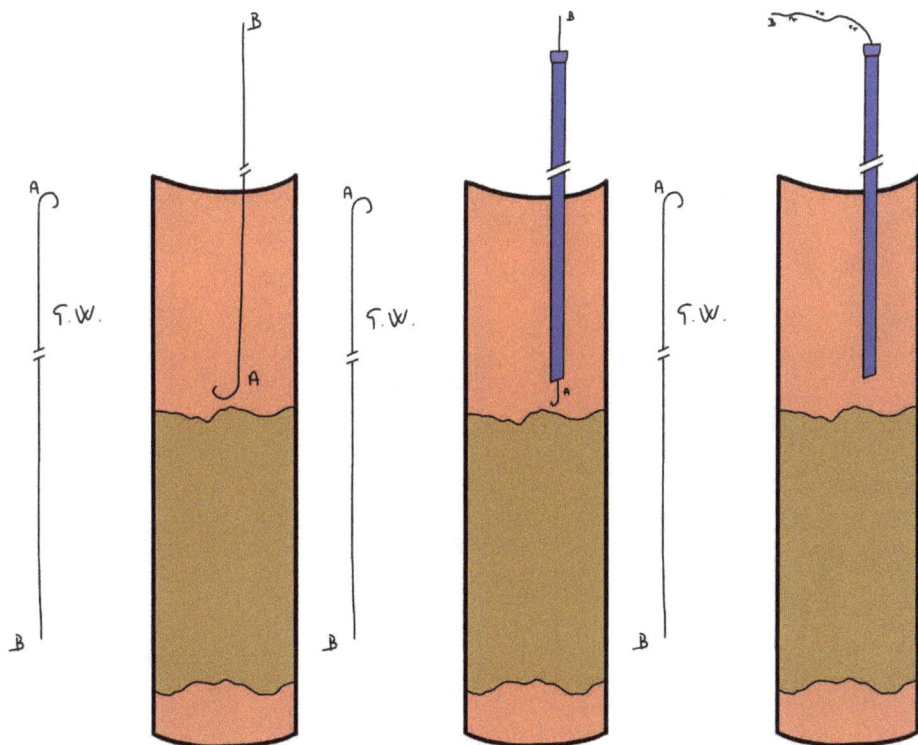

Figures 1.17–1.17b How to pierce the proximal cap of a CTO with the posterior end of a guidewire.

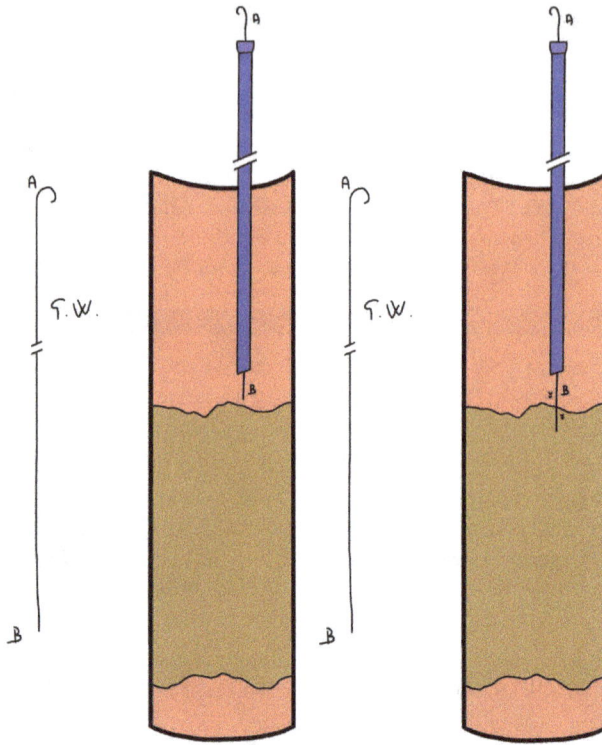

Figures 1.17c–1.17d (Continued)

This maneuver is usually sufficient to pierce the cap. Once this occurs, complete the procedure as follows.

1. Advance the catheter over the 1–2 cm of guidewire that has penetrated the CTO (Figure 1.17e).

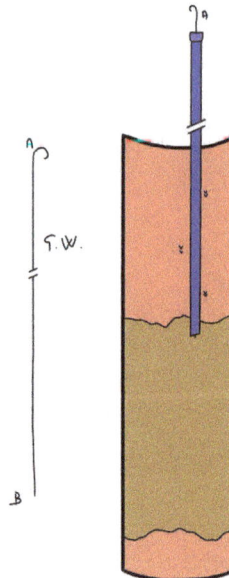

Figure 1.17e (Continued)

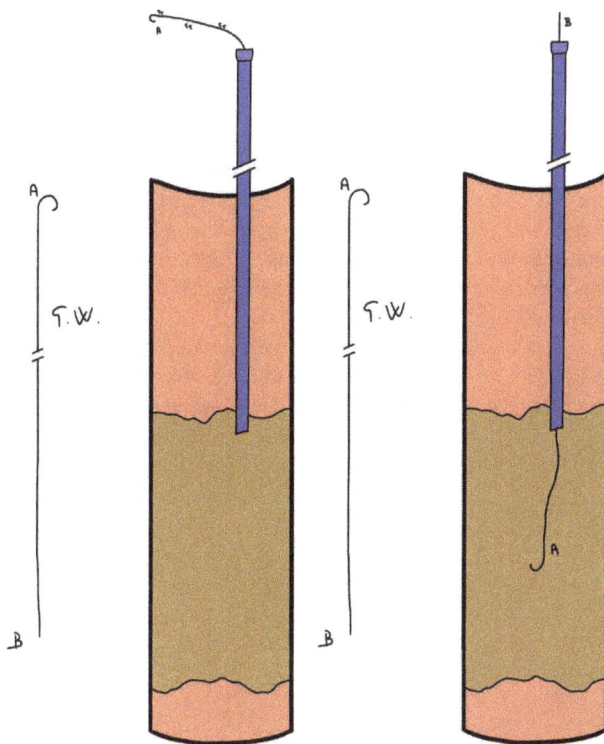

Figures 1.17f–1.17g (Continued)

2. Remove the guidewire from the catheter and reinsert it in the correct orientation – or replace it with another guidewire, depending on the situation (Figures 1.17f–1.17g).

TIP #17

Guidewire Bending

Bending the tip of a 0.018 or 0.014 guidewire is an incredibly useful skill that can assist in numerous situations. However, not all guidewires are suitable for bending. Those typically used for this purpose are medium/low tip-load guidewires, such as the Boston V18 and similar models (tip load < 10–12 g), which have a *shapeable* tip. With time and experience, operators will learn to determine the appropriate angle and length of the bend depending on the situation.

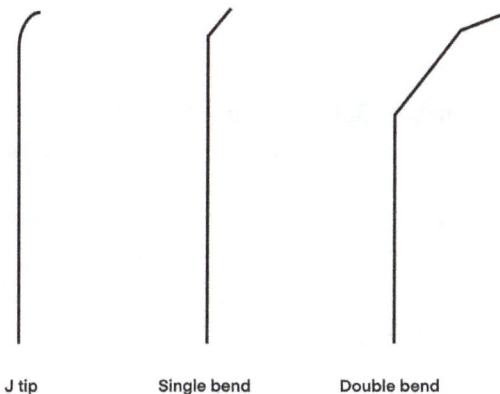

J tip   Single bend   Double bend

Figure 1.18 J curve, Single bend, and Double bend.

- **J-curve** (Figure 1.18): This can be created using the fingertips or the shaft of a needle. The motion used to bend the guidewire is similar – though gentler – to the motion used to curl a ribbon. The tip of the guidewire should be passed between the fingertips (or along the needle shaft) while applying light pressure in a pulling motion.
  The J-curve represents the basic shape, suitable for generic guidewire applications: navigating vessels, providing support in place of catheters or devices, buddy wiring, etc.
- **Single bend** (Figure 1.18): This is typically performed on the first few millimeters of the guidewire using a stylet. The guidewire is inserted into the stylet, leaving only the tip segment exposed. Gentle pressure is then applied to the exposed segment using the fingertip of the index finger.
  This type of curve is particularly useful for various techniques of endoluminal CTO recanalization, such as sliding or drilling.
- **Double bend** (Figure 1.18): To a guidewire already bent as described in the previous point, a second bend can be applied – again using a stylet – a few centimeters further along the same direction (in parallax). The second bend generally acts as a shoulder, allowing the guidewire to rest against wall prominences and thereby directing it toward otherwise hard-to-reach areas (e.g., toward a highly angulated vessel or one with an ostial stenosis – Figure 1.18a).

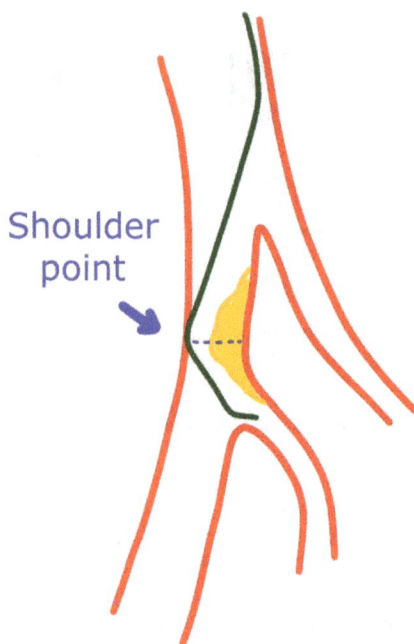

Shoulder point

Figure 1.18a Guidewire bending.

TIP #18

Buddy Wire Technique: This technique involves positioning a second guidewire parallel to the one being used. It serves several purposes.

1. **Preservation of adjacent vessels:** When treating the ostium of an arterial branch via PTA, and the procedure risks compromising an adjacent patent branch (e.g., treating the tibio-peroneal trunk and the ostium of the peroneal artery while aiming to preserve and secure access to the posterior tibial artery), the buddy wire can be advanced into the vessel to be preserved (Figures 1.19–1.19a). After PTA, if the procedure compromises the ostium of the secondary branch where the buddy wire is positioned, the buddy wire can be used to perform the necessary bailout maneuvers.

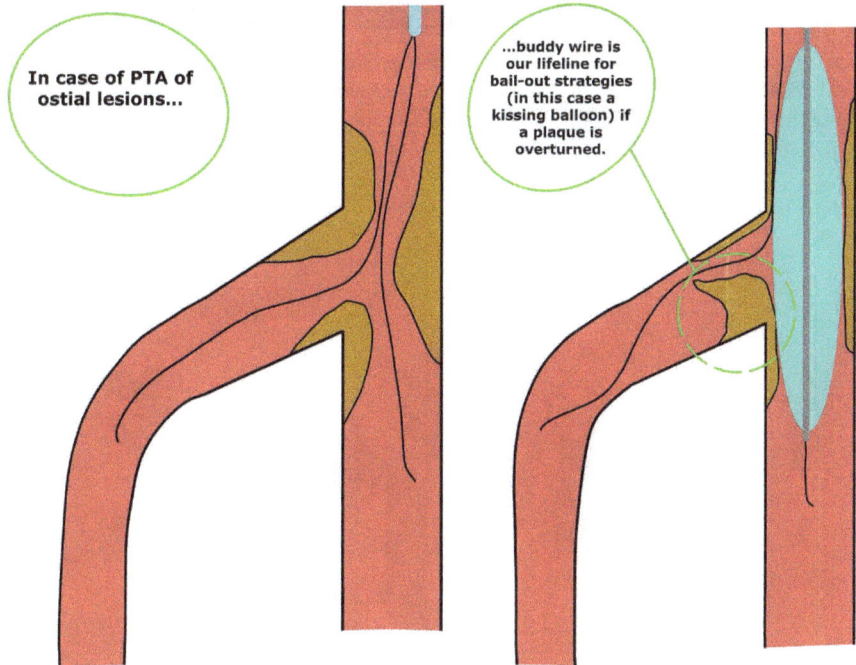

Figures 1.19–1.19a Applications of the Buddy Wire Technique

2. **Providing stability:** It enhances stability during PTA or stent deployment in highly tortuous anatomies or in severely calcified stenoses.

3. **Facilitating device advancement:** The buddy wire provides additional support to help advance the system in highly tortuous anatomies (Figures 1.19b–1.19c).

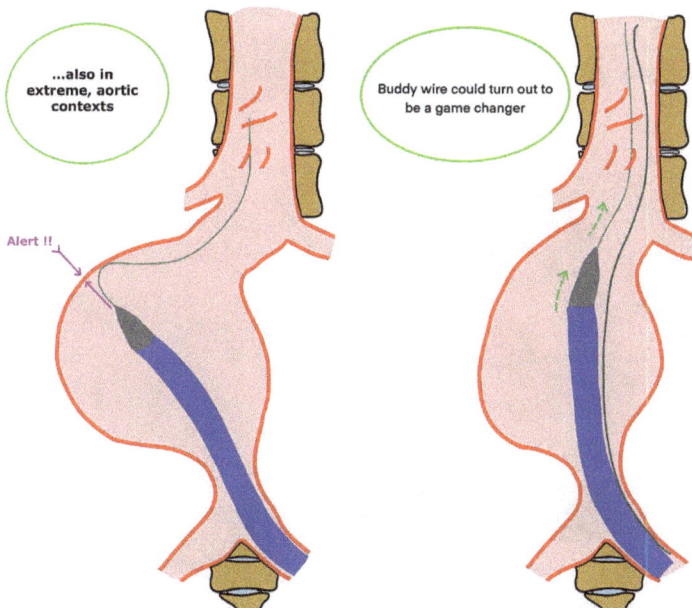

Figures 1.19–1.19c (Continued)

A clever tip borrowed from interventional cardiology can be helpful when ostial engagement of a vessel is difficult due to stenoses obstructing guidewire passage. This technique is particularly useful for stenoses located on the superior wall of the ostium of the anterior tibial artery (Figure 1.20).

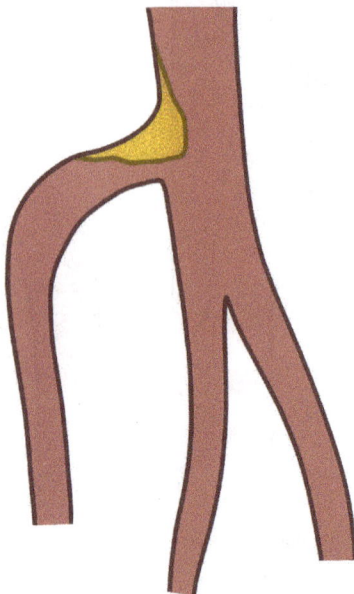

Figure 1.20 How to gain a challenging arterial ostium using the Reverse Wire Technique.

The main guidewire is advanced into the arterial tree and allowed to progress into infrapopliteal branches following the usual technique. A reverse-curved bend is applied to the tip of a second guidewire (Figure 1.20a). This second guidewire is then inserted into a Bern or Straight catheter, leaving only the curved segment exposed (Figure 1.20b).

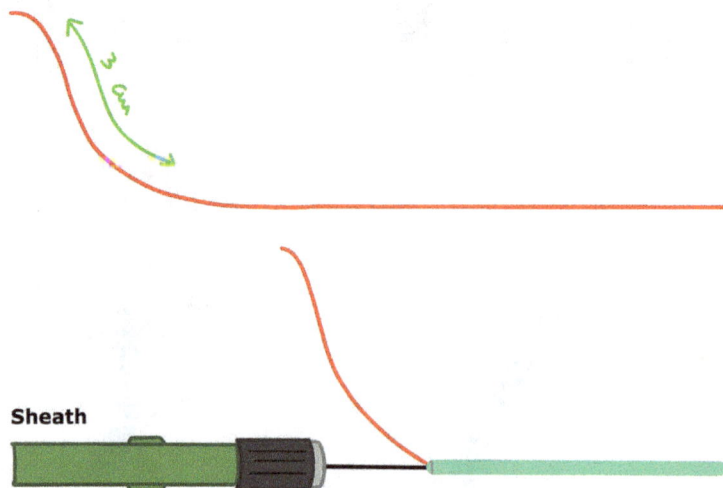

Sheath

Figures 1.20a and 1.20b (Continued)

Hold the catheter and the guidewire together with your fingers (Figure 1.20c) and advance the catheter over the main guidewire, allowing it to slide along it. In this way, the curved segment of the second guidewire, flipped backward into the arterial flow, will advance together with the catheter.

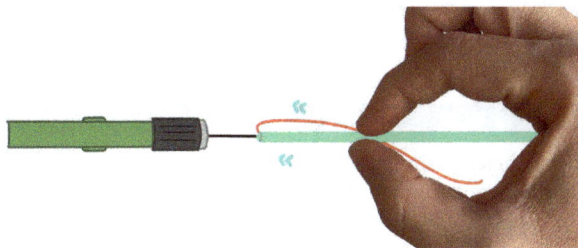

Figure 1.20c (Continued)

Progress the catheter beyond the ostial segment to be catheterized (Figure 1.20c). At this point, a careful and coordinated retraction/rotation movement of the catheter/second guidewire system will allow the second guidewire to easily engage the desired arterial ostium (Figures 1.20d–1.20f).

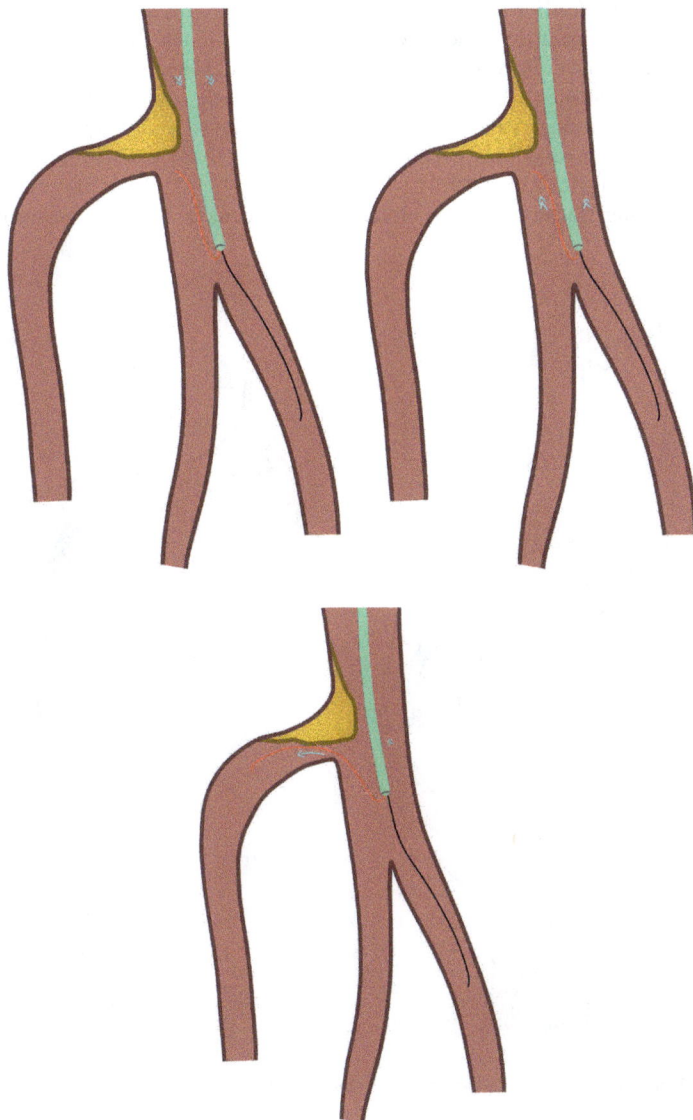

Figures 1.20d–1.20f (Continued)

TIP #20

To advance a Bern-type catheter or similar in highly tortuous, diseased, or curvilinear anatomies (or simply when the catheter does not progress), the following tips may be helpful.

- **Use catheters with the smallest possible curvature:** A Bern is preferable to a Cobra, and a Straight catheter is preferable to a Bern.
- **Opt for low-profile, high-support catheters:** A supportive catheter is preferable to a Bern in challenging anatomies.
- **Use higher-support guidewires:** These facilitate advancement.
- **Favor advancing catheters and other devices within introducers or guiding catheters whenever possible:** This approach minimizes the potential for damage (e.g., microdissections or microemboli) caused by the back-and-forth movement of devices within the arterial lumen.
- **Use rotational advancement for catheters on their guidewire:** Rotate the proximal end of the catheter repeatedly in a clockwise direction, mimicking the motion of counting a stack of banknotes. Once the catheter is "charged" with this twisting motion, grip the section emerging from the introducer with your fingers and push it forward into the vessel while keeping the guidewire stationary with the other hand. In most cases, this technique will effectively advance the catheter several centimeters (Figures 1.21–1.21b).
- **Employ the "Flossing" Technique where indicated:** This technique will be addressed in subsequent sections.

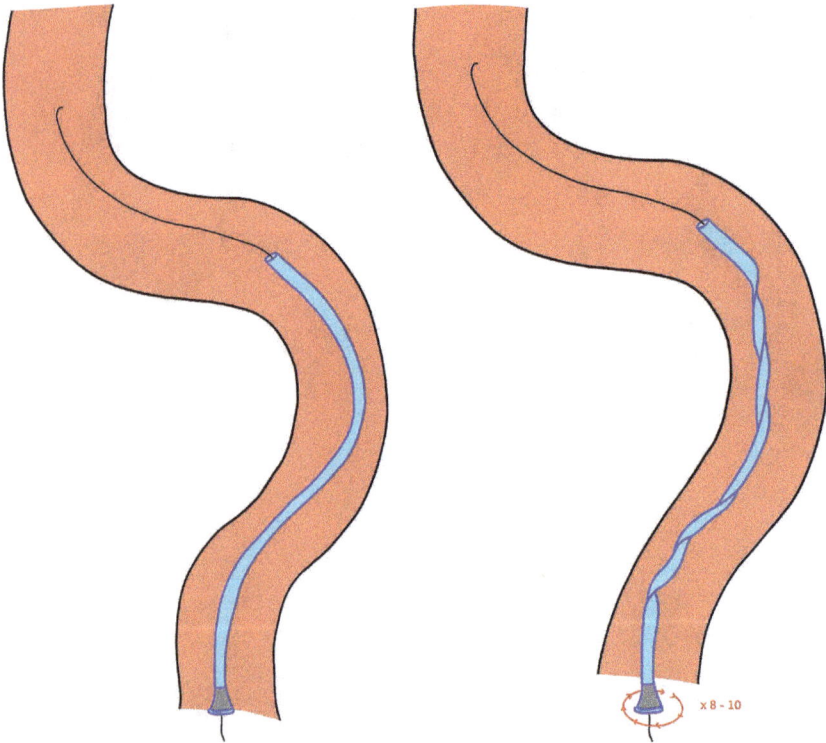

Figures 1.21–1.21a How to advance a catheter in challenging anatomies using a twisting maneuver.

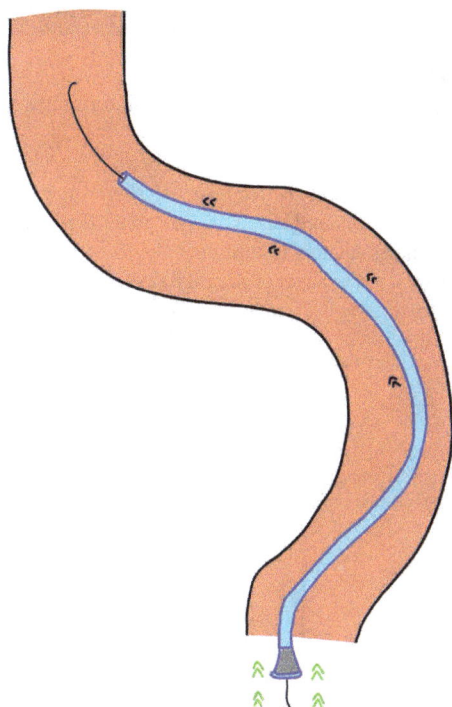

Figure 1.21b (Continued)

TIP #21

When deploying a self-expanding stent, the catheter should initially be kept stationary, ensuring that it is not pulled back from the desired implantation position. The first stent struts should then be released very, very (did I mention very?) slowly, until the first 1–2 cm of the device emerge and anchor to the artery.

From this point onward, the stent will be securely attached to the vessel wall, allowing the catheter to be held under tension for the remainder of the deployment. This ensures the stent is fully extended and prevents overlapping of its struts.

Micrometric stent deployment systems provide greater precision and control during release compared to *pull-back* systems.

TIP #22

Always remember that the larger the diameter of the catheters used, the greater the likelihood of thrombus formation around them, especially during long procedures, in highly diseased arterial segments, or in BTK vessels.

For this reason, it is advisable to always use catheters with the smallest possible French size (4 Fr or less in most circumstances), along with appropriate systemic heparinization and repeated flushing of the catheters with heparinized saline solution.

TIP #23

When removing a guidewire from a Pigtail or UF catheter, the curvature of their shaping is relatively blunt. Therefore, if only a few centimeters are involved – such as during proper positioning for an aortography in the context of an EVAR procedure – the catheter can be gently retracted or advanced without the need to reintroduce the guidewire.

However, when catheters need to be completely removed from the introducer, it is always a good practice to do so over a guidewire.

Differences between guiding catheters and long sheaths.

- Guiding catheters have an external reinforcement that provides rigidity, allowing catheters and balloons to pass smoothly over long distances.
- Guiding catheters do not have a hemostatic valve or side port.
- The French size of guiding catheters is measured based on their outer diameter, whereas long sheaths (like all introducers) are measured based on their inner diameter.
- Guiding catheters do not include a dilator. To minimize the shoulder discrepancy between the guiding catheter and the guidewire it travels over, it should be advanced with a straight or slightly angled catheter protruding a few centimeters beyond its tip (Mother and Child Technique, Figure 1.22).

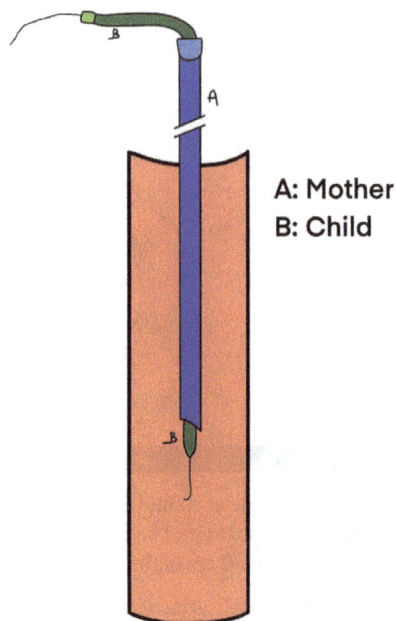

A: Mother
B: Child

Figure 1.22 The Mother and Child Technique

The **Mother and Child Technique** introduced in the previous tip also provides the following.

1. **Increased stability and support**, especially in tortuous anatomies.
2. **Improved trackability** (the ability to travel along both straight and curved paths on a guidewire).
3. **Reduced vessel trauma:** The caliber discrepancy between the guidewire and the Mother catheter can cause damage to the vessel wall, which may be "scraped" by the catheter. The Child catheter, inserted into the Mother catheter, helps prevent this by softening and gradually tapering the shoulder of the Mother catheter.

When working through a contralateral femoral access, standard catheters, such as Bern, typically reach only as far as the infrageniculate popliteal artery.

Additionally, in most cases, a crossover access does not allow the execution of a pedal plantar loop due to limitations in length and *pushability*. If an ultradistal procedure is required, it is advisable to assess the feasibility of an antegrade access, which is always preferable for infrainguinal procedures unless contraindications – often manageable – are present.

Homemade Snare

If a snare device is not available, a homemade version can be created in various ways. The method described here is simple and requires a balloon compatible with a 0.014" guidewire (2–3 mm diameter; 20–30 mm length), a 0.014" guidewire with a soft tip, and a guiding catheter (or a long sheath).

Steps

• Insert the guidewire into the balloon, allowing 20–30 mm of the wire to protrude beyond the balloon tip (Figure 1.23).

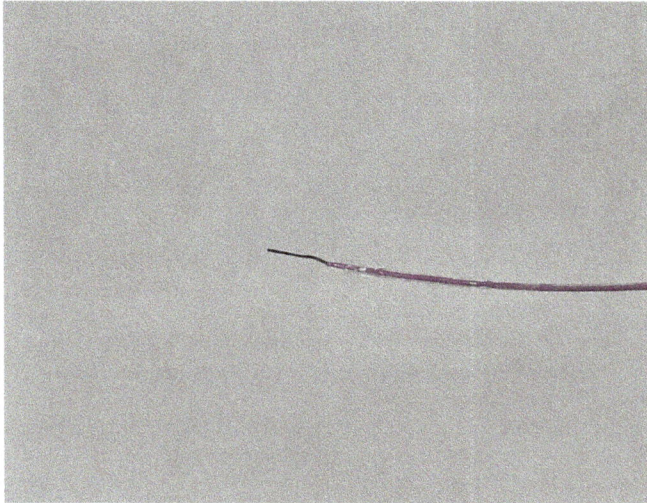

Figures 1.23–1.23c Homemade Snare (Technique A)

• Bend the protruding 20–30 mm of the guidewire backward, folding it over the balloon (Figure 1.23a). The assembled system is then inserted into the guiding catheter and advanced approximately 10–20 mm from its distal end (Figure 1.23b).

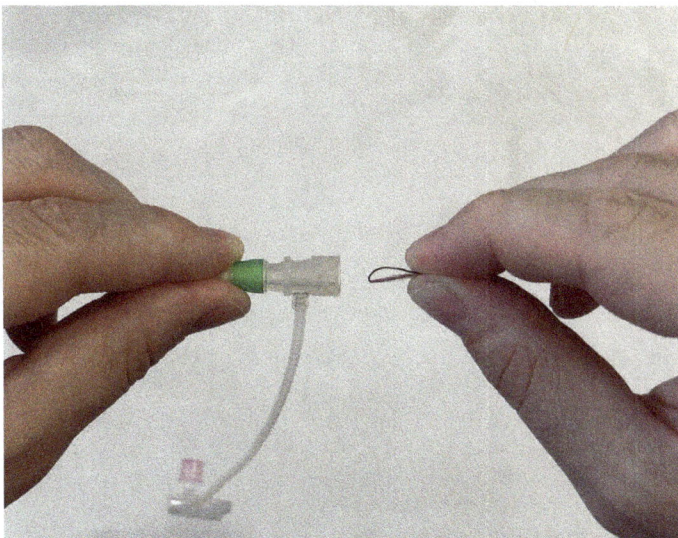

Figure 1.23a (Continued)

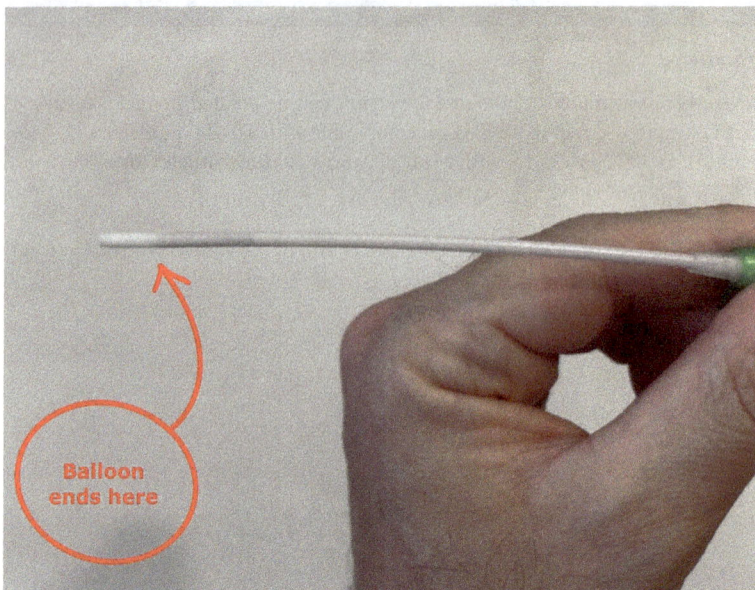

Figure 1.23b (Continued)

- When ready for use, inflate the balloon – without allowing it to emerge from the guiding catheter – up to 10–12 atm. This traps the folded segment of the guidewire against the inflated balloon inside the guiding catheter.
- At this point, manual advancement of the guidewire creates a snare with an adjustable diameter (Figure 1.23c).

Simple and elegant – try it to see for yourself!

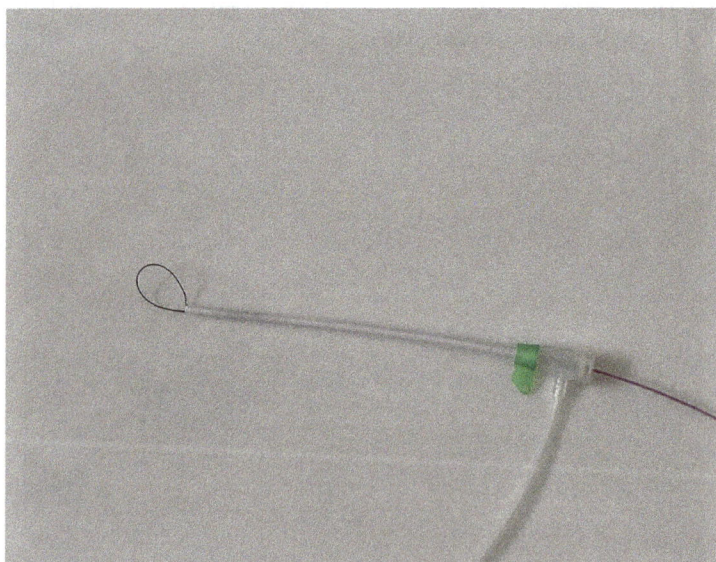

Figure 1.23c (Continued)

Homemade Snare (Alternative Method)

This alternative method uses a 0.014″ guidewire folded in half (Figure 1.24). The distal ends of the folded guidewire are inserted into a straight catheter or the dilator of a long introducer (Figures 1.24a–1.24c).

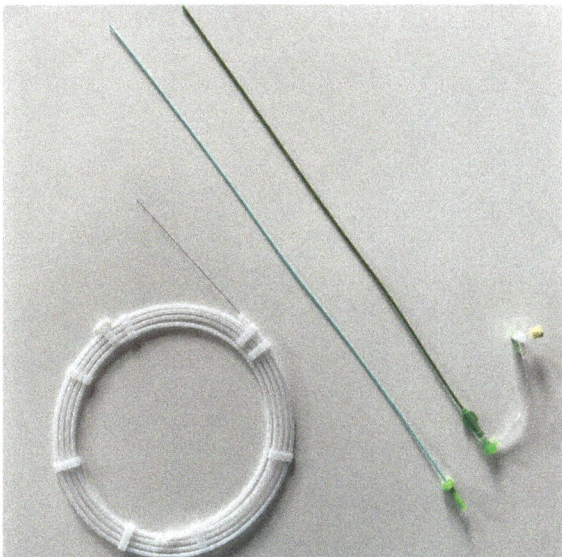

Figure 1.24 Homemade Snare (Technique B)

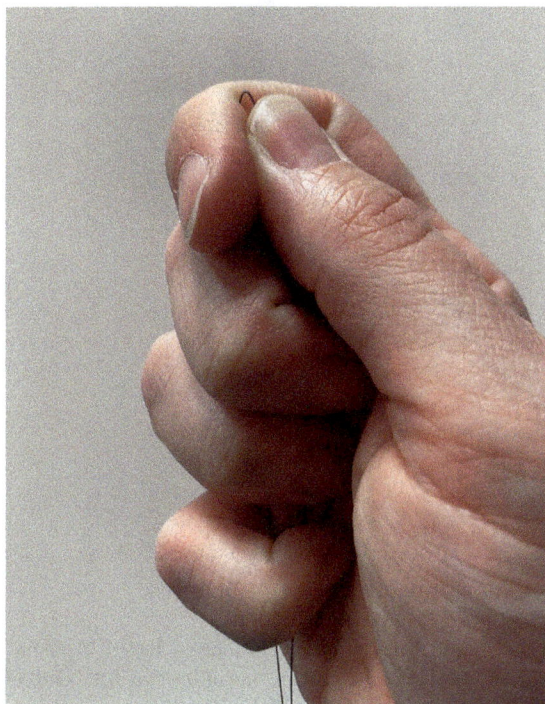

Figure 1.24a (Continued)

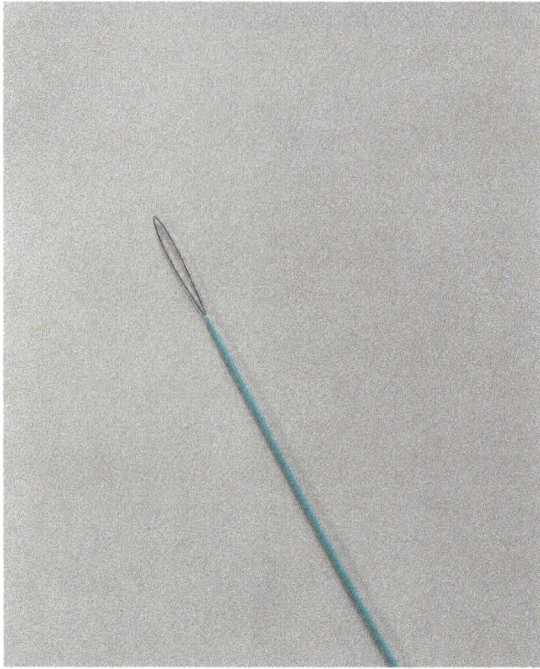

Figure 1.24b (Continued)

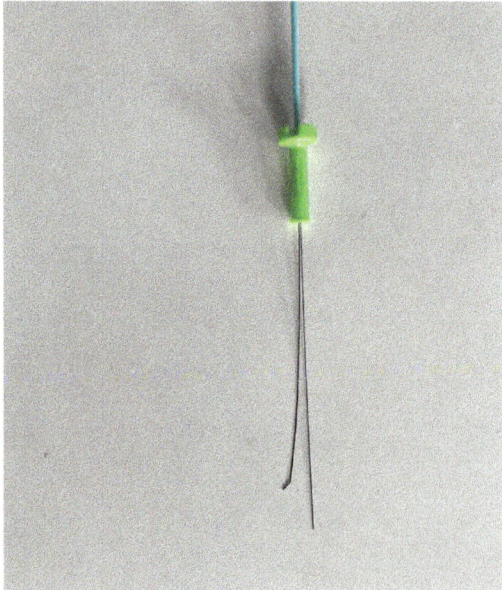

Figure 1.24c (Continued)

Steps

- Insert the assembled system into the introducer. The loop of the 0.014″ guidewire (the snare) can be enlarged or reduced by retracting or advancing one of the two distal ends of the guidewire while holding the other end steady with your fingers (Figures 1.24d–1.24e).
- Once the object to be retrieved is captured, tighten the snare loop by retracting the guidewire end and advancing the dilator or catheter in which it is housed.

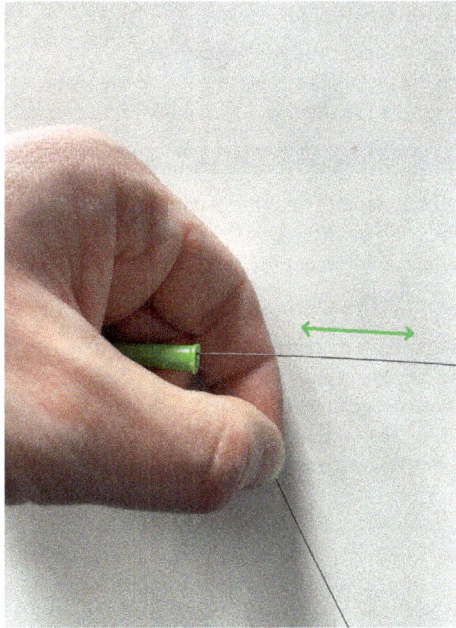

Figure 1.24d (Continued)

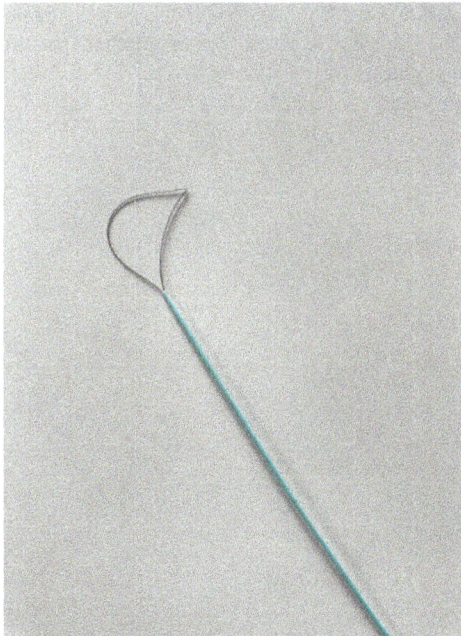

Figure 1.24e (Continued)

TIP #29

In the stenting of pre-occlusive stenoses and/or chronic occlusions – particularly when deploying a balloon-mounted stent – the lesion should always be pre-dilated. Pre-dilation ensures the safe positioning of the stent, preventing its dislodgement from the catheter during passage through the lesion.

After pre-dilation, the following steps should be taken.

- **Cross the lesion** with a long introducer or guiding catheter.
- **Advance the stent** through the introducer, centering it over the lesion.
- **Retract the introducer** to expose the stent, and then deploy it in the desired position.

TIP #30

During an infrainguinal POBA, outcomes in terms of patency and complication rates favor **long inflations** (ideally 120–180 seconds). Short inflations (30–60 seconds) are associated with higher rates of extensive dissections, stent usage, reinterventions, and residual stenoses >30%.

Additional Tips for Better Post-POBA Outcomes

- **Perfect balloon-to-vessel diameter matching:** The ratio should be 1:1. Tools like Doppler ultrasound, CTA, and IVUS can help determine the appropriate diameter.
- **Avoid excessive balloon pressures unless necessary:** Adhere to the manufacturer's guidelines and keep inflation pressures within the nominal range indicated in the instructions for use (IFU).
- **Thorough and correct use of vessel preparation techniques:** These will be discussed in more detail in the next section.
- **Gradual deflation strategy:** Although there is no clear evidence on this, my approach during balloon catheter deflation includes a slow and gradual reduction of pressure during the last 20–30 seconds of inflation. This is achieved by gently rotating the manometric syringe piston, gradually decreasing the pressure to zero. Rapid and sudden deflation may cause a vacuum effect in the vessel, potentially leading to endothelial dissections. Try releasing the manometric syringe slowly (reducing the pressure by approximately 1–2 atm every 5 seconds). Over time, you will notice the advantages of this method, which is completely free of complications. All it takes is a bit of patience – you will not regret it!
- **Managing post-POBA dissections:** If a dissection is observed on the post-POBA angiogram, remain calm (and keep the guidewire in place). Before opting for stenting – which is best avoided in critical areas such as the popliteal artery – attempt to resolve the complication with a low-pressure PTA (4–5 atm) maintained for 3–4 minutes.

TIP #31

Manual compression is the most effective form of hemostasis for percutaneous access.

An empirical rule suggests maintaining manual compression by applying finger pressure along the artery for 2–3 minutes per French. For example, for a 6 Fr introducer, at least 12–18 minutes of compression is required; for a 5 Fr introducer, at least 10–15 minutes, and so on.

Pressure is applied starting upstream from the puncture site and extending with the fingers to a point downstream along the artery. Essentially, the hands (and fingers) should be positioned side by side along this longitudinal axis of the vessel.

Ideally, an ultrasound check should be performed after compression and after the removal of the bandage, which typically occurs 6–12 hours later.

TIP #32

I personally consider relative contraindications to manual compression to include significantly obese patients and patients who are non-compliant with compression maneuvers or the subsequent bandaging. In such cases, the use of closure devices may be a safer option.

TIP #33

After compression, the access site should be covered with a layer of gauze approximately 8–10 cm thick, and an elastic adhesive bandage, such as Tensoplast, should be applied.

To Apply the Bandage

1. Start from the contralateral iliac crest and bring the bandage across to the puncture site.
2. Pass the bandage under the thigh of the punctured artery.
3. Wrap it again over the puncture site and then around the back.
4. Finish by bringing the bandage across the groin on the side of the puncture, securing it with TNT adhesive strips.

This method is effective and should remain in place for 6–12 hours.

TIP #34

If the use of closure devices is necessary for retrograde accesses, the most commonly used devices are the following.

- **Femoseal by Terumo:** Simple, fast, and reliable.
- **AngioSeal by Terumo:** Shares a mechanism similar to the previous device but is slightly more complex to implant.
- **ProGlide by Abbott.**

TIP #35

For antegrade accesses, the only devices indicated for use are **MynxGrip** and **MynxControl**. These are fully extravascular devices, with no intraluminal components, making them very safe. We have never experienced complications with their use, even when testing them in a variety of challenging situations.

This type of device can also be used for retrograde accesses. However, personally, I prefer the closure systems mentioned in the previous tip for retrograde accesses. The Mynx platform, unlike the others, does not travel over a guidewire and can therefore face difficulties advancing retrogradely toward the iliac axis, which is notoriously tortuous. The lack of a guidewire for the Mynx to travel on means that, in some cases, it may encounter resistance against the arterial wall, making it impossible to advance the closure system fully into the artery.

With the exception of the challenges mentioned for retrograde accesses, the Mynx platform delivers excellent results in antegrade accesses.

TIP #36

For large arterial accesses (EVAR, FEVAR, etc.), the safest and most tested closure system remains the **ProGlide by Abbott**. In these cases, two ProGlide devices should be used according to the **Preclose Technique**, which is well described and illustrated on the manufacturer's website.

We routinely perform percutaneous aortic endograft implantation, and ProGlide has consistently ensured hemostasis with a very low complication rate. During implantation – whether using one or multiple ProGlide devices – it is recommended to keep the guidewire in the artery until adequate hemostasis is confirmed. This precaution allows for the insertion of an additional device or replacement of a broken suture if needed.

Recently introduced to the market – and with a mechanism of action somewhat similar to the AngioSeal – is the **Manta system by Teleflex**, whose prospects in terms of efficacy and complication rates are promising.

REFERENCES

1. Modarai B, Haulon S, Ainsbury E, et al. Editor's choice – European society for vascular surgery (ESVS) 2023 clinical practice guidelines on radiation safety. *Europ J Vasc Endovas Surg.* 2023; 65(2): 171–222.

2. Biagioni LC, Pereira L, Nasser F, et al. Comparison between antegrade common femoral artery access and superficial femoral artery access in infrainguinal endovascular interventions. *J Vasc Surg.* 2021; 74(3): 763–770.

3. Li Y, Esmail A, Donas KP, et al. Antegrade vs crossover femoral artery access in the endovascular treatment of isolated below-the-knee lesions in patients with critical limb ischemia. *J Endovasc Ther.* 2017; 24(3): 331–336.

4. Wheatley BJ, Mansour MA, Grossman PM, et al. Complication rates for percutaneous lower extremity arterial antegrade access. *Arch Surg.* 2011; 146(4): 432–435.

5. Seto AH, Abu-Fadel MS, Sparling JM, et al. Real-time ultrasound guidance facilitates femoral arterial access and reduces vascular complications: FAUST (femoral arterial access with ultrasound trial). *JACC Cardiovasc Interv.* 2010; 3(7): 751–758.

6. Xenogiannis I, Varlamos C, Keeble TR, et al. Ultrasound-guided femoral vascular access for percutaneous coronary and structural interventions. *Diagnostics.* 2023; 13(12): 2028.

7. Nguyen P, Makris A, Hennessy A, et al. Standard versus ultrasound-guided radial and femoral access in coronary angiography and intervention (SURF): A randomised controlled trial. *EuroIntervention.* 2019; 15(6): e522–e530.

8. Franz RW, Tanga CF, Herrmann JW. Treatment of peripheral arterial disease via percutaneous brachial artery access. *J Vasc Surg.* 2017; 66(2): 461–465.

9. Wu J, Xu J, Yu Q, et al. Transbrachial artery as single or combined approach for complex interventions in patients with peripheral artery disease. *Ann Vasc Surg.* 2024; 102: 209–215.

10. Alvarez-Tostado JA, Moise MA, Bena JF, et al. The brachial artery: A critical access for endovascular procedures. *J Vasc Surg.* 2009; 49(2): 378–385.

11. Mordhorst A, Yan TD, Hoskins N, et al. Percutaneous proximal axillary artery versus femoral artery access for endovascular interventions. *J Vasc Surg.* 2022; 76(1): 165–173.

12. Bertoglio L, Mascia D, Cambiaghi T, et al. Percutaneous axillary artery access for fenestrated and branched thoracoabdominal endovascular repair. *J Vasc Surg.* 68(1): 12–23.

13. Wittig T, Sabanov A, Schmidt A. Feasibility and safety of percutaneous axillary artery access in a prospective series of 100 complex aortic and aortoiliac interventions. *J Clin Med.* 2023; 12(5): 1959.

14. Lorenzoni R, Ferraresi R, Manzi M, et al. Guidewires for lower extremity artery angioplasty: A review. *EuroIntervention.* 2015; 11(7): 799–807.

15. Burzotta F, Trani C, Mazzari MA, et al. Use of a second buddy wire during percutaneous coronary interventions: A simple solution for some challenging situations. *J Invasive Cardiol.* 2005; 17(3): 171–174.

16. Hildick-Smith D, Arunothayaraj S, Stankovic G, et al. Percutaneous coronary intervention of bifurcation lesions. *EuroIntervention.* 2022; 18(4): e273–e291.

17. Di Mario C, Ramasami N. Techniques to enhance guide catheter support. *Catheter Cardiovasc Interv.* 2008; 72(4): 505–512.

18. Takahashi S, Saito S, Tanaka S, et al. New method to increase a backup support of a 6 French guiding coronary catheter. *Catheter Cardiovasc Interv.* 2004; 63(4): 452–456.

19. Yokoi K, Sumitsuji S, Kaneda H, et al. A novel homemade snare, safe, economical and size-adjustable. *EuroIntervention.* 2015; 10(11): 1307–1310.

20. Zhang T, Zhang Y, Feng T, et al. Effectiveness and safety of a novel modified homemade snare in retrograde percutaneous coronary intervention for chronic total occlusion lesions: A retrospective cohort study. *J Thorac Dis.* 2024; 16(5): 3272–3281.

21. Zorger N, Manke C, Lenhart M, et al. Peripheral arterial balloon angioplasty: Effect of short versus long balloon inflation times on the morphologic results. *J Vasc Interv Radiol.* 2002; 13(4): 355–359.

22. Horie K, Tanaka A, Taguri M. Impact of prolonged inflation times during plain balloon angioplasty on angiographic dissection in femoropopliteal lesions. *J Endovasc Ther.* 2018; 25(6): 683–691.

TIPS & TRICKS IN INFRAINGUINAL PATHOLOGY

Toolkit A – **Tips & Tricks in CTO Recanalization**   **42**
  • Tips 1 to 8

Toolkit B – **Tips & Tricks in Complex Recanalization**   **52**
  • Tips 9 to 18

Toolkit C – **CTO Crossing Algorithm**   **65**
  • Tip 19

Toolkit D – **Tips & Tricks in Vessel Preparation**   **68**
  • Tips 20 to 26

Toolkit E – **Tips & Tricks for the Use of Drug-Coated Balloons**   **78**
  • Tips 27 to 29

Toolkit F – **Anastomotic PTA and PTA of Stenotic Patches**   **80**
  • Tips 30 to 31

Toolkit G – **Tips & Tricks in the Endovascular Treatment of Acute Arterial Lesions** **81**
  • Tips 32 to 37

Toolkit H – **Tips & Tricks in Popliteal Aneurysms**   **86**
  • Tips 38 to 39

DOI: 10.1201/9781003567080-2

(TO CROSSING ALGORITHM

To date, there is still no standardization of the correct approach to a CTO, and it is likely not an over-statement to say that every experienced operator has their own particular approach and personal algorithm for managing these complex lesions.

SO, HOW SHOULD ONE PROCEED?

I will attempt to provide some guidelines based on the evidence available in the literature and on what I have learned through my clinical practice.

Let us begin by clarifying some basic concepts.

TIP #1

Angiography

As P. Schneider asserts in his *Endovascular Skills*, angiography should be strategic, not diagnostic.

An initial assessment can be performed using fluoroscopy without contrast injection, allowing evaluation of the arterial wall quality. Extremely calcified walls – representing the most challenging CTOs to cross – are clearly visible due to the characteristic double calcium rail marking their boundaries.

For a proper angiographic evaluation of a CTO, long acquisitions are necessary to allow contrast to flow distally beyond the lesion through the collateral networks developed around it. The following aspects should be assessed.

- **Lesion Length:** Determine the extent of the occlusion.
- **Precise Point of Distal True Lumen Reconstruction:** Identify where the true lumen resumes distally.
- **Presence and Quality of Collateral Circulation:** Collaterals should ideally be preserved. This is why, as will be discussed shortly, in cases of a subintimal approach, distal re-entry into the true lumen should occur as close as possible to the distal cap. Losing critical collaterals could potentially result in acute or subacute ischemia in the event of reocclusion.
- **Feasibility and Navigability of Collaterals:** Assess if collateral vessels can be navigated, which may be necessary during advanced techniques such as transcollateral recanalization (discussed later).
- **Target Pedal Artery in CLTI:** When dealing with chronic limb-threatening ischemia (CLTI), prioritize identifying the leg vessel that directly supplies the foot. Remember, the goal is to alleviate symptoms or heal the ischemic lesion, not to achieve aesthetically pleasing images of restored arterial pathways. Attempting to recanalize all three leg arteries can sometimes worsen renal function; increase cardiac complications; prolong operative, anesthetic, and radiation exposure times; and raise costs – all without providing a proven functional benefit.
- **Proximal and Distal Cap Morphology:** Understanding Cap Morphology helps predict the success or failure of a specific recanalization technique, leading directly to the next tip.

TIP #2

The CTOP Classification

When selecting the appropriate approach to a femoropopliteal lesion, it is important – as mentioned earlier – to carefully observe the morphology of the proximal and distal caps during angiography. In this regard, the concept of "Cap Morphology," introduced by Saab et al., can be highly useful (Figure 2.1). According to their proposed classification, CTOs can be divided into the following four types based on the shape of the proximal and distal caps.

- **Type I:** Proximal cap concave, distal cap convex.
- **Type II:** Both proximal and distal caps concave.

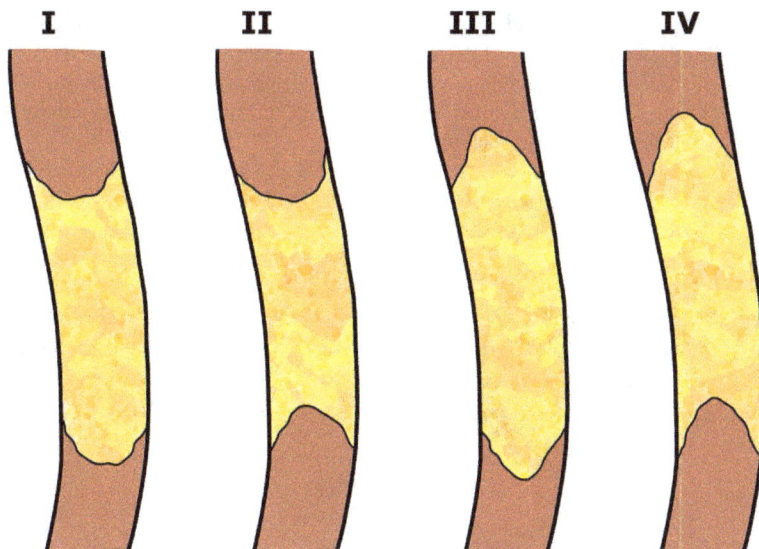

Figure 2.1 The chronic total occlusion (CTOP) crossing approach based on Plaque Cap Morphology classification.

- **Type III:** Both proximal and distal caps convex.
- **Type IV:** Proximal cap convex, distal cap concave.

Type I CTOs are generally easily recanalized using an antegrade endoluminal approach. Type IV CTOs are often successfully recanalized using a retrograde technique. Type II and Type III CTOs are complex lesions that frequently require advanced techniques (as will be described shortly). These often necessitate dual antegrade/retrograde access or advanced subintimal techniques. Type III lesions are the most challenging of all.

The value of the CTOP classification lies in its ability to predict the effectiveness of advanced recanalization techniques, which may be needed after the failure of initial antegrade endoluminal and subintimal attempts.

Personally, I find this classification particularly useful in Type IV lesions: in these cases, if antegrade endoluminal or subintimal attempts fail – both of which should always be the initial strategies – it can be useful to proceed directly with a retrograde approach.

***

BASIC CHARACTERISTICS OF GUIDEWIRES

The market for CTO guidewires (and catheters) is vast and constantly growing. While each company has its own unique formula for designing guidewires for specific uses, these devices share a set of fundamental characteristics that define their performance and differentiate them. These key features are as follows.

- **Pushability:** This refers to the amount of force required to advance a guidewire through a CTO (i.e., the ease with which it progresses once it penetrates the lesion). It depends on how readily the guidewire navigates the target lesion.
- **Trackability:** In the context of combined guidewire/catheter use, trackability describes the catheter's ability to travel over the guidewire through tortuous anatomies or CTOs. This property depends on the lateral supportive force of the guidewire, as well as the vertical supportive force (or column strength) of the catheter.

- **Torquability:** This refers to the guidewire's responsiveness to rotational movements applied by the operator. It represents the ability of the guidewire to transmit rotational movements from the proximal end to the distal tip without loss of motion. Ideally, the transmission ratio should be 1:1 (i.e., for every 360° rotation applied by the operator to the guidewire, there should be a corresponding 360° rotation of the distal tip).
- **Steerability:** Often confused with torquability, steerability instead refers to the guidewire's ability to respond precisely to the operator's manipulations, allowing it to be directed and oriented along the desired path.
- **Lubricity:** This property measures the guidewire's ability to minimize friction between its surface and the inner walls of the CTO. Lubricity is typically achieved through polymer coatings and hydrophilic coatings.
- **Penetrability:** This describes the guidewire's ability to penetrate the lesion, specifically the proximal cap of a CTO. Penetrability is directly related to the guidewire's tip load: the greater the tip load,* the higher the penetrability.

(*Note:* Tip load refers to the force in grams required to deflect the distal 10 mm of a guidewire laterally by 2 mm.)

***

GUIDEWIRE ESCALATION

This is the algorithm for a correct use of the guidewires typically used in the endovascular treatment of CTOs. It involves the sequential use of guidewires with progressively more aggressive physical characteristics and increasing tip loads. The goal is to navigate a guidewire through a completely occluded arterial segment. The choice of guidewire and the progression toward stiffer options depend on the lesion's response and the anatomical characteristics of the affected vascular segment.

1. **First phase:** The procedure usually begins with guidewires of low tip load (0.5–3 g) and high flexibility. These wires feature atraumatic tips and excellent navigability within the vessel and the CTO, making them ideal for managing less calcified lesions.

2. **Second phase:** If the first attempt fails, the next step involves guidewires with a medium tip load (3–18 g). These wires are characterized by greater rigidity and a tapered, conical tip designed to enhance penetration through occluded segments that are more fibrotic or moderately calcified.

3. **Third phase:** For CTOs with high structural resistance – often found in older lesions – guidewires with a high tip load (20–40 g) are employed. These wires are designed to penetrate extremely calcified or fibro-calcific lesions.

    Guidewires must be used with caution, advanced only over short distances, and kept straight within the arterial lumen. Although they are often more effective than softer wires, they carry a higher risk of vessel perforation.

TIP #3

The use of a supportive catheter is highly beneficial for crossing a CTO and providing support to the guidewire, regardless of the technique employed (whether endoluminal in its various forms or subintimal).

Regardless of the guidewire used to cross the lesion (commonly a 0.018" or 0.014"), a supportive catheter compatible with a 0.035" guidewire is stiffer and offers greater support than those designed for 0.018" or 0.014" guidewires. Personally, I prefer this option, as it also allows me to switch platforms (e.g., from 0.018" to 0.035") as needed, without requiring additional catheter exchanges.

As an alternative to a supportive catheter, a low-profile balloon can be advanced over the guidewire.

***

ENDOLUMINAL GUIDEWIRE MANIPULATION TECHNIQUES

In what follows, I will list the techniques used to manipulate guidewires, organized according to a principle of **handling escalation**, which generally progresses in parallel with the Guidewire Escalation described earlier.

SLIDING

This technique is typically used with low tip-load and high-lubricity guidewires. It involves a synchronized maneuver of gentle forward advancement, combined with slow and smooth rotation of the guidewire. The purpose of this approach is to cross the CTO by engaging the microchannel often present within it (Figures 2.2–2.2c). This method allows the operator to remain endoluminal and ensures the process is as atraumatic as possible.

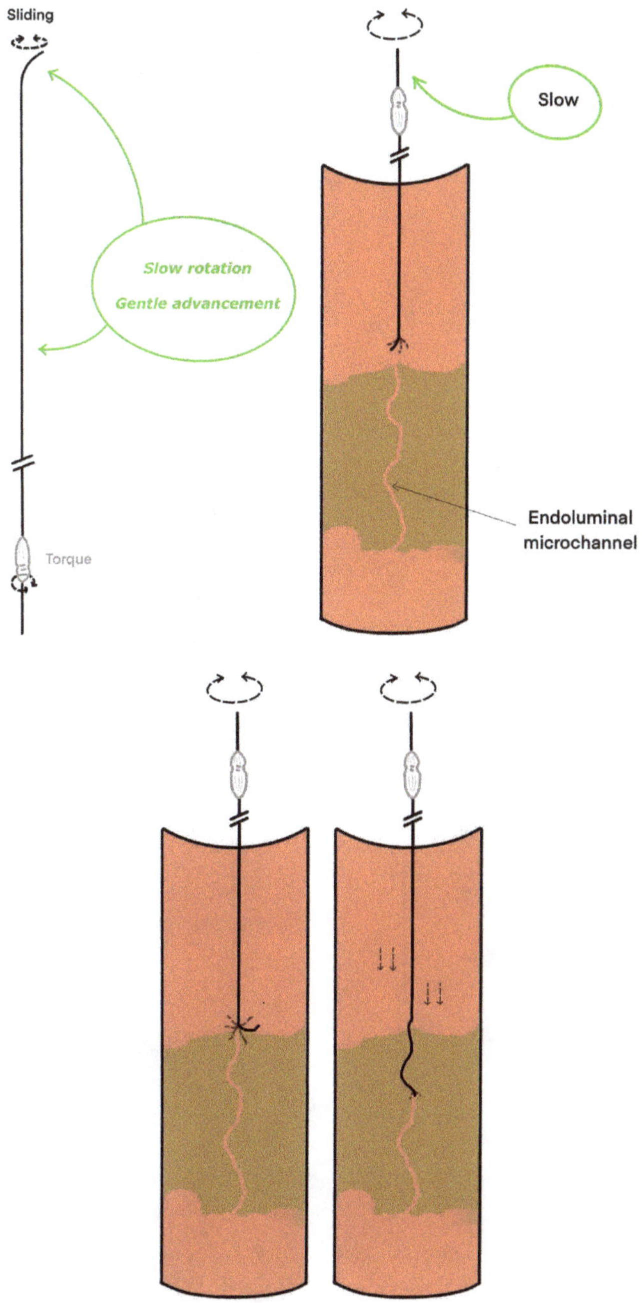

Figures 2.2–2.2c The Sliding Technique

DRILLING

This technique requires low/moderate tip-load guidewires with high torquability. It involves applying rapid rotational movements, both clockwise and counterclockwise, combined with firm but controlled forward pressure. Even in the absence of a microchannel that can be engaged using the sliding technique, this method creates a pathway by progressively advancing the guidewire through the more recent and less resistant areas of the CTO (Figures 2.3–2.3c). The drilling technique is effective for crossing fibrotic or moderately calcified CTOs.

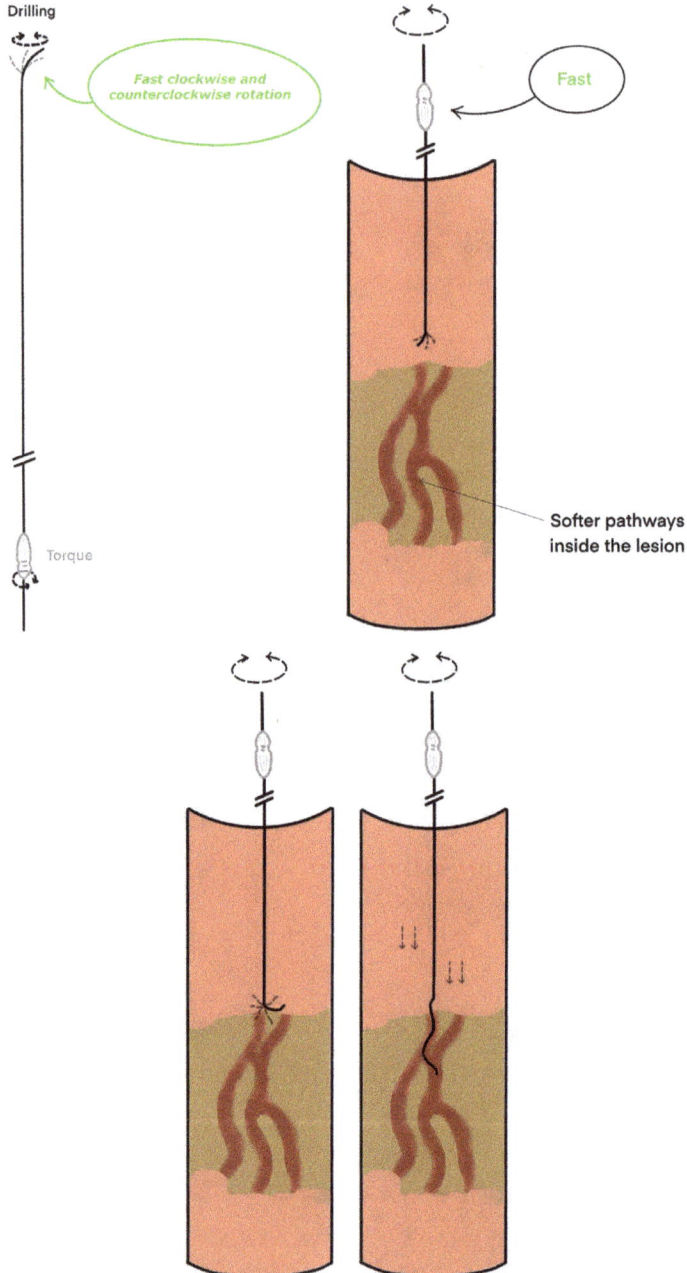

Drilling

Fast clockwise and counterclockwise rotation

Fast

Torque

Softer pathways inside the lesion

Figures 2.3–2.3c The Drilling Technique

PERFORATING

In more severe and calcified CTOs, the previously described techniques are ineffective. In such cases, a more aggressive approach is required, utilizing high tip-load guidewires (with increased penetrability). In the perforating technique, the guidewire is advanced against the proximal cap of the CTO without rotation: essentially, it is used almost like a needle to pierce through the lesion (Figure 2.4).

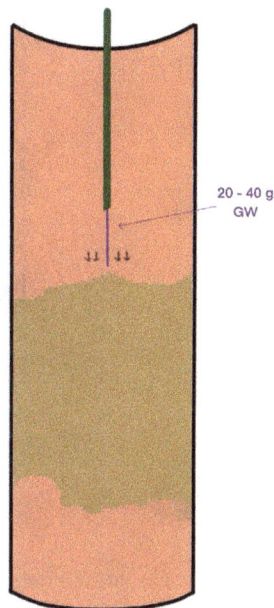

20 - 40 g
GW

Figure 2.4 The Perforating Technique

For femoropopliteal lesions, 0.018" guidewires with tip loads of up to 30–40 g are typically used. For infrapopliteal lesions, 0.014" guidewires with tip loads of up to 20–30 g are generally preferred (though this is not a strict rule, and with experience, operators will determine the most suitable weight for each case).

Given the characteristics of the guidewires used, there is a higher risk of vessel perforation. The following tips should be considered.

- Use the perforating technique only for short occlusions located in straight vessel segments.
- The guidewire must remain straight and centered within the vessel. If it deviates laterally (toward the vessel wall), it is advisable to stop, retract, and attempt to reposition centrally or abandon the technique and choose another approach (Figures 2.4a–2.4b).
- Multiple projections may be necessary to confirm that the guidewire remains centered within the CTO during advancement.

TIP #4

We have already mentioned the possibility of perforating the proximal cap using the posterior end of a standard 0.035" hydrophilic guidewire (refer to the corresponding tip and Figures 1.17–1.17g); its perforative capability is excellent.

This maneuver is off-label and should therefore be performed with caution and only by experienced hands. However, it can be a decisive solution in many situations.

***

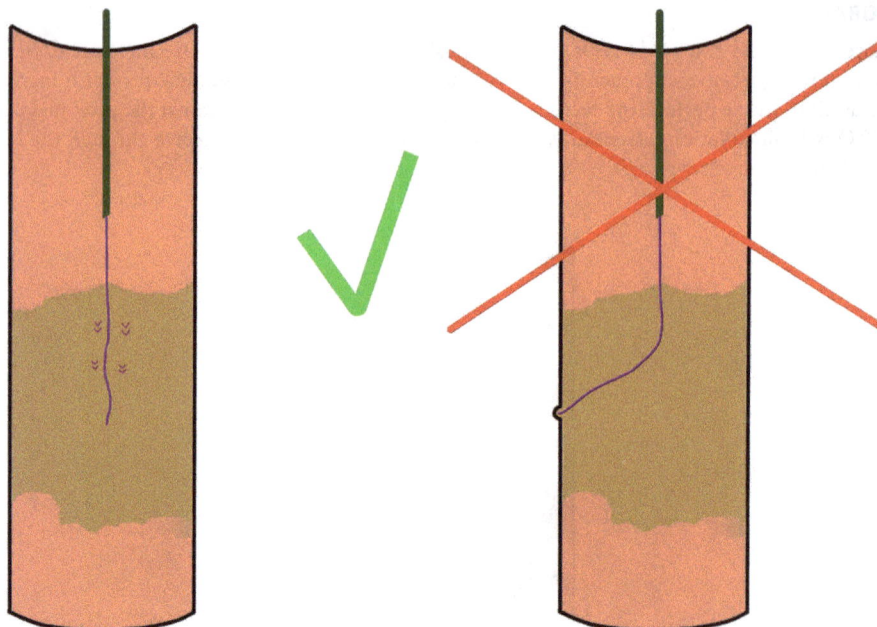

Figures 2.4a–2.4b (Continued)

THE SUBINTIMAL TECHNIQUE

If the endoluminal approach fails, a subintimal recanalization should be attempted. In the femoropopliteal segment, workhorse guidewires such as the V18 (Boston Scientific) or similar (with low-to-moderate tip load) are typically used.

For the infrapopliteal segment, guidewires such as the V14–V18 or similar are commonly employed.

(*Note:* I must admit that, sometimes, I use a 0.035" stiff hydrophilic guidewire in the infrapopliteal vessels to perform the subintimal technique in long, straight, and calcified segments. It is highly effective and can yield great results, but it should be used with caution and by experienced hands.)

TIP #5

Entering the subintimal plane is easier than an inexperienced surgeon might expect; in fact, it often becomes the natural and preferential path for a low-to-moderate tip-load guidewire when endoluminal attempts fail.

However, if the guidewire does not naturally engage this pathway and the subintimal technique is chosen, the correct maneuver involves orienting the catheter toward the vessel wall – just adjacent to the proximal cap of the CTO – and gently advancing the guidewire with moderate force (Figure 2.5). This action creates a dissection between the intima and media layers, effectively entering the subintimal plane.

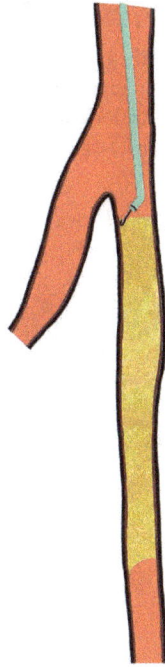

Figure 2.5 The Subintimal Technique

It is easy to recognize when the guidewire has entered the subintimal plane, as its tip forms a character-istic loop (Figure 2.5a).

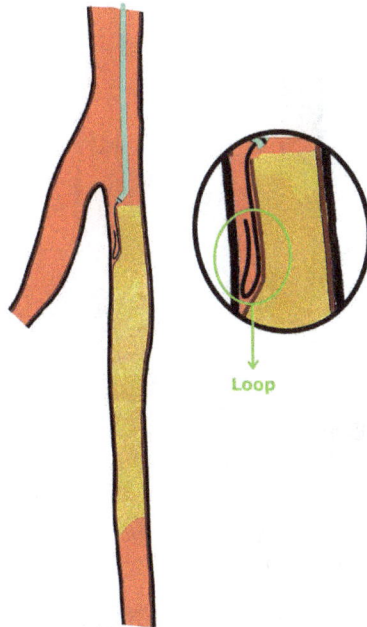

Loop

Figure 2.5a (Continued)

TIP #6

In the subintimal plane, it is crucial to keep the loop formed by the guidewire as small as possible. To achieve this, the catheter should be advanced incrementally behind the guidewire as it progresses. If the guidewire is pushed forward carelessly, the loop will grow larger, causing the subintimal chamber to expand excessively. This enlargement makes re-entry into the distal lumen significantly more challenging.

The correct technique involves alternating small advancements of a few centimeters of the guidewire with corresponding advancements of the catheter (Figure 2.5b). This process is repeated until the distal cap is reached, beyond which re-entry into the true lumen is required.

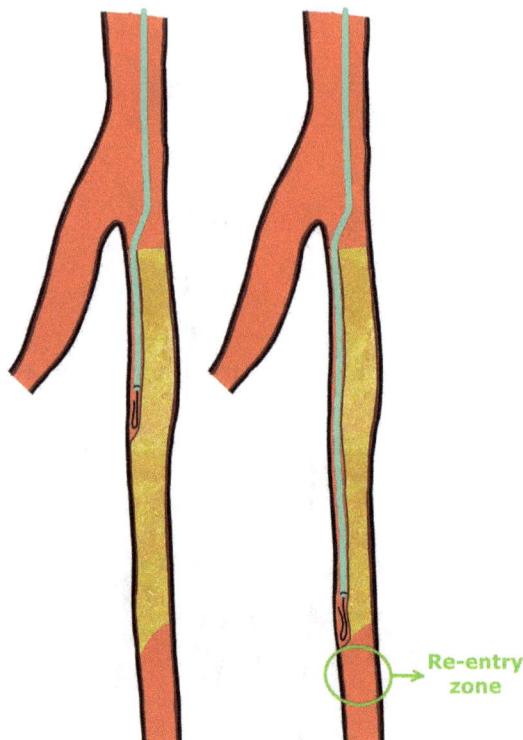

Figures 2.5b–2.5c (Continued)

In many cases, the guidewire will naturally tend to re-enter the distal lumen at the level of the distal cap. The tactile sensation upon re-entering the lumen is distinctive, as the guidewire advances with minimal resistance and moves within the vessel without further expansion of the loop at its tip.

As a general rule, once convinced of a correct re-entry into the lumen, it is advisable to inject a small amount of contrast to confirm the position.

TIP #7

Sometimes re-entry proves to be more challenging than expected. The most important rule in such cases is to **absolutely avoid extending the dissection plane beyond the distal cap** (Figure 2.5c). Re-entry must occur immediately after the distal cap. If re-entry is performed too far distally – several centimeters beyond the end of the CTO – the result will be the loss of important collateral branches during angioplasty dilation.

Re-entry should therefore be attempted as closely as possible to the distal cap, using patient and minimal rotational and forward movements of the guidewire (similar to the sliding technique). The goal is to engage that tiny microchannel that allows re-entry. At this stage, it is helpful to magnify the fluoroscopic image and carefully observe the movements of the guidewire tip. Focus on areas where the guidewire appears to engage a microchannel. The following tips may be helpful.

- **Try different guidewires**, as long as they remain within the low-to-moderate tip-load range. Hydrophilic guidewires (or those with hydrophilic distal segments) are often more effective, as they glide more easily through microchannels.
- **Be patient**.
- **Limit the duration of this attempt** – A few minutes should suffice. If re-entry is not successful, it is necessary to switch to another re-entry technique.

TIP #8

If the previous attempts fail, and before resorting to advanced techniques or expensive re-entry devices, it is possible to attempt re-entering the true lumen using a **high tip-load 0.018" guidewire** (20–30 g) with a pre-bent tip at approximately 35–40°. This bent tip, carefully directed beyond the distal cap, can assist in perforating the medial-intimal layer separating the guidewire from the true lumen (Figure 2.6).

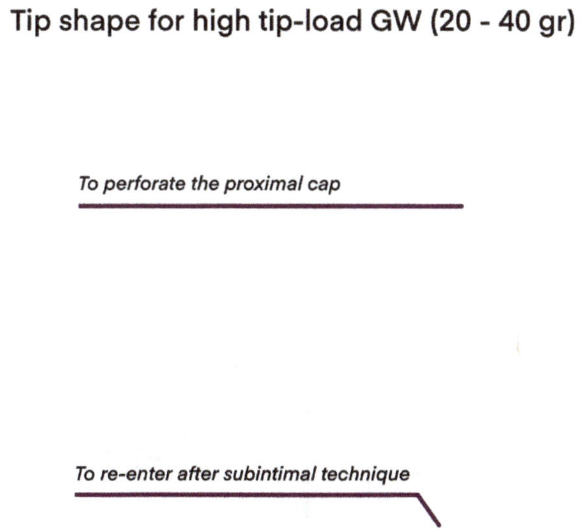

Tip shape for high tip-load GW (20 - 40 gr)

To perforate the proximal cap

To re-enter after subintimal technique

Figure 2.6 Tip shapes and purpose for high tip-load guidewires.

When employing this approach, it is essential to obtain multiple vessel projections to confirm the correct orientation of the guidewire tip toward the vessel lumen. The risk of perforation in this situation is significant.

We will propose a series of technical strategies aimed at mastering even the most complex CTOs using only catheters and guidewires.

ADVANCED SUBINTIMAL TECHNIQUES

These strategies are primarily aimed at ensuring re-entry in cases where it proves challenging with standard techniques (a situation that occurs in 25–40% of cases). Specifically, the superficial femoral artery, due to its dimensions and characteristics, is particularly well suited for the application of the SAFARI (Subintimal Arterial Flossing with Antegrade–Retrograde Intervention) and Double Balloon techniques.

TIP #9

Crush Balloon Technique: A small-diameter balloon (3.5–4 mm is usually sufficient for re-entry at the level of the superficial femoral artery) inflated in the subintimal plane near the re-entry zone can help tear the dissecting membrane separating the true lumen from the false lumen (Figures 2.7–2.7b).

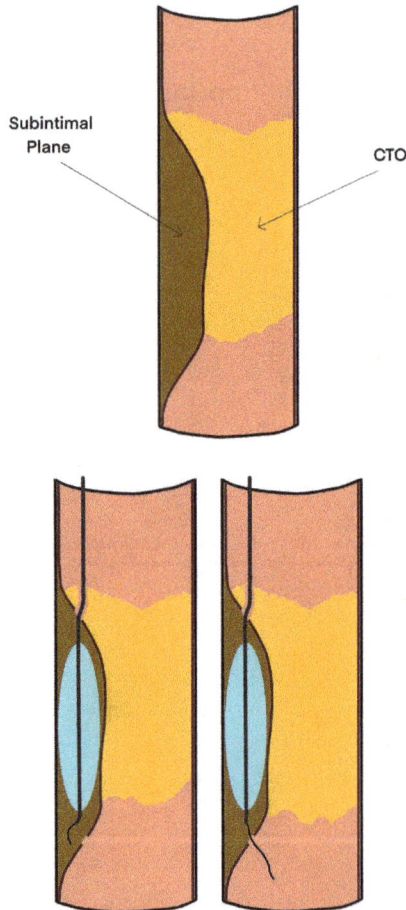

Figures 2.7–2.7b The Crush Balloon Technique

TIP #10

Parallel Wire Technique: With the first guidewire left in the subintimal plane, a second 0.014" or 0.018" guidewire with a moderate-to-high tip load can be inserted in parallel to probe the CTO via the endoluminal route. The first guidewire in the subintimal plane acts as a marker to direct the second guidewire intraluminally. Additionally, it helps prevent the second guidewire from repeatedly entering the false lumen, which often occurs once a subintimal plane has already been created (Figure 2.8).

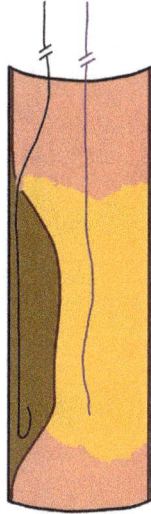

Figure 2.8 The Parallel Wire Technique

TIP #11

SAFARI Technique: In this technique, the subintimal plane is accessed through both an antegrade approach and a second, distal retrograde access, typically using a 0.018" guidewire.

Through both access points, a 3 mm or 4 mm balloon is inflated in the subintimal plane to create a "working room" where the two subintimal planes (antegrade and retrograde) can be brought together (Figures 2.9–2.9a).

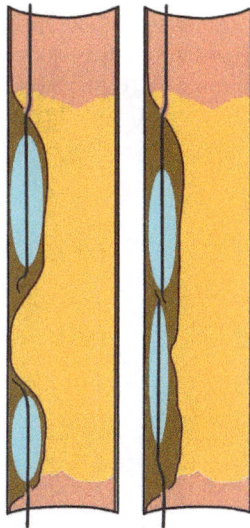

Figures 2.9–2.9a The SAFARI Technique

Once the rendezvous of the two planes is achieved, the guidewire from the retrograde access is directed into the antegrade catheter (Figures 2.9b–2.9c), from which it is externalized via the femoral sheath.

With the guidewire under control, the antegrade catheter can then be advanced into the true lumen beyond the subintimal plane using the Flossing Wire Technique.

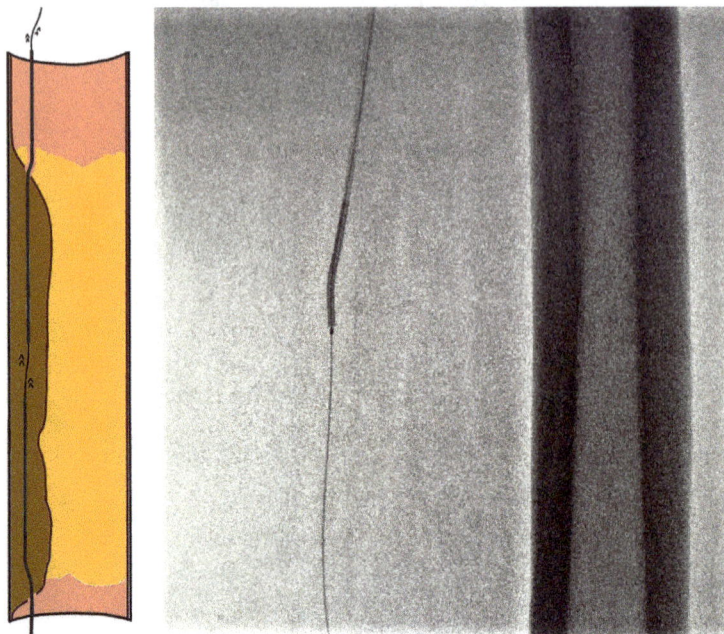

Figures 2.9b–2.9c (Continued)

TIP #12

Double Balloon: Two **PTA balloons**, with nominal diameters matching the arterial diameter, are inserted into the subintimal plane – one via the antegrade access and the other through a distal retrograde access.

The balloons are advanced toward each other but without their tips meeting; a gap of approximately 5 mm between their ends is sufficient (Figure 2.10). After removing the guidewires from both balloons, they are simultaneously inflated for a few seconds (Figure 2.10a). This maneuver often causes the rupture of the dissecting membrane separating them (Figure 2.10b).

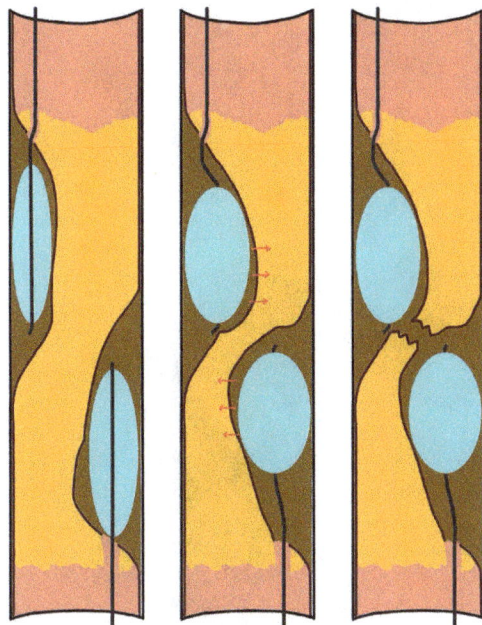

Figures 2.10–2.10b The double Balloon Technique

Once the membrane is ruptured, consider the following.

- If the retrograde balloon was fully inflated along its length in the subintimal plane, distal access can be gained using the **Flossing Wire Technique** (Figure 2.10c), as described in the SAFARI Technique.
- If the proximal portion of the retrograde balloon emerges into the true distal lumen, the proximal guidewire can simply be advanced into the space created by the retrograde balloon, securing access to the distal lumen.

This technique is effective when the balloon diameters are nominal relative to the vessel diameter. Initial hesitation is common; however, the theoretical risk of vessel rupture remains very low – provided that the balloons do not overlap during inflation.

RETROGRADE RECANALIZATION TECHNIQUES

The general principle underlying retrograde access is based on the assumption that the distal cap of a CTO is typically "softer" – primarily composed of thrombus and therefore easier to penetrate – compared to the proximal cap, which tends to have a harder, fibrocalcific composition.

Retrograde access can be achieved at any level of the vascular tree. Described access points include the posterior tibial artery, dorsalis pedis artery, anterior tibial artery, peroneal artery, superficial femoral artery (SFA), popliteal artery, plantar arch, and even digital arteries.

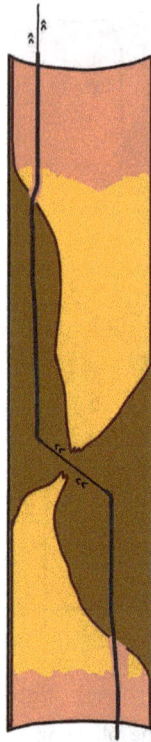

Figure 2.10c (Continued)

TIP #13

Retrograde puncture of tibial, peroneal, or dorsalis pedis arteries.

- **Preventing arterial spasm**: Administer a small volume of intra-arterial nitroglycerin (or isosorbide dinitrate, or another nitrate) through the anterograde catheter, as closely as possible to the retrograde access site. Additionally, infiltrate the subcutaneous area around the access site with lidocaine and nitrates. These compounds should be highly diluted and used under strict anesthetic monitoring.

Preparation of the Nitroglycerin Solution

1. Draw 1 cc (0.33 mg) of nitroglycerin into a 10 cc syringe and dilute it with 9 cc of saline.
2. Remove 8 cc of the solution, leaving 2 cc. Then add 4 cc of saline to bring the total volume to 6 cc.
3. Each cc will contain 100 mcg. Inject 2 cc (200 mcg) at a time, every 10–15 minutes, while carefully monitoring blood pressure and heart rate.
4. This solution should be injected locally, either intra-arterially or as subcutaneous infiltration at the retrograde puncture site.

- **Ultrasound-Guided Puncture:** Perform the puncture under ultrasound guidance, as described previously. For distal vessels that are more superficial (e.g., the posterior tibial artery at the malleolus), a **hockey stick probe** may be beneficial due to its better surface insonation and adaptability to the ankle and foot anatomy.
- **Fluoroscopic Puncture:** If using fluoroscopy, employ multiple projections and inject contrast proximally to visualize the distal artery to be punctured. Use digital zoom or magnification for enhanced precision. In some cases, visible arterial wall calcifications on fluoroscopy can serve as a mapping

guide for the puncture. Avoid parallax between the needle and the vessel during puncture. Ideally, the artery should be visualized longitudinally, with the needle fully aligned along the longitudinal axis of the vessel for optimal accuracy and efficacy (Figures 2.11–2.11a).

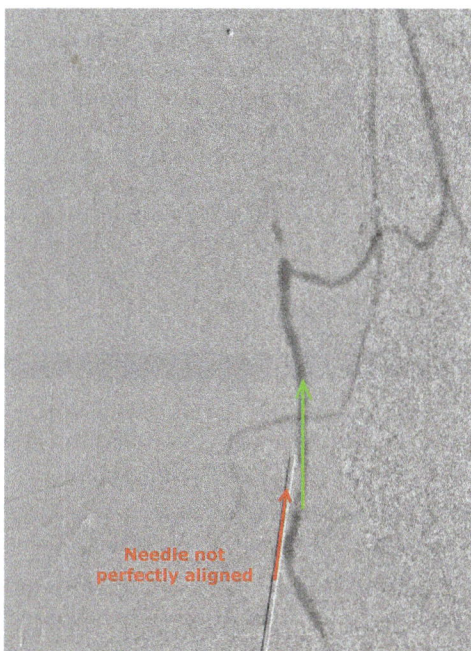

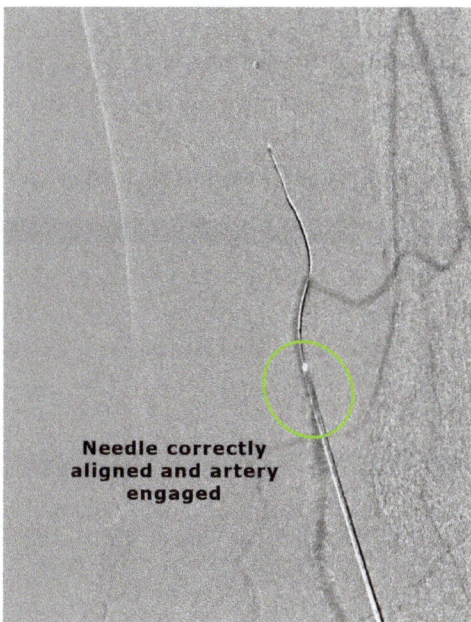

Figures 2.11–2.11a Needle orientation in retrograde access.

- **Choice of Needle:** Use a 21G needle compatible with a 0.018" guidewire or a retrograde-specific system, such as the Cook system. Alternatively, a 22G pediatric arterial needle (compatible with a 0.018" guidewire) can be used. Avoid standard angiographic needles, as they are too traumatic for distal vessels.
- **Advancing the Guidewire:** Once access is achieved, advance a Boston V18 guidewire, engaging the lesion from the distal cap, which is generally easier to penetrate endoluminally than the proximal cap. Avoid bending the guidewire tip.
- **Recanalization and Flossing Wire Technique:** After recanalizing the lesion retrogradely, capture the distal guidewire through the common femoral sheath or a catheter. As previously described in the SAFARI Technique, externalize the distal guidewire from the femoral access and use the **Flossing Wire Technique** to advance the antegrade catheter distally. In selected cases, the procedure may be completed entirely through the retrograde access.
- **Sheathless Technique:** To minimize the caliber of the retrograde access, use a sheathless approach for retrograde recanalization. This reduces trauma to the vessel and simplifies hemostasis. If guidewire support is needed, a supportive catheter or a low-profile balloon is typically used.
- **Achieving Hemostasis:** At the end of the procedure, achieve hemostasis at the puncture site by performing PTA of the artery for approximately 3 minutes (or longer if necessary). Always perform a follow-up angiography to confirm successful hemostasis.

TIP #14

Popliteal artery access is relatively simple to perform; however, it is recommended to use ultrasound-guided puncture as a standard approach at this level to avoid puncturing the vein, which could lead to the formation of an arteriovenous fistula (AVF).

A disadvantage of puncturing the infragenicular popliteal artery is related to the patient's position. Some operators prefer positioning the patient prone, at least during the retrograde phase.

Personally, I avoid this access site unless absolutely necessary. When I perform the puncture, I position the leg externally rotated and slightly flexed, which helps expose the popliteal artery.

TIP #15

Accessing the SFA, especially at the Hunter's canal, may require the use of long needles – up to 15 cm in length and 21G – due to the depth of the artery at this level.

In some cases, these long needles can be supported by employing a telescopic technique, where they are inserted coaxially into a shorter 18G needle that acts as a stabilizing support through the tissue.

The telescopic technique can be applied in any situation when the target artery is particularly deep.

TIP #16

It is possible to perform a retrograde puncture of the SFA through a previously implanted stent. The stent struts can serve as a mapping guide.

However, the occlusion must terminate at a level **proximal** to the chosen site for retrograde puncture.

ALTERNATIVE TECHNIQUES

TIP #17

Transcollateral Technique: This technique is highly useful when the occluded artery can be accessed retrogradely via a navigable collateral branch. The procedure requires a microcatheter and a 0.014" guidewire (Figures 2.12–2.12c).

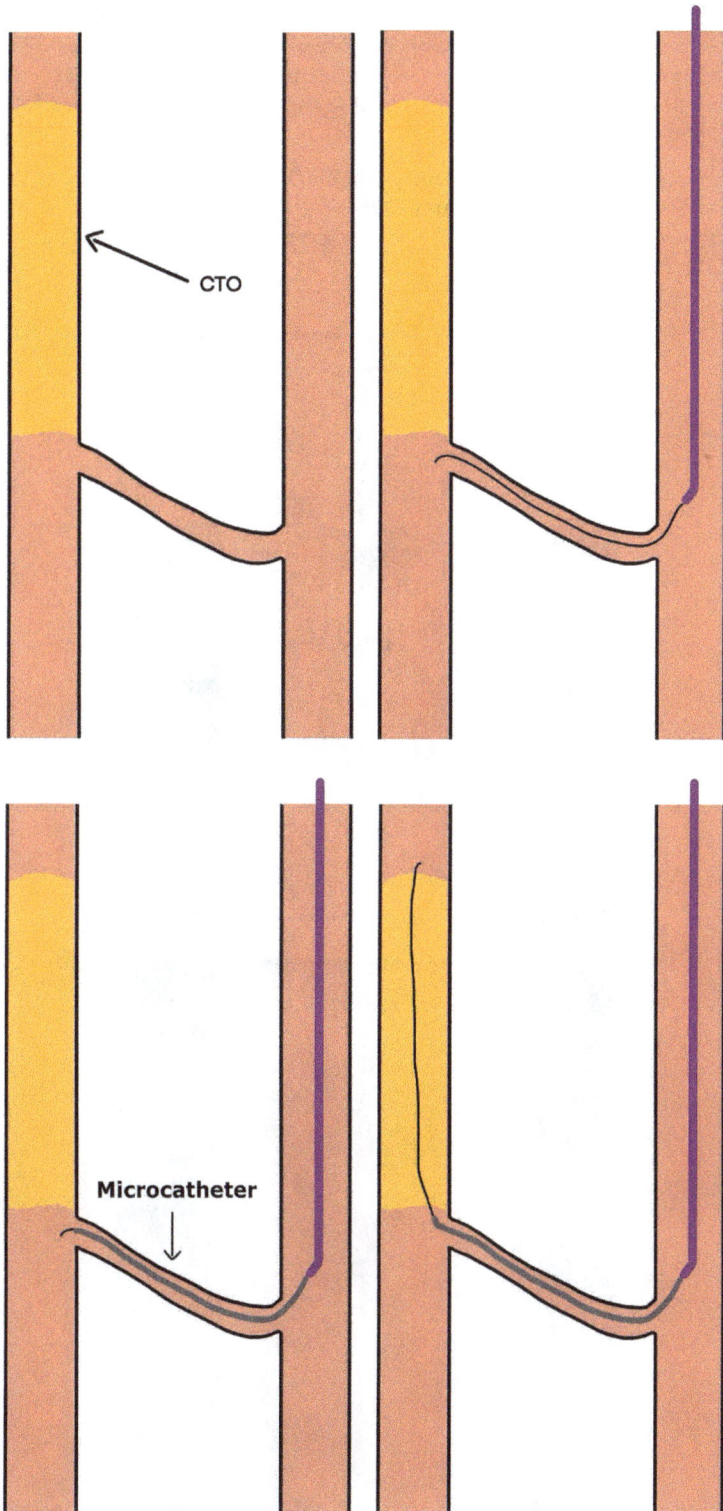

Figures 2.12–2.12c The Transcollateral Technique

For example, if during a procedure you reach the peroneal artery with a catheter and guidewire, and this artery is connected through a well-developed collateral to a distal portion of posterior tibial artery that is occluded proximally, the collateral branch can be used to reach the posterior tibial artery. From there, you can retrogradely recanalize the proximal segment of the artery, similar to a pedal plantar loop (Figures 2.12d–2.12e).

Once the guidewire has successfully recanalized the CTO retrogradely, a PTA catheter is advanced over the wire to perform angioplasty (Figures 2.12f–2.12g). at this point, to access the distal posterior tibial artery through the standard antegrade pathway, a catheter is advanced antegradely through the recanalized CTO (Figure 2.12h).

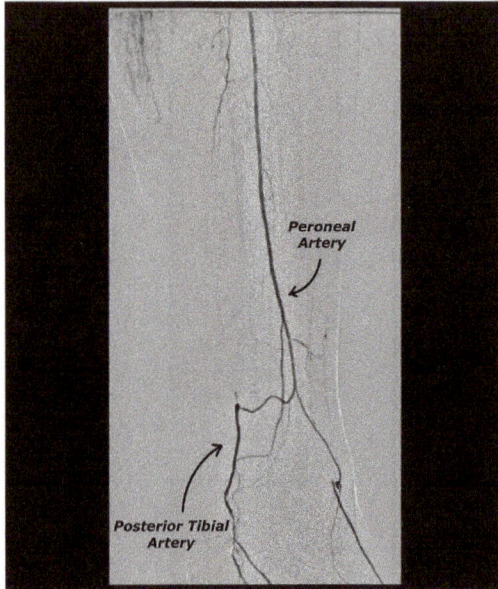

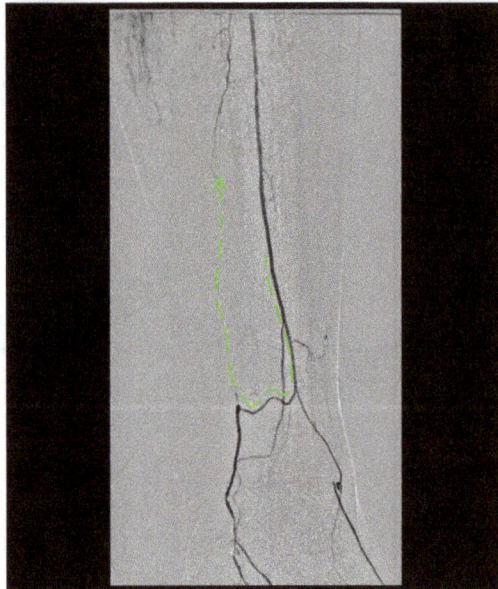

Figures 2.12d–2.12e (Continued)

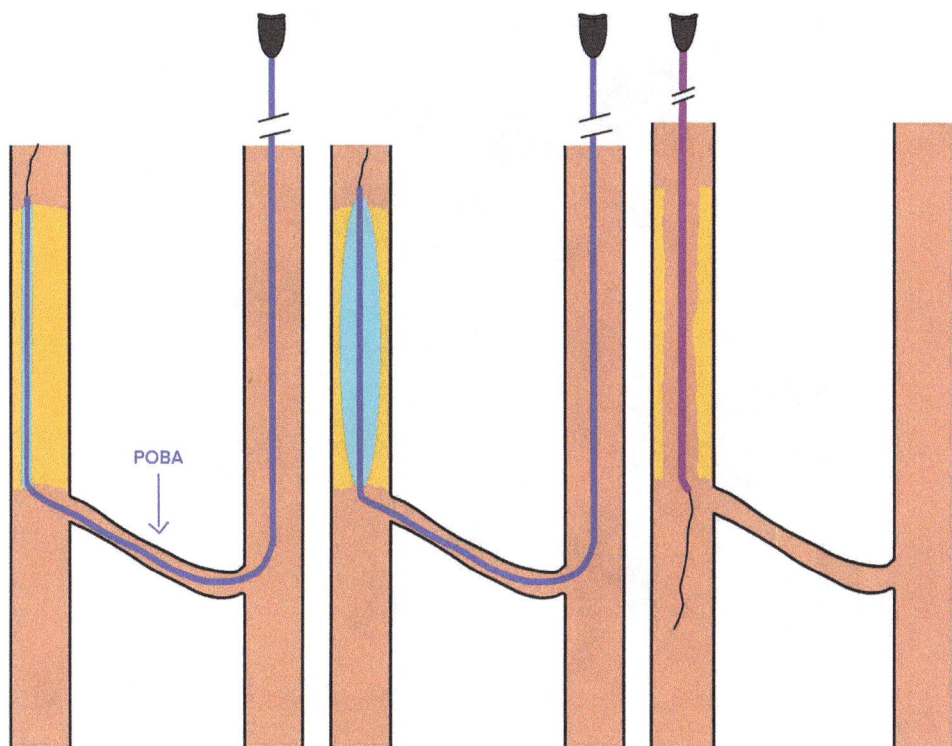

Figures 2.12f–2.12h (Continued)

This technique can be used not only for tibial arteries but also for the superficial femoral artery (via branches of the deep femoral artery) or the popliteal artery (via genicular arteries).

The use of vasodilators (as described in earlier tips) and appropriate heparinization is critical to preserve the navigated collateral branch and ensure procedural success.

TIP #18

Pedal Plantar Loop (Figure 2.13): The pedal plantar loop can be reached not only for its direct recanalization (Figure 2.13a) but also as a route for retrograde recanalization of the arteries connected to it. For example, the pedal plantar loop can be navigated starting from the posterior tibial artery to retrogradely recanalize the anterior tibial artery, or vice versa (Figure 2.13b).

If the loop is patent and used solely as a collateral route for retrograde recanalization of proximal branches, it must not be ballooned to avoid disrupting the hemodynamics of the forefoot.

It is important to note that in nearly half of cases, the pedal plantar anatomy is incomplete, and a navigable loop is absent. (Figure 2.13c illustrates the classification of pedal plantar loop variations as described by Kawarada. Navigation is possible only in the Kawarada type 1 pedal plantar loop)

IMAGING CONSIDERATIONS

Proper visualization of this vascular region requires the use of appropriate **lateral** and **anteroposterior projections**. The following two standard projections, as suggested by Manzi et al., are typically necessary.

- **Lateral Projection:** This should include the heel and the proximal forefoot. Additionally, the base of the fifth metatarsal should be "unsuperimposed" in this view (Figure 2.13d).

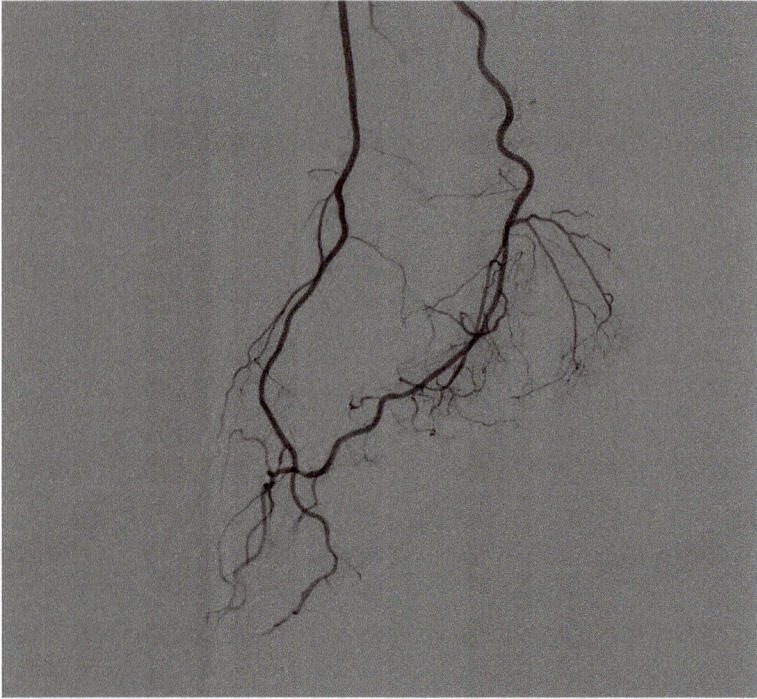

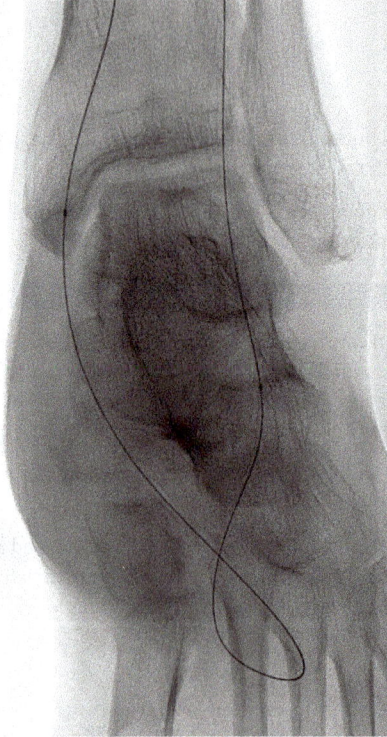

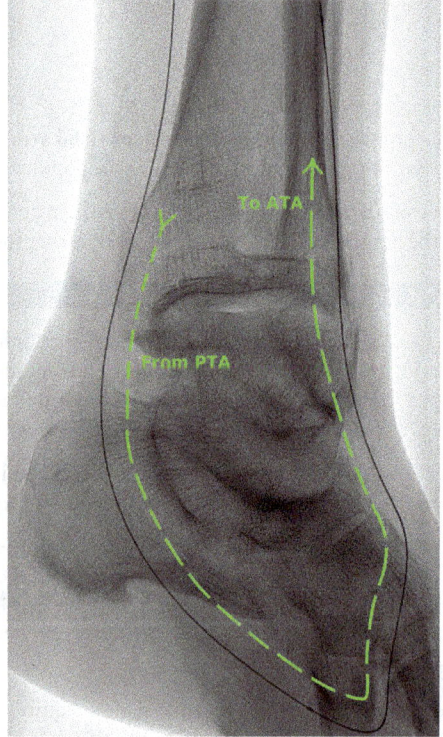

Figures 2.13–2.13b The Pedal Plantar Loop

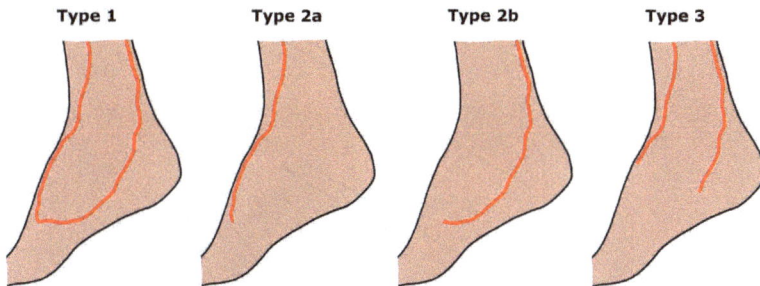

Pedal Arch Classification sec. Kawarada

Type 1: Complete pedal-plantar loop (dorsalis pedis and lateral plantar artery patent)
Type 2a: Incomplete loop - only dorsalis pedis is patent
Type 2b: Incomplete loop - only lateral plantar artery is patent
Type 3: Incomplete loop - both dorsalis pedis and lateral plantar artery occluded

Figure 2.13c The Kawarada Classification of Pedal Plantar Loop Types

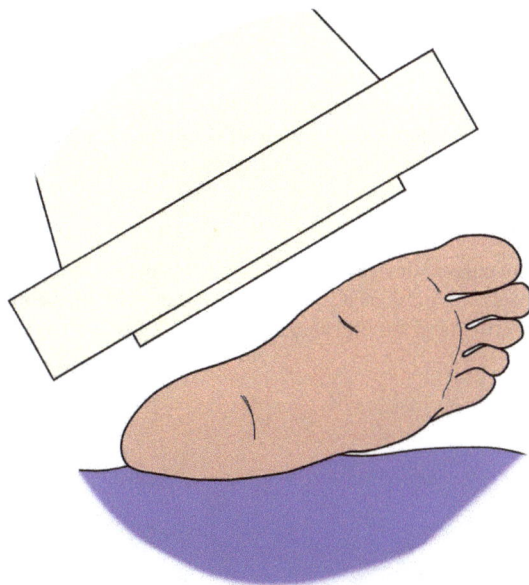

Figure 2.13d Frontal and lateral fluoroscopic orientation during the Pedal Plantar Loop Technique.

- **Anteroposterior Projection:** This should include the proximal portion of the first intermetatarsal space and the entire forefoot (Figure 2.13e).

Angiography in these two projections is performed by injecting a slow mixture (2–3 cc/sec) of 8–10 cc of contrast and heparinized saline (at an approximately 1:1 ratio). This mixture minimizes burning sensations in the foot caused by the contrast, which can provoke involuntary patient movements during image acquisition. Long acquisitions are required to allow the contrast to reach the foot via collateral circulation, when injected from the femoral sheath.

RECANALIZATION TIPS

In our experience, forefoot circulation is effectively recanalized using 0.014" guidewires with high flexibility, soft atraumatic tips, and excellent torquability, such as Boston PT Graphix or Abbott BMW coronary guidewires.

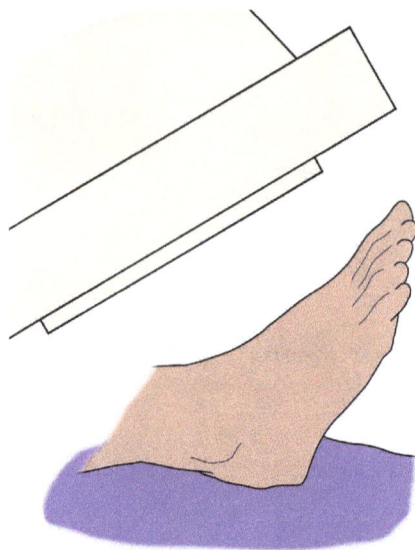

Figure 2.13e (Continued)

As with other techniques, the appropriate use of nitrates is essential while navigating the loop with guidewires and catheters to prevent acute occlusion of the loop. Such an event could result in severe hemodynamic instability of the limb.

ACCESS CONSIDERATIONS

Due to the shaft lengths of current devices, this technique is generally not feasible via crossover femoral access. Antegrade access is crucial, as it provides the system with pushability that is impossible to achieve via retrograde contralateral femoral access.

Concluding the discussion on CTO Management Techniques, let us come back to the following questions posed at the beginning of this section.

- *How should one proceed during a CTO recanalization?*
- *What algorithm should be followed?*

As emphasized earlier, no evidence-based standardized method exists to date. The debate remains open and highly active. It could almost be said that there is a unique strategy for every operator facing a CTO. Nevertheless, some general principles can be outlined. I have attempted to summarize our approach in Figure 2.14. Let us decode it together and sketch an algorithm that could work well in most scenarios.

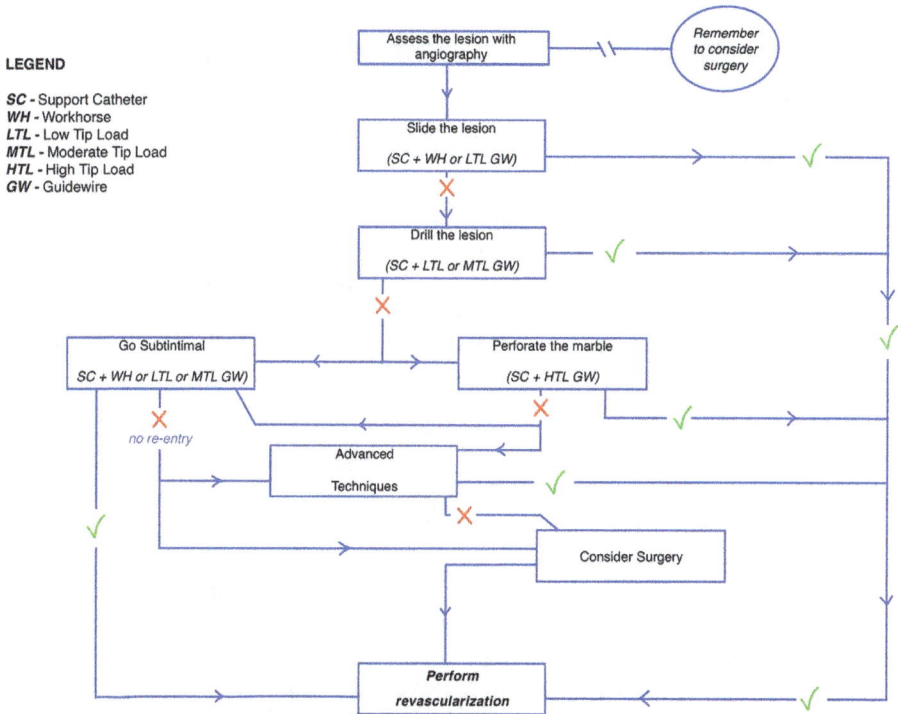

Figure 2.14 The CTO Crossing Algorithm

1. **Perform a comprehensive angiography:** The first and most critical step is always to execute a high-quality angiography, following the criteria described at the beginning of this section.

2. **Start with antegrade endoluminal recanalization:** Once the lesion is characterized, it is generally advisable to begin with antegrade endoluminal recanalization attempts, following the principles of guidewire escalation and handling escalation. Start by attempting to cross the CTO using the Sliding Technique, then progress to the Drilling Technique, utilizing the appropriate guidewires. A few minutes of patient attempts with each technique (and those described later) are sufficient. Our rule of thumb is to spend about 2–3 minutes per technique.

3. **Decide between perforation and subintimal techniques:** If previous techniques fail, decide whether to continue with endoluminal techniques – attempting to perforate the cap using the perforating technique – or switch to a subintimal approach.

    a) For short CTOs in a straight arterial segment, endoluminal perforation is often effective.
    b) For long and complex CTOs, transitioning to a subintimal technique is often unavoidable.

4. **Transition to advanced techniques if needed:** Failure of both endoluminal perforating and subintimal techniques warrants the use of advanced techniques described in the previous chapter.

   a) *A key tip to remember* – Highlighted in the CTOP classification – is that Type IV CTOs identified on angiography often respond well to retrograde recanalization.

   b) Depending on the specific scenario, it is essential to develop the experience and observational skills to determine which advanced technique is best suited to the lesion's morphology and the current position of guidewires and catheters.

5. **Consider surgical options when necessary:** Always remember to evaluate the feasibility of surgical intervention in cases of repeated failures with the proposed techniques. This reminder should not be taken lightly, as it serves to ensure that potential surgical landing zones are not compromised by an overly persistent attempt to complete the procedure endovascularly.

By adhering to these principles, the operator can systematically approach even the most challenging CTOs while preserving future options for surgical management if needed.

TIP #19

How to cross a CTO with a PTA catheter.

How often have you crossed a challenging CTO with a guidewire, only to find that you cannot advance the PTA catheter through the lesion? This frustrating scenario has occurred to me countless times.

In what follows, I outline some **tips based on experience** to overcome this particularly troublesome issue.

1. **Use an antegrade access whenever possible:** Antegrade puncture always simplifies the procedure and should be the default approach whenever feasible. In obese patients, when antegrade access at the common femoral artery level can be extremely challenging, puncturing the proximal superficial femoral artery may be a practical alternative. While unconventional, it is highly effective. However, at this level, the lack of posterior support from the femoral head can increase access-related complications. To minimize risks, observing the following.

   a) **Always use ultrasound guidance** and puncture a healthy segment at the artery's ostium. If the arterial wall quality is poor, this approach should be abandoned.

   b) **Achieve hemostasis** using a closure device. Currently, the only approved device for antegrade access is the Cordis MynxControl or MynxGrip, which delivers optimal results in these conditions.

2. **Use a support catheter for wire exchange:** After crossing the lesion with a guidewire and failing to advance the PTA catheter, place a support catheter along the CTO to exchange the recanalization wire for a more supportive one.

3. **Increase support with a long sheath:** If additional stability is required, consider using a long, reinforced sheath, positioned just proximal to the CTO's proximal cap.

4. **Select ultra–low-profile balloons:** Choose unused PTA catheters with ultra-low profiles and robust support characteristics. Personally, I find Abbott Armada catheters effective for the SFA and Medtronic Nanocross catheters ideal for infrapopliteal vessels.

5. **Proceed gradually:** For the most resistant lesions, start with balloons of smaller diameter and length (e.g., 2 mm × 20 mm) and progress step by step. Advance the balloon, inflate it briefly (a few seconds will suffice to clear the way), deflate it, and move forward incrementally (Figures 2.15–2.15a). Repeat this process until the entire lesion is crossed. This approach often allows subsequent placement of the desired PTA catheter.

6. **Try coronary CTO balloons:** If peripheral balloons fail, consider using coronary CTO balloons as an alternative.

7. **Manually manipulate the artery:** In certain regions, manual manipulation of the patient can help straighten particularly tortuous arterial segments. For instance, in the posterior tibial artery at the retromalleolar passage, forced hyperextension of the foot can partially straighten the vessel (Figures 2.16–2.16a). This maneuver can facilitate catheter advancement in some cases.

8. **Use dual access and Flossing Wire Technique:** In most challenging scenarios, employing a dual antegrade/retrograde access allows the use of the Flossing Wire Technique. The guidewire tension created by this technique enables the PTA catheter to cross the lesion in nearly all cases.

9. **Vessel preparation – the last resort:** While vessel preparation techniques generally serve other purposes (as will be discussed in the next toolkit), they can solve difficulties when all other strategies have failed.

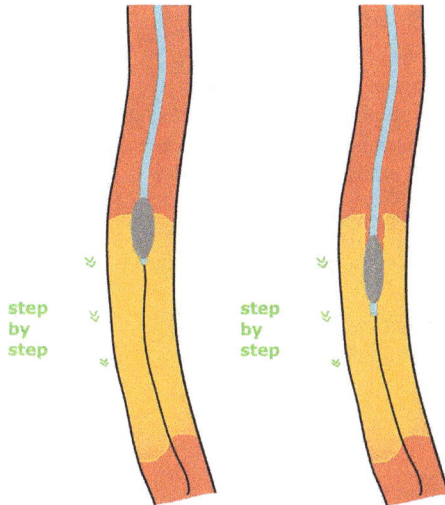

Figures 2.15–2.15a Step-by-step approach for advancing the PTA catheter through a CTO.

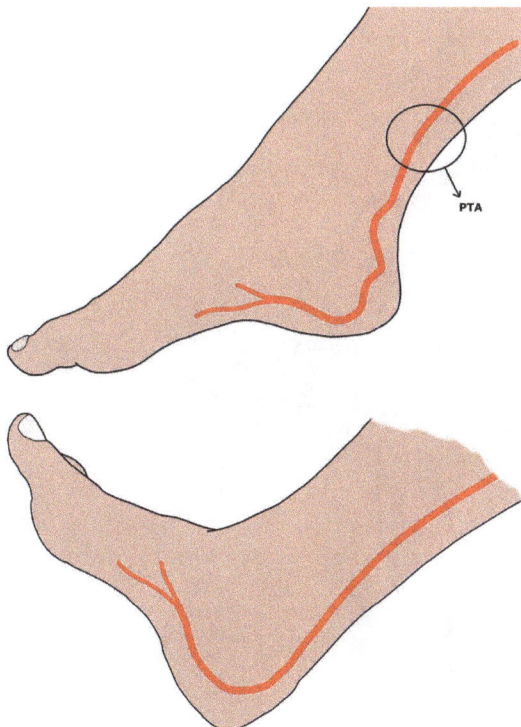

Figures 2.16–2.16a Hyperextending the foot to straighten the posterior tibial artery at the retromalleolar passage.

In many stenotic and occlusive lesions, proper pre-treatment of the plaque can significantly improve post-procedural outcomes. Vessel preparation aims to modify the consistency and structure of the plaque, enhancing the long-term patency of treated arteries, especially in cases with extensive calcification.

The objectives of **vessel preparation** are the following.

- Reduce the risk of extensive dissections following PTA.
- Optimize the quality of the lumen achieved by PTA.
- Improve drug penetration in cases where drug-coated balloons are planned.
- Minimize the risk of restenosis, reocclusions, and/or elastic recoil.
- Lower the rate of bailout stent implantation.

RATIONALE FOR VESSEL PREPARATION

The importance of vessel preparation, particularly in complex lesions, has become increasingly evident in recent years due to several factors:

1. **Wall injury from traditional PTA:** Any standard PTA (POBA – Plain Old Balloon Angioplasty) causes some degree of arterial wall damage, often resulting in dissections of varying severity. This outcome is almost expected, as it stems from the rupture and fragmentation of atherothrombotic material caused by barotrauma (Figures 2.17–2.17a).

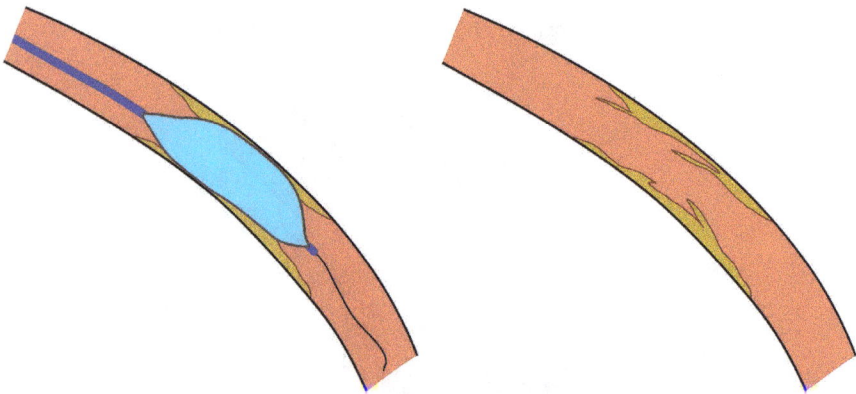

Figures 2.17–2.17a Wall injury from traditional PTA.

2. **Pressure distribution and the "dogbone effect":** During balloon inflation, the pressure within traditional balloons is evenly distributed. However, this does not produce a uniform response in the different regions of the treated vessel. Traditional PTA catheters classically create a phenomenon known as the **"dogbone effect"** on the treated vessel (Figure 2.18).

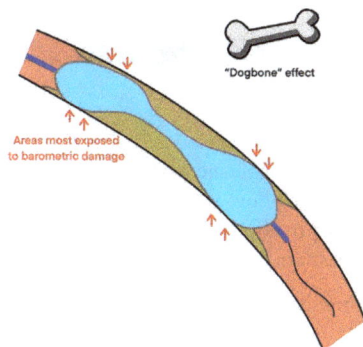

Figure 2.18 The Dogbone Effect

a) This occurs because, to dilate a stenosis or occlusion, the balloon's ends must be positioned in healthy arterial segments. These healthy segments experience much greater barometric damage than the central part of the lesion, where the PTA catheter encounters the resistance of a hardened CTO. Conversely, in the healthy, non-stenotic areas beyond the CTO edges, the balloon meets minimal resistance (Figure 2.18).

b) In these healthy zones, the atmospheric pressure applied during dilation – while effective at expanding the lesion's central portion (Figures 2.18a–2.18b) – often causes endothelial damage, resulting in post-PTA dissections that may be severely flow-limiting (Figure 2.18c).

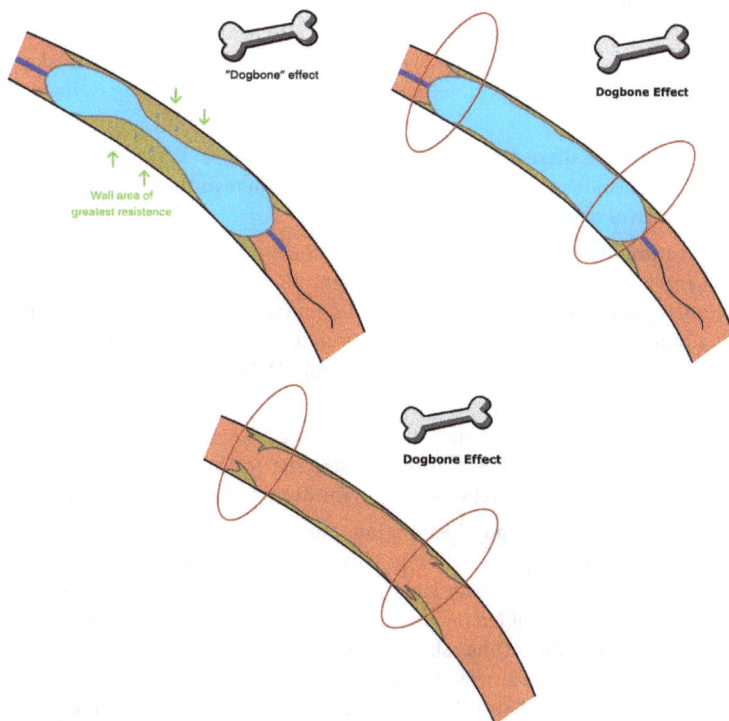

Figures 2.18a–2.18c (Continued)

3. **Challenges in highly calcified lesions:** Highly calcified lesions often do not respond adequately to simple PTA. Extensive calcification also poses a significant barrier to the absorption of antiproliferative drugs when DCBs are used.

4. **Restenosis and recoil risks:** When treating restenosis – particularly those caused by neointimal hyperplasia – the risk of early recoil following POBA is high.

TIP #20

Preliminary Tips

Before considering the use of costly devices specifically designed for vessel preparation, it is worth revisiting some simple concepts that can enable successful treatment of even the most stubborn stenotic-occlusive lesions. These strategies often allow avoidance of advanced technologies while optimizing angiographic outcomes and reducing bailout stenting, particularly in critical areas like the popliteal artery, where stent occlusion rates remain unacceptably high in most cases.

Following are the **Ten Commandments for Effective Vessel Preparation**, achieved solely with guidewires and PTA catheters.

1. **Balloon diameter matching:** The balloon diameter must perfectly match the vessel diameter, maintaining a 1:1 ratio. Preoperative mapping with ultrasound or measurement of the artery diameter via CT angiography can ensure this match. If available, IVUS provides even more precise measurements.

2. **Slow inflation:** Inflate the balloon slowly to its nominal pressure – no higher.

3. **Prolonged inflation:** Maintain inflation for **150–180 seconds** with constant pressure throughout this time.

4. **Gradual deflation:** Deflate the balloon slowly. My method involves reducing pressure by *2 atm every 5 seconds*. While there is no strong evidence supporting this practice, clinical outcomes have consistently favored this approach.

5. **Buddy wiring at bifurcations:** When performing angioplasty near arterial bifurcations (e.g., at the popliteal trifurcation), consider using a *buddy wire* in the branch that will not be treated. Occasionally, plaque displacement from angioplasty may cause acute occlusion of an ostial branch. The buddy wire allows for bailout maneuvers, such as a *Kissing Balloon Technique*, to restore vessel patency.

6. **Address flow-limiting dissections:** If angioplasty results in a dissection requiring treatment, first perform another low-pressure angioplasty for 4–5 minutes at 3–4 atm maximum. This simple intervention resolves many dissections effectively.

7. **Not all dissections require treatment:** Minor dissections of the vessel wall are an expected outcome of angioplasty and do not necessarily compromise the procedure. Treatment is warranted for *flow-limiting dissections* or those with specific characteristics, such as spiral dissections, long dissections, or multiple short dissections in succession. If there is doubt about the significance of a dissection, use intraoperative ultrasound or, preferably, **IVUS** which is the most sensitive diagnostic modality.

8. **Spot stenting over Full Metal Jacket:** If bailout stenting is unavoidable, particularly in the superficial femoral artery, avoid *Full Metal Jacket* (stenting the entire artery length). In nearly all cases, *spot stenting* (placing a short stent only in the dissected area) is sufficient (Figure 2.19).

9. **Special considerations for the popliteal region:** The popliteal artery is unique due to the biomechanical stress caused by knee joint motion. This stress accounts for the high rates of stent occlusion and fracture in this area. Many endovascular surgeons, myself included, believe that the popliteal region should be *avoided for stenting* whenever possible. If stenting is absolutely necessary, the **Supera Stent (Abbott)** has shown superior patency rates in the popliteal territory. Its unique mesh design, high radial strength, and exceptional flexibility make it the preferred choice at this level. Do not forget that – despite the persistence often characteristic of endovascular operators – **open surgery** is a feasible option in most cases of endovascular failure.

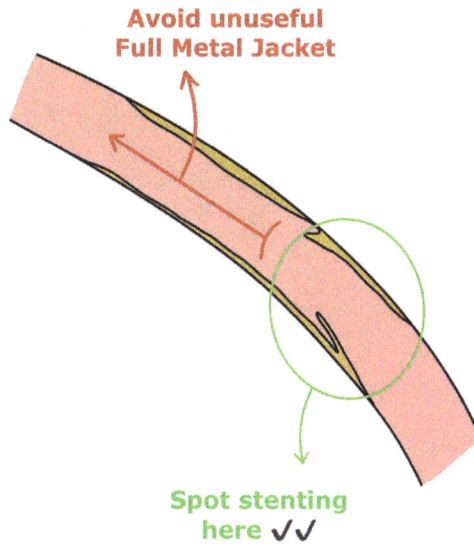

Figure 2.19 Spot Stenting vs. Full Metal Jacket

10. **Advanced devices as a last resort:** If the aforementioned tips fail or advanced vessel preparation is deemed necessary, transitioning to dedicated devices becomes essential.

WHICH VESSEL PREPARATION?

The devices currently used for vessel preparation include the following.

1. **Cutting balloons**
2. **Scoring balloons**
3. **Atraumatic balloons**
4. **Atherectomy devices**
5. **Shockwave therapy**

TIP #21

Cutting balloons (Figure 2.20) have metal blades on their surface designed to precisely and selectively cut through plaque. They are generally indicated for use in the endovascular treatment of stenoses in arteriovenous fistulas for hemodialysis, as well as for restenoses in arteries previously treated surgically or endovascularly – particularly when the restenosis is highly resistant, fibrotic, and prone to recoil.

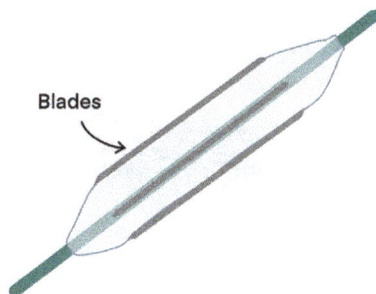

Figure 2.20 Cutting balloons.

Specifically, in cases of **post-TEA restenosis** of the common femoral artery caused by neointimal hyperplasia, which is a fibrotic and highly resistant type of stenosis, cutting balloons can effectively rupture the hyperplastic zone. This rupture allows the arterial wall to yield adequately during the subsequent POBA. Additionally, it enhances drug uptake when drug-coated balloons are used, which is typically recommended for these lesions.

For post-TEA restenosis of the common femoral artery, where an "endovascular-first" approach is almost always the preferred choice, the sequence is as follows.

- **Cutting balloon**, undersized relative to the vessel's nominal diameter (balloons 3 mm or 4 mm in diameter are sufficient).
- **POBA**, using a balloon with a nominal diameter matching the vessel.
- **DCB**.

TIP #22

Scoring balloons (Figure 2.21) are semi-compliant balloons wrapped with scoring elements made of polymer or nitinol, which can have a helical configuration (e.g., **AngioSculpt**, Philips) or run parallel to the catheter's longitudinal axis (e.g., **UltraScore**, BD). This design significantly increases the pressure exerted at the points where the metallic mesh contacts the plaque, leading to controlled plaque rupture.

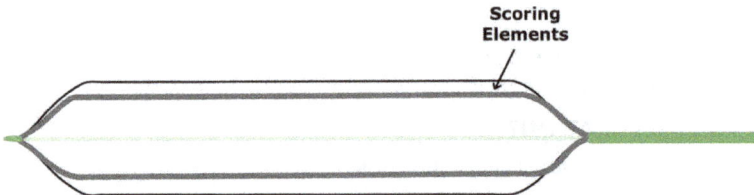

Figure 2.21 Scoring balloons.

This mechanism of action differs from that of atraumatic balloons (e.g., **Chocolate**, Medtronic), which will be described shortly, and from cutting balloons, as previously discussed, where the metallic elements are actual blades.

Scoring balloons are typically indicated for **ostial stenoses**, such as at the origin of the superficial femoral artery, where it is critical to minimize the extent of post-PTA dissection. Controlled plaque rupture at these sites also enhances drug uptake when using DCBs.

TIP #23

Atraumatic balloons (e.g., **Chocolate**, Medtronic – Figure 2.22) are semi-compliant balloons encased in a nitinol mesh designed to deliver balanced PTA with minimal and uniform vessel trauma. The Chocolate balloon minimizes the long dissections typical of POBA by creating controlled and localized microdissections along the treated artery. These microdissections are generally benign and non–flow-limiting.

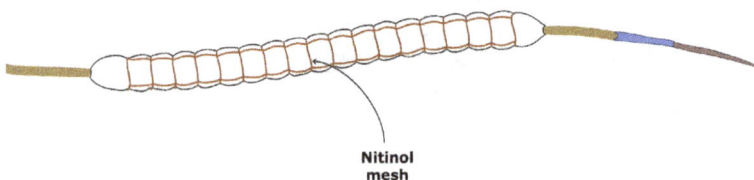

Figure 2.22 Atraumatic balloons.

The Chocolate balloon differs from scoring balloons in that the nitinol mesh does not directly contact the plaque. Instead, the balloon emerges through the mesh as atraumatic pillows that compress the plaque effectively without significantly altering its consistency.

Given its properties, this balloon is particularly useful in popliteal CTOs, which are a significant challenge for traditional POBA. In this region, it is critical to avoid long dissections that might necessitate bailout stenting.

The use of DCBs following the Chocolate balloon is recommended to optimize outcomes.

TIP #24

When dealing with particularly tenacious, long, calcified, or coraliform stenotic-occlusive lesions, **atherectomy devices** provide an excellent option for debulking atherothrombotic material, achieving results beyond what can be achieved with the compression offered by PTA balloons. However, it is worth emphasizing that plaque pre-treatment using atherectomy devices still lacks robust supporting evidence. Additionally, their use prolongs procedure time, requires larger sheath sizes, and comes with significantly higher costs.

Several types of devices are currently available on the market, including the following.

1. **Directional (excisional) atherectomy:** Directional atherectomy devices, such as the *Hawk systems* from Medtronic, allow the operator to direct the cutting edge toward the plaque. In the Hawk system, the plaque is excised by a rotating blade and collected in a conical reservoir, which must be emptied after several passes. A distal filter is mandatory due to the risk of embolization. These devices are particularly useful in vessel preparation of the common femoral artery in patients unfit for open surgery, thanks to the operator's ability to precisely control the amount of tissue removed. Soft and mixed lesions respond best to directional atherectomy. The most effective technique involves performing multiple passes along the lesion, orienting the cut in 4–8 directions. Operator expertise is critical to avoid complications and reduce the risk of embolization. Specifically, the reservoir collecting the excised debris must be emptied before it becomes full. If not, the excised material may overflow and embolize distally instead of being collected.

2. **Rotational atherectomy:** Rotational atherectomy devices differ from other debulking systems by utilizing a high-speed rotational burr along a fixed axis, enabling selective fragmentation of the lesion without altering the device's central trajectory. Examples include the *Jetstream* (Boston Scientific) and *Rotarex* (BD). The **Jetstream** achieves plaque debulking with a crown located at its tip, equipped with cutting blades that rotate at speeds of approximately 70,000 rpm. If necessary, adjunctive lateral blades positioned behind the catheter tip can be deployed to create a larger lumen. This system is designed to target plaque exclusively, deflecting and sparing healthy elastic tissue. An aspiration port near the catheter tip collects debris into an external reservoir during the procedure. In addition to its use in the superficial femoral artery and tibial vessels, the Jetstream is particularly valuable for treating the popliteal artery and in-stent restenosis or reocclusions. The use of a distal filter is also recommended. The **Rotarex** device combines rotational atherectomy with active aspiration, allowing real-time removal of debris into an external reservoir. The device consists of a blunt-tipped, rotating outer housing with an internal metallic helix that spins at 40,000–60,000 rpm, generating negative pressure to aspirate fragments during the procedure. Compatible with 6–8 Fr sheaths, it can treat vessels with diameters ranging from 3–8 mm. A key advantage of the Rotarex is its versatility, allowing it to address both fresh thrombotic lesions and chronic occlusions, including **CTOs**. This all-in-one device is suitable for both elective and acute settings.

3. **Orbital atherectomy:** The *Diamondback 360* from Cardiovascular Systems employs a diamond-coated crown that fragments plaque through orbital, eccentric rotation around its axis. This mechanism enables circumferential plaque removal, effectively smoothing the arterial wall. Unlike rotational systems, the Diamondback 360 does not include an aspiration mechanism, increasing the risk of distal embolization. However, the debris generated is microscopically small,

with 99% of particles being smaller than a red blood cell. The device is designed specifically for debulking calcified and fibrocalcific plaques while sparing the healthy, elastic arterial wall. To prevent arterial overheating, which could cause thermal damage, continuous infusion of a cold saline and Rota-Glide mixture is recommended during the procedure. Evidence is growing to support its use in infrapopliteal segments.

4. **Laser atherectomy:** Laser atherectomy devices, such as the ***Turbo-Elite*** from Philips, vaporize plaque using ultraviolet laser light through photochemical and photomechanical mechanisms, rather than photothermal action. This approach minimizes damage to healthy tissue and generates subcellular-sized debris.

    In addition to treating de novo lesions in the superficial femoral artery, laser atherectomy is particularly effective for in-stent restenosis or reocclusions. Uniquely among atherectomy devices, laser atherectomy is also indicated for the recanalization of CTOs that cannot be crossed with a guidewire, making it an invaluable option for managing the most resistant lesions.

TIP #25

Intravascular Lithotripsy

This unique device is designed to overcome even the most calcified stenotic-occlusive lesions, which may be resistant to atherectomy devices, through the use of intravascular lithotripsy, which fractures the calcified plaque. The ***Shockwave system*** (Shockwave Medical) consists of an OTW balloon equipped with emitters along its surface that generate electro-hydraulic sonic waves.

The balloon's diameter should have a 1.1:1 ratio to the nominal diameter of the vessel being treated (e.g., a 5.5 mm balloon is suitable for a 5 mm superficial femoral artery). The balloon is inflated to 4 atm to establish contact with the lesion and then activated. The sonic waves penetrate the calcium in the plaque, fracturing it while sparing healthy tissue. After modifying the plaque's calcium consistency, further PTA using the integrated balloon ensures optimal plaque remodeling.

In addition to enabling effective PTA in calcium-dominated lesions, the fracturing of calcium enhances drug uptake when a drug-coated balloon is used. Indeed, calcium impedes the absorption of antiproliferative drugs present in drug-coated devices.

The Shockwave device can be utilized at all anatomical levels and has demonstrated excellent results with a low complication rate, even during subintimal recanalization. However, the device's high cost remains a significant drawback.

Recently, some operators have begun employing lithotripsy with positive outcomes in the following.

- **Vessel preparation for coral reef aortic plaques and iliac lesions** prior to aortoiliac endovascular reconstruction.
- **Pre-treatment of severely diseased and calcified iliac axes** during EVAR procedures.
- During **carotid stenting procedures**, particularly for heavily calcified stenoses.

TIP #26

The use of distal filters in infrainguinal pathology and vessel preparation.

The use of distal filters is particularly recommended – especially in the treatment of the femoropopliteal segment – when employing directional or rotational atherectomy devices (Figure 2.23). On the other hand, the debris produced by laser and orbital atherectomy devices is subcellular in size, rendering it harmless and smaller than the filter mesh diameter, making the use of a filter unnecessary in these cases.

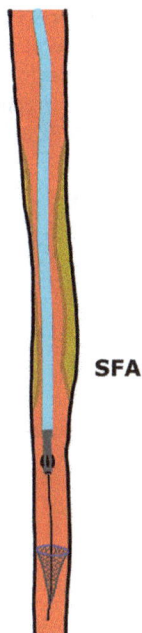

During rotational or escissional atherectomy of an infrainguinal CTO

N.B. *(leave your filter some cms beyond)*

SFA

Figure 2.23 When to use a distal filter during infrainguinal interventions.

The filters most commonly used in conjunction with atherectomy devices are the *SpiderFx* (Medtronic) and the *Emboshield NAV6* (Abbott).

Figures 2.23a–2.23d illustrate other potential uses of distal filters during infrainguinal procedures, specifically:

1. Placement in the deep femoral artery is crucial during an endarterectomy of the femoral trifurcation when the superficial femoral artery is occluded (Figure 2.23a).

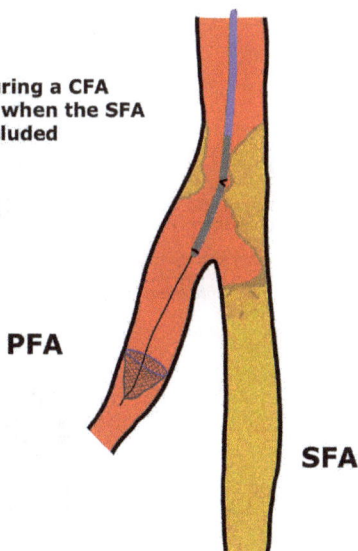

In PFA, during a CFA atherectomy, when the SFA is occluded

PFA

SFA

Figure 2.23a (Continued)

2. In cases of femoral trifurcation endarterectomy whereby the superficial femoral artery is patent, it is possible – though off-label and recommended only for experienced operators – to perform a second percutaneous antegrade access in a healthy segment of the distal superficial femoral artery. Through this access, a second filter can be introduced to protect the femoropopliteal distal segment from embolization (Figure 2.23b).

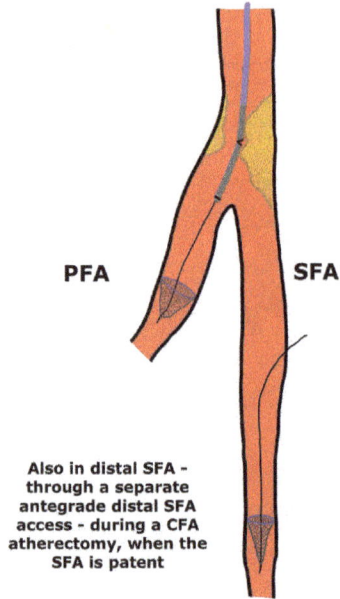

PFA　　　　**SFA**

Also in distal SFA - through a separate antegrade distal SFA access - during a CFA atherectomy, when the SFA is patent

Figure 2.23b (Continued)

3. The use of a filter is also beneficial in the treatment of occlusions characterized by fresh thrombosis (Figure 2.23c). The following signs may suggest such a lesion.

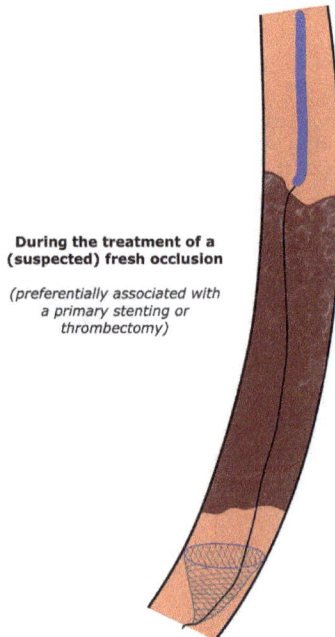

During the treatment of a (suspected) fresh occlusion

(preferentially associated with a primary stenting or thrombectomy)

Figure 2.23c (Continued)

a) Easy passage of the guidewire.
b) Acute or sudden onset of symptoms.
c) Thrombotic appearance of the lesion on ultrasound or CT angiography.

4. Finally, distal filters are particularly advantageous in the endovascular treatment of popliteal aneurysms, especially when the aneurysmal sac contains thrombotic material (Figure 2.23d).

During an endovascular treatment of a popliteal aneurysm

N.B. *(when the aneurysmal sac is full of thrombus)*

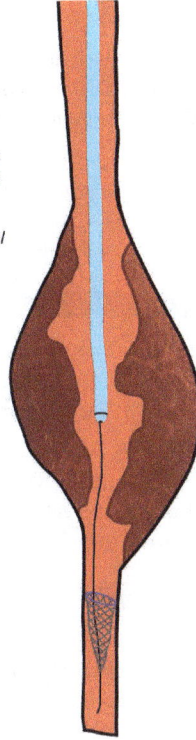

Figure 2.23d (Continued)

For more than a decade, the use of **drug-coated balloons (DCBs)** has revolutionized the treatment of peripheral vascular disease. The necessity for such platforms arises from the persistently high rate of early post-procedural restenosis. This phenomenon occurs due to arterial wall damage induced by barotrauma, which triggers proliferative mechanisms in smooth muscle cells – the primary agents responsible for the cellular reproduction that underlies neointimal hyperplasia. This progressive thickening of the arterial wall caused by neointimal hyperplasia ultimately results in early restenosis.

The rationale for using drug-coated devices is tied to the antimitotic and antiproliferative properties of the drug embedded in the device – typically **Paclitaxel**, with **Sirolimus** being a more recent addition. These properties inhibit the cellular reproductive processes that drive neointimal hyperplasia and subsequent restenosis.

Given these considerations, ideally, every endovascular procedure involving angioplasty – which inherently induces arterial barotrauma – can benefit from the concurrent use of a DCB. These devices are indicated for both de novo lesions and restenoses (including in-stent restenosis).

TIP #27

The use of DCBs should be preceded by a procedural step focused on adequate vessel preparation, as outlined earlier. This preparation optimizes the quality of the arterial wall surface that comes into contact with the drug, thereby enhancing its uptake.

It is also important to note that high calcium content within a lesion can significantly impair drug absorption at that site. Therefore, in cases of severely calcified lesions, adequate debulking of the stenotic-occlusive segment through atherectomy or effective modification of lesion consistency via lithotripsy are critical steps to ensure the efficacy of DCBs in highly calcified arterial contexts.

TIP #28

The appropriate matching between the diameter of the DCB and the vessel should follow a ratio of 1.1:1 (Figure 2.24). For instance, for a superficial femoral artery with a diameter of 5 mm, a 5.5 mm balloon is the preferred choice. This ensures that the entire surface of the balloon effectively contacts the vessel wall.

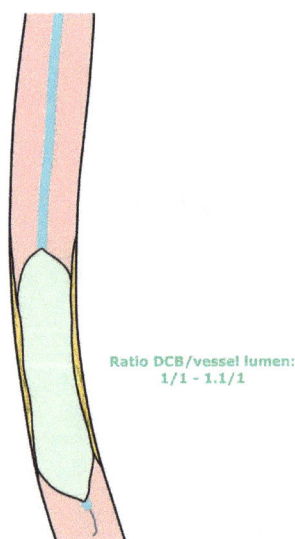

Ratio DCB/vessel lumen:
1/1 - 1.1/1

Figure 2.24 The DCB ratio: 1:1:1.

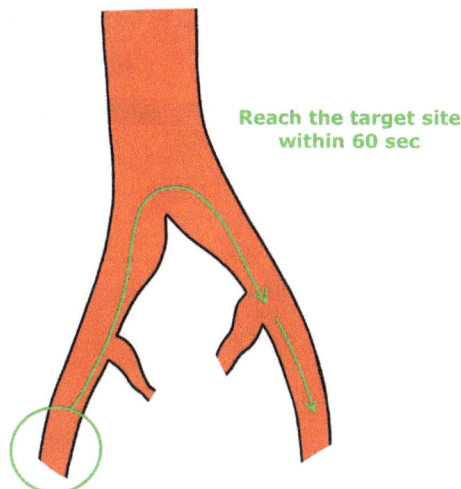

Reach the target site within 60 sec

Hurry Up!!

Figure 2.24a The correct strategy for successful DCB deployment.

It is important to emphasize that the optimal method for measuring vessel diameter is IVUS (Intravascular Ultrasound), and the measurement technique should consider the diameter of the artery based on the external elastic membrane (rather than lumen-to-lumen measurements). Employing these techniques has been associated with a significantly lower rate of restenosis compared to other measurement methods.

TIP #29

Once deployed into the bloodstream, the **DCB must reach the target site within 60 seconds** at most; otherwise, the drug may be lost into circulation, significantly reducing the device's efficacy if positioning takes longer (Figure 2.24a). If it takes more than 2 minutes to reach the desired site, the drug will have completely dispersed, rendering the device ineffective.

To mitigate this issue, the use of long sheaths or guiding catheters positioned immediately upstream of the lesion to be treated can be advantageous. These tools allow the device to travel within a controlled environment, minimizing its exposure to blood flow during its over-the-wire advancement, thereby preserving drug integrity.

TIP #30

In the case of an anastomotic stenosis (particularly involving a prosthetic graft), it is generally advisable to avoid performing PTA directly on the anastomosis unless absolutely necessary. Instead, the focus should be on dilating only the native artery, the graft, or both, separately and in succession (Figures 2.25–2.25c).

The use of a **DCB** following POBA is highly recommended to optimize outcomes.

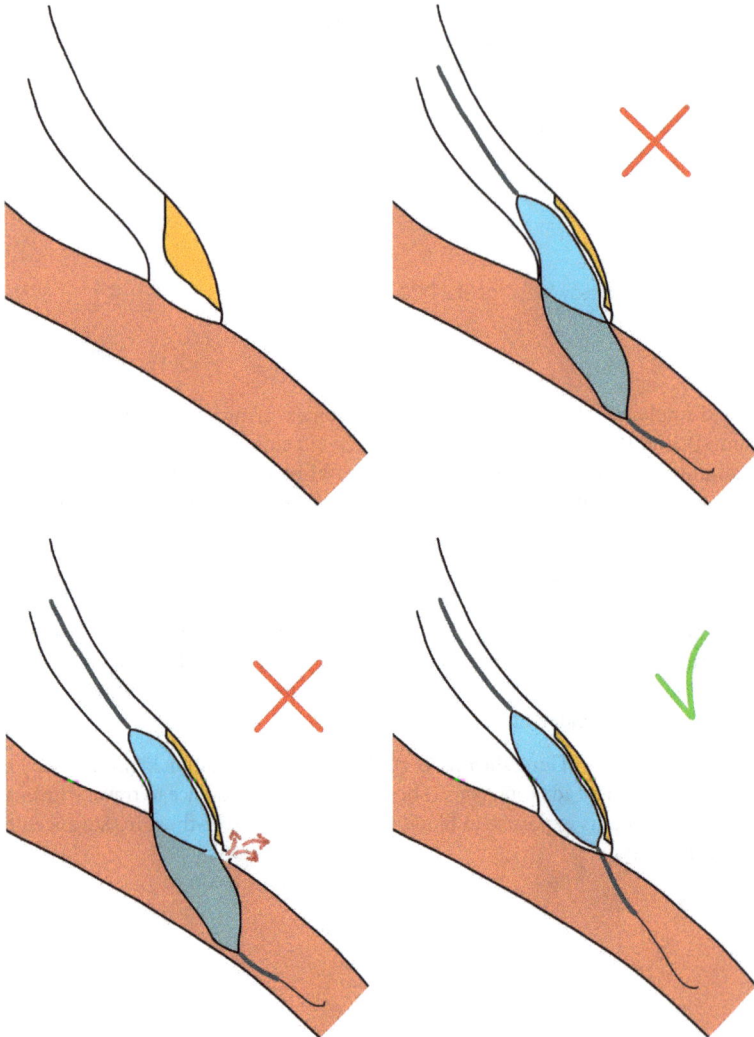

Figures 2.25–2.25c Performing a correct anastomotic PTA.

TIP #31

Restenosis at the level of prosthetic material, such as femoral patches, can typically be treated with balloon angioplasty starting approximately 3 months after the open surgical procedure. By this time, the prosthetic material will have been incorporated into the surrounding fibrotic tissue (the "prosthetic rind"), which helps prevent complications such as hemorrhage or pseudoaneurysm formation.

I deliberately omitted the term *"acute ischemia"* from the title of this section, as this is a technical volume focused not on arterial pathologies in a broad sense, but specifically on the lesions that cause them and, consequently, on the methods to address them. Additionally, it is important to consider that an acutely developed lesion does not necessarily result in acute ischemia. In patients with underlying atherosclerotic disease, for instance, acute thrombosis of a vessel often leads to symptoms resembling those of chronic occlusive arterial disease, such as claudication or the onset of CLTI.

It is also not uncommon, during an elective endovascular procedure in a patient with chronic PAD, to encounter acute, fresh lesions. These require first to be recognized and then treated appropriately, as the risk of complications – most notably distal embolization – can significantly worsen the underlying disease.

Finally, though rare, intraoperative management of thrombosis or embolization may become necessary, requiring prompt recognition and resolution to avoid further complications.

TIP #32

The first step, therefore, is to recognize and distinguish a **fresh lesion** from a **chronic lesion**. This can be achieved through the following methods.

1. A **detailed patient history**. Investigating the onset and progression of symptoms is crucial. Determining whether symptoms appeared gradually or suddenly can provide valuable insights. For example, a patient reporting the sudden onset of calf claudication within the past month likely has a recent thrombosis of the superficial femoral artery.

2. **Preoperative diagnostics**. In most cases, preoperative imaging can differentiate between fresh and chronic lesions. A fresh, thrombotic lesion typically appears hypo/anechoic on duplex ultrasound, in contrast to older, fibrocalcific lesions, which present as heterogeneous hypo/isoechoic masses with calcified spots. Purely calcified lesions, on the other hand, are identified by acoustic shadows that hinder normal vessel visualization on color Doppler. The occlusion of an artery with otherwise normal-appearing walls is almost certainly recent.

3. A **thorough angiographic evaluation**, both at the start and at the conclusion of the procedure, is essential.

4. The **ease of crossing the lesion with a guidewire**. If the guidewire traverses the occlusion with exceptional ease – "like cutting butter with a knife" – the lesion is likely fresh and carries a high risk of embolization. In such cases, **primary stenting** of the entire obliterated segment is much safer than performing a simple PTA.

TIP #33

In our experience, for stenting or primary stenting of fresh lesions, we find it more practical and safer to use self-expanding, closed-cell stents. These stents should be positioned at least 15–20 mm beyond the distal edge of the lesion and at least 10–15 mm proximal to it. This technique effectively cages the thrombus, reducing the risk of distal embolization during the deployment and expansion of the device (Figures 2.26–2.26c).

To ensure precision, it is highly recommended to use micrometric-release stents. Stents with a pullback mechanism, on the other hand, carry the risk of jumping forward during deployment, which could leave the proximal portion of the thrombus uncovered and therefore prone to embolization.

Post-deployment PTA of the stent should only be performed if necessary (i.e., in cases of suboptimal results), with inflation pressures limited to 4–6 atm. This minimizes the risk of thrombus prolapse through the stent struts.

Using balloon-mounted stents in this setting presents a significant risk: during expansion, the proximal and distal ends of the thrombus, not yet encased within the stent, may be squeezed upward or downward, leading to fragmentation and an increased risk of embolization.

GW easily
crosses the lesion

"Fresh" Thrombotic Lesion

Ensure that the proximal and
distal landing zones extend
far beyond the lesion, to avoid
squeezing it out

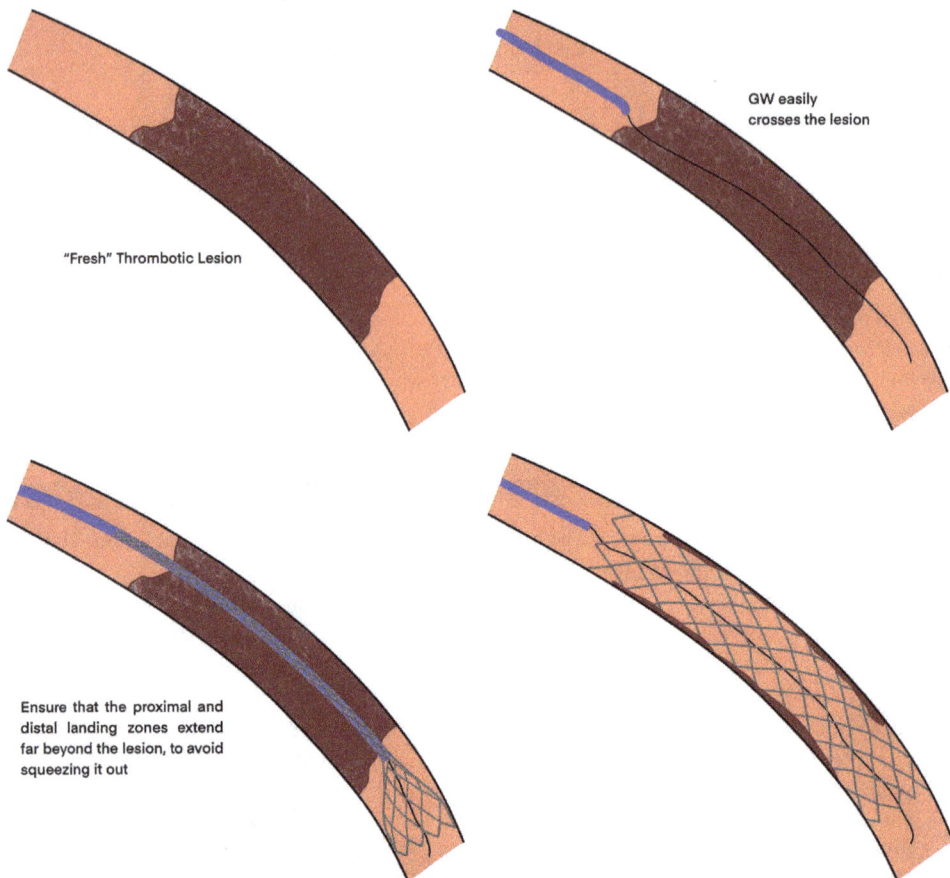

Figures 2.26–2.26c Primary stenting of a fresh arterial occlusion.

TIP #34

Some authors suggest performing primary stenting using self-expanding covered stents (e.g., Gore Viabahn) to prevent thrombus prolapse through the stent struts. However, their superior efficacy compared to uncovered stents has not been conclusively demonstrated.

A significant additional risk following the use of these devices is the potential coverage of important collateral branches. If this occurs, the clinical progression to acute ischemia in the event of graft occlusion can be severe and should not be underestimated.

TIP #35

The hybrid surgical techniques described for the treatment of chronic lesions (which will be detailed in subsequent sections) are also useful in addressing acute lesions. However, their effectiveness in an emergency setting has yet to be definitively demonstrated. In such cases, the endovascular step can complement the open procedure by addressing lesions located proximally or distally to the surgical site.

The key addition to consider when using these techniques for acute lesions, compared to atherosclerotic lesions, is that the endovascular phase may also include thromboembolectomy using a Fogarty catheter guided over a wire and under fluoroscopic guidance. This approach significantly improves the outcomes of the traditional blind Fogarty Technique, whereby the catheter is inserted and advanced without visual control. For instance, when addressing the femoral trifurcation, the following steps are typically taken.

1. **Isolation of the femoral trifurcation:** Vessel loops and proximal and distal clamps are placed. An introducer sheath is inserted into the artery to perform an angiogram, identifying the extent of the occlusion requiring treatment (Figure 2.27).

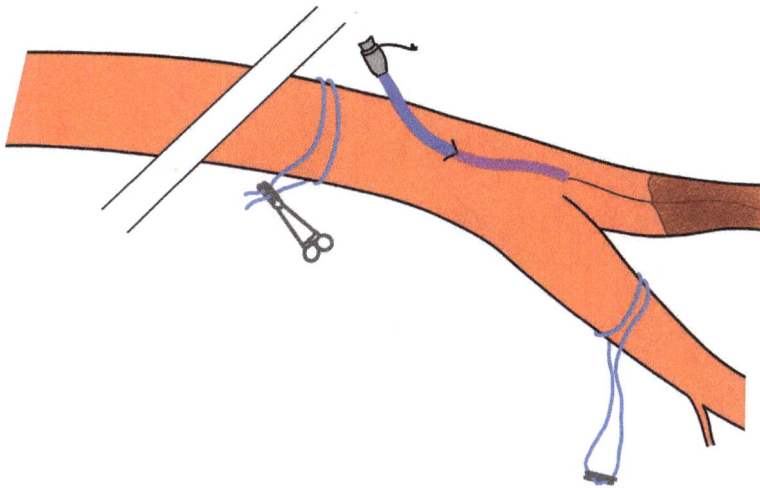

Figure 2.27 The hybrid surgical approach for treating acute lesions.

2. **Guidewire advancement:** A guidewire is advanced under fluoroscopic guidance to cross the thromboembolic lesion. This can be done in an **antegrade direction** (toward the SFA) or **retrograde direction** (toward the iliac axis), depending on the location of the occlusion.

3. **Clamp placement:** The clamp on the side opposite the treatment site is secured. For example, if treating the SFA, the iliac clamp is secured, and vice versa.

4. **Arteriotomy and re-insertion of the introducer:** The introducer sheath is temporarily removed to perform an arteriotomy. It is then reinserted into the artery.

5. **Insertion of the Fogarty catheter:** The Fogarty catheter is advanced over the guidewire under fluoroscopic visualization until the balloon passes well beyond the thrombotic lesion.

6. **Thromboembolectomy:** The introducer sheath is withdrawn, and thromboembolectomy is performed by extracting the thrombus (Figures 2.27a–2.27b).

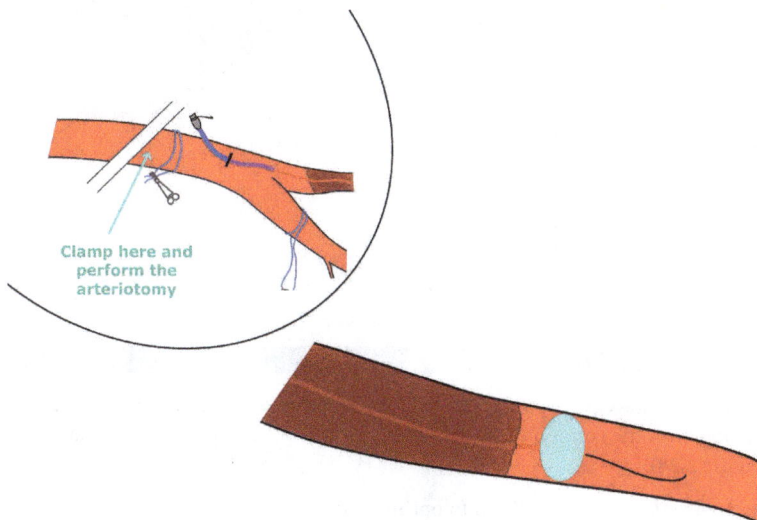

Clamp here and perform the arteriotomy

Figure 2.27a (Continued)

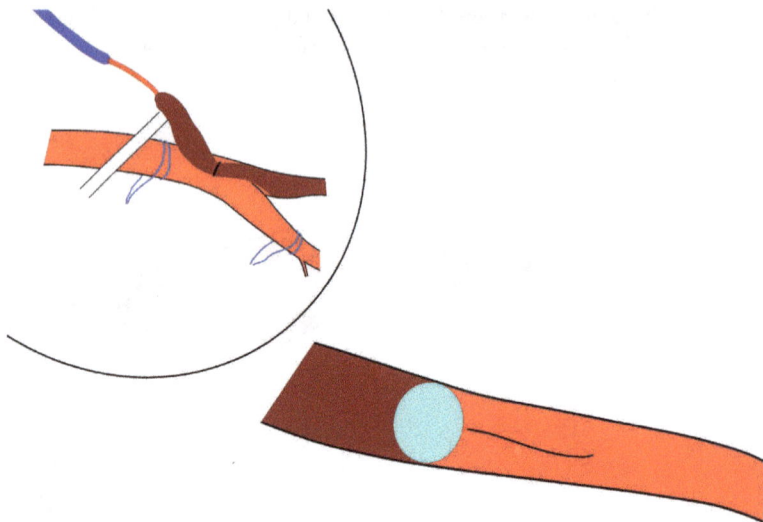

Figure 2.27b (Continued)

7. **Completion angiography:** After completing the necessary number of passes to ensure full removal of the thromboembolic material, a follow-up angiogram is performed. Any underlying chronic lesions are then treated (Figure 2.27c).

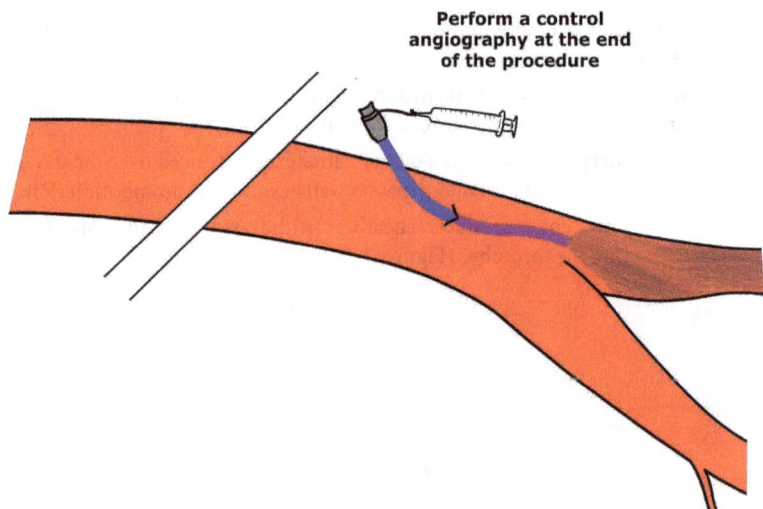

Perform a control
angiography at the end
of the procedure

Figure 2.27c (Continued)

TIP #36

In certain cases, a dual access approach, such as the *Rendezvous Technique,* may be required. This involves isolating both the common femoral artery and the infragenicular popliteal artery at the trifurcation (Figure 2.28).

Through the popliteal artery, in addition to optimizing proximal thromboembolectomy if needed, it becomes possible to perform Fogarty thrombectomy distally. This is achieved by sequentially advancing the Fogarty catheter into each tibial vessel.

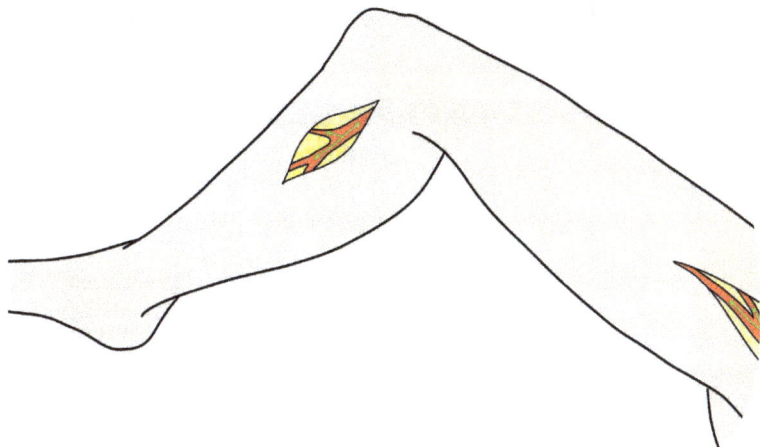

Figure 2.28 The Rendezvous Technique during a hybrid thromboembolectomy.

TIP #37

As an alternative to the two previous (and more economical) methods of treating fresh arterial lesions, there is the possibility of mechanical thromboaspiration conducted using dedicated devices (Boston AngioJet, BD Rotarex, Indigo Penumbra) – whose ease of use and clinical efficacy have now made them indispensable tools to have in one's material inventory.

Due to the frequent and concomitant use of thrombolytic drugs, the only precautions to keep in mind when planning an approach with these devices *ab initio* are the following.

• The use of a femoral crossover access, which is easier to manage compared to antegrade access.
• The use of a percutaneous closure system at the end of the procedure.
• The placement of a distal filter.

A precise and careful post-procedural angiography, which, especially in atherosclerotic patients where the acute event may have been caused by thrombosis on an atheromatous plaque, will in many cases reveal the chronic lesion – which will need to be treated.

TIP #38

Although open surgery remains the gold standard for treating popliteal aneurysms and is, unsurprisingly, our first choice, with endovascular treatment reserved for truly exceptional cases, if we must treat a popliteal aneurysm using an endovascular technique, the following tips apply.

- In our experience, Viabahn stent grafts are the best choice for this application.
- The diameter difference between the proximal and distal arteries should not exceed 4 mm.
- Perform multiple angiographic projections, including with the knee flexed and externally rotated, to determine the optimal stent positioning and the best overlap zone. Dynamic limb testing during final angiography is essential to verify proper stent positioning and the absence of endoleaks.
- Under no circumstances should a single stent terminate in the region where the artery kinks during knee flexion. It is better to use a slightly longer stent to avoid landing in this area.
- If overlap is necessary, position a longer graft distally, overlapped by a shorter, larger-diameter graft proximally. This configuration improves sealing and better excludes the aneurysmal sac.
- Avoid excessive overlap, as stent fractures are more likely to occur at the overlap zone; 15–20 mm is sufficient. Before implanting the second (proximal) stent graft, balloon the distal sealing zone of the first stent graft. Complete ballooning for post-implantation modeling should be performed at the end of the procedure on both grafts.
- Oversize the covered stent by 10–15% relative to the proximal and distal arterial diameters.

TIP #39

Anatomical criteria for endovascular feasibility in the treatment of popliteal aneurysms.

- A **proximal and distal healthy landing zone** of at least **20 mm** in length, with good quality and free of parietal thrombus.
- Vessel **tortuosity less than 45°**.
- An aneurysm diameter (**D**) of less than **5 cm** to minimize the risk of stent-graft displacement or excessive kinking within the aneurysmal sac.
- At least **two patent distal vessels** for adequate outflow.

REFERENCES

1. Korosoglou G, Schmidt A, Lichtenberg M, et al. Best crossing of peripheral chronic total occlusions: A systematic algorithm and an interdisciplinary position statement. *Vasa*. 2023 May; 52(3): 147–159.

2. Korosoglou G, Schmidt A, Lichtenberg M, et al. Crossing algorithm for infrainguinal chronic total occlusions. *JACC: Cardiovasc Interv*. 2023 Feb; 16(3): 317–331.

3. Schneider PA. Principles of arteriography. In: *Endovascular Skills: Guidewire and Catheter Skills for Endovascular Surgery*. 4th ed. Boca Raton, FL: CRC Press; 2020. pp. 113–121.

4. Saab F, Jaff MR, Diaz-Sandoval LJ, et al. Chronic total occlusion crossing approach based on plaque cap morphology: The CTOP classification. *J Endovasc Ther*. 2018 Jun; 25(3): 284–291.

5. Turkyilmaz S, Kavala AA. The relationship between plaque cap morphology and access technique in lower extremity chronic total occlusion. *Vascular*. 2019 Apr; 27(2): 135–143.

6. Solimeno G, Salcuni M, Capparelli G, et al. Technical perspectives in the management of complex infrainguinal arterial chronic total occlusions. *J Vasc Surg*. 2022 Feb; 75(2): 732–739.

7. Lorenzoni R, Ferraresi R, Manzi M, et al. Guidewires for lower extremity artery angioplasty: A review. *EuroIntervention*. 2015 Nov; 11(8): 799–807.

8. Mishra S. Language of CTO interventions – focus on hardware. *Indian Heart J*. 2016 Jul–Aug; 68(4): 450–463.

9. Laksono S, Pasciolly RMRJ, Munirwan H, et al. Choosing the appropriate catheter and wire in peripheral intervention. *AsiaIntervention*. 2022 Oct; 8(2): 162–170.

10. Ferraresi R, Palena LM, Mauri G, et al. Tips and tricks for a correct "endo approach". *J Cardiovasc Surg*. 2013 Dec; 54(6): 685–711.

11. Huang HL, Chou HH, Wu TY. Endovascular sharp recanalization for calcified femoropopliteal artery occlusion. *Case Rep Cardiol*. 2012: 1–5.

12. Bolia A, Miles KA, Brennan J, et al. Percutaneous transluminal angioplasty of occlusions of the femoral and popliteal arteries by subintimal dissection. *Cardiovasc Intervent Radiol*. 1990 Nov; 13(6): 357–363.

13. Yilmaz S, Sindel T, Yegin A, et al. Subintimal angioplasty of long superficial femoral artery occlusions. *J Vasc Interv Radiol*. 2003 Aug; 14(8): 997–1010.

14. Desgranges P, Boufi M, Lapeyre M, et al. Subintimal angioplasty: Feasible and durable. *Eur J Vasc Endovasc Surg*. 2004 Aug; 28(2): 138–141.

15. Pernès JM, Auguste M, Borie H, et al. Infrapopliteal arterial recanalization: A true advance for limb salvage in diabetics. *Diagn Interv Imaging*. 2015 May; 96(5): 423–434.

16. Spinosa DJ, Harthun NL, Bissonette EA, et al. Subintimal arterial flossing with antegrade – retrograde intervention (SAFARI) for subintimal recanalization to treat chronic critical limb ischemia. *J Vasc Interv Radiol*. 2005 Jan; 16(1): 37–44.

17. Ozen M, Zhu F, Ma C, et al. Outcomes of subintimal arterial flossing with antegrade – retrograde intervention on patients with critical limb ischemia and tissue loss. *Vasc Med*. 2021 Apr; 26(2): 207–209.

18. Zhuang KD, Tan SG, Tay KH. The "SAFARI" technique using retrograde access via peroneal artery access. *Cardiovasc Intervent Radiol*. 2012 Aug; 35(4): 927–931.

19. Kaushal A, Roche-Nagle G, Tan KT, et al. Outcomes at a single center after subintimal arterial flossing with antegrade-retrograde intervention for critical limb ischemia. *J Vasc Surg*. 2018 May; 67(5): 1448–1454.

20. Schmidt A, Bausback Y, Piorkowski M, et al. Retrograde recanalization technique for use after failed antegrade angioplasty in chronic femoral artery occlusions. *J Endovas Ther*. 2012 Feb; 19(1): 23–29.

21. Ysa A, Lobato M, Patrone L, et al. Tips and tricks for simple and complex below-the-ankle punctures. *J Endovasc Ther*. 2024 Mar 5. doi: 10.1177/15266028241234506.

22. Palena LM, Manzi M. Extreme below-the-knee interventions: Retrograde transmetatarsal or transplantar arch access for foot salvage in challenging cases of critical limb ischemia. *J Endovas Ther*. 2012 Dec; 19(6): 805–811.

23. Hua WR, Yi MQ, Min TL, et al. Popliteal versus tibial retrograde access for subintimal arterial flossing with antegrade – retrograde intervention (SAFARI) technique. *Eur J Vasc Endovasc Surg*. 2013 Aug; 46(2): 249–254.

24. Rogers RK, Dattilo PB, Garcia JA. Retrograde approach to recanalization of complex tibial disease. *Cathet Cardio Intervent*. 2011 May; 77(6): 915–925.

25. Montero-Baker M, Schmidt A, Bräunlich S, et al. Retrograde approach for complex popliteal and tibioperoneal occlusions. *J Endovasc Ther*. 2008 Oct; 15(5): 594–604.

26. Choi JH, Ryu YS, Suh J, et al. Successful recanalization of a long superficial femoral artery occlusion by retrograde subintimal angioplasty after a failed antegrade subintimal approach. *Korean Circ J*. 2008; 38(10): 557–560.

27. Ruzsa Z, Nemes B, Bánsághi Z, et al. Transpedal access after failed anterograde recanalization of complex below-the-knee and femoropopliteal occlusions in critical limb ischemia. *Cathet Cardio Intervent*. 2014 May; 83(6): 997–1007.

28. Gür S, Oğuzkurt L, Gürel K, et al. US-guided retrograde tibial artery puncture for recanalization of complex infrainguinal arterial occlusions. *Diagn Interv Radiol*. 2013 Mar–Apr; 19(2): 134–140.

29. Zander T, Gonzalez G, De Alba L, et al. Transcollateral approach for percutaneous revascularization of complex superficial femoral artery and tibioperoneal trunk occlusions. *J Vasc Interv Radiol*. 2012 May; 23(5): 691–695.

30. Fusaro M, Agostoni P, Biondi-Zoccai G. "Trans-collateral" angioplasty for a challenging chronic total occlusion of the tibial vessels: A novel approach to percutaneous revascularization in critical lower limb ischemia. *Cathet Cardio Intervent*. 2008 Feb; 71(2): 268–272.

31. Shimada Y, Kino N, Yano K, et al. Transcollateral retrograde approach with rendezvous technique for recanalization of chronically occluded tibial arteries. *J Endovasc Ther*. 2012 Oct; 19(5): 620–626.

32. Kuroki MT, Parikh UM, Chandra V. How I do it: Pedal access and pedal loop revascularization for patients with chronic limb-threatening ischemia. *J Vasc Surg Cases Innov Tech*. 2023 Sep; 9(3): 101236.

33. Kawarada O, Fujihara M, Higashimori A, et al. Predictors of adverse clinical outcomes after successful infrapopliteal intervention. *Cathet Cardio Intervent*. 2012 Nov; 80(5): 861–871.

34. Voûte MT, Stathis A, Schneider PA, et al. Delphi consensus study toward a comprehensive classification system for angioplasty-induced femoropopliteal dissection. *JACC: Cardiovasc Interv*. 2021 Nov; 14(21): 2391–2401.

35. Salamaga S, Stępak H, Krasiński Z. Supera stent implantation for the treatment of isolated popliteal artery disease – systematic review and evaluation of current endovascular strategies. *Pol Przegl Chir*. 2022 Aug 12; 95(4): 47–53.

36. Lee JY, Kye MS, Kim J, et al. Cutting balloon angioplasty for severe in-stent restenosis after carotid artery stenting: Long-term outcomes and review of literature. *Neurointerv*. 2024 Mar 1; 19(1): 24–30.

37. Böhme T, Noory E, Beschorner U, et al. Combined treatment of dysfunctional dialysis access with cutting balloon and paclitaxel-coated balloon in real world. *Vasa*. 2023 Jul; 52(4): 284–289.

38. Spiliopoulos S, Karamitros A, Reppas L, et al. Novel balloon technologies to minimize dissection of peripheral angioplasty. *Expert Rev Med Devices*. 2019 Jul 3; 16(7): 581–588.

39. Shirai S, Mori S, Yamaguchi K, et al. Impact of chocolate percutaneous transluminal angioplasty balloon on vessel preparation in drug-coated balloon angioplasty for femoropopliteal lesion. *CVIR Endovasc*. 2022 Sep 1; 5(1): 46.

40. Katsanos K, Spiliopoulos S, Reppas L, et al. Debulking atherectomy in the peripheral arteries: Is there a role and what is the evidence? *Cardiovasc Intervent Radiol*. 2017 Jul; 40(7): 964–977.

41. Bhat TM, Afari ME, Garcia LA. Atherectomy in peripheral arterial disease: A review. *J Invasive Cardiol*. 2017; 29(4): 135–144.

42. Wardle BG, Ambler GK, Radwan RW. Atherectomy for peripheral arterial disease (review). *Cochrane Database of Systematic Reviews*. 2020; 9: Art. No. CD006680. doi: 10.1002/14651858. CD006680.pub3.

43. Saucy F, Probst H, Trunfio R. Vessel preparation is essential to optimize endovascular therapy of infrainguinal lesions. *Front. Cardiovasc. Med*. 2020; 7: 558129. doi: 10.3389/fcvm.2020.558129.

44. Ormiston W, Dyer-Hartnett S, Fernando R, et al. An update on vessel preparation in lower limb arterial intervention. *CVIR Endovasc*. 2020; 3: 86. doi: 10.1186/s42155-020-00175-6.

45. Albaghdadi M, Young MN, Al-Bawardy R, et al. Outcomes of atherectomy in patients undergoing lower extremity revascularisation. *EuroInterv*. 2023 Dec; 19(11): e955–e963.

46. Ponukumati AS, Suckow BD, Powell CJ, et al. Outcomes of rotational atherectomy in complex lesions of the superficial femoral artery. *J Vasc Surg*. 2021 Jan; 73(1): 172–178.

47. Shammas N. JETSTREAM atherectomy: A review of technique, tips, and tricks in treating the femoropopliteal lesions. *Int J Angiol*. 2014 Sep 17; 24(2): 81–86.

48. Bai H, Fereydooni A, Zhang Y, et al. Trends in utilization and outcomes of orbital, laser, and excisional atherectomy for lower extremity revascularization. *J Endovasc Ther*. 2020; 29(3): 389–401.

49. Misuraca L, Buonpane A, Trimarchi G, et al. Covered endovascular reconstruction of aortic bifurcation facilitated by intravascular lithotripsy with shockwave balloon: A case report. *Cureus*. 2024 Aug 14; 16(8): e66874.

50. Wong CP, Chan LP, Au DM, et al. Efficacy and safety of intravascular lithotripsy in lower extremity peripheral artery disease: A systematic review and meta-analysis. *Eur J Vasc Endovasc Surg*. 2022 Mar; 63(3): 446–456.

51. Giannopoulos S, Speziale F, Vadalà G, et al. Intravascular lithotripsy for treatment of calcified lesions during carotid artery stenting. *J Endovasc Ther*. 2021 Feb; 28(1): 93–99.

52. Saratzis A, Jane Messeder S, Thulasidasan N, et al. Shockwave intravascular lithotripsy use in the femoro-popliteal segment: Considerations from an expert Pan-European panel regarding best-care practice. *J Endovasc Ther*. 2024 Aug 12. doi: 10.1177/15266028241266417.

53. Koeckerling D, Raguindin PF, Kastrati L, et al. Endovascular revascularization strategies for aortoiliac and femoropopliteal artery disease: A meta-analysis. *Eur Heart J*. 2023 Mar 14; 44(11): 935–950.

54. Amlani V, Falkenberg M, Nordanstig J. The current status of drug-coated devices in lower extremity peripheral artery disease interventions. *Prog Cardiovasc Dis*. 2021 Mar; 65: 23–28.

55. Basavarajaiah S, Kalkat H, Bhatia G, et al. How to perform a successful drug-coated balloon angioplasty? Tips and tricks. *Cathet Cardio Intervent*. 2023 Dec; 102(7): 1238–1257.

56. Cina CS. Endovascular repair of popliteal aneurysms. *J Vasc Surg*. 2010; 51(4): 1056–1060.

57. Sousa RS, Oliveira-Pinto J, Mansilha A. Endovascular versus open repair for popliteal aneurysm: A review on limb salvage and reintervention rates. *Int Angiol*. 2020; 39(5): 381–389.

58. Noory E, Böhme T, Beschorner U. Early results after exclusion of popliteal aneurysms with an endoprosthesis. *Cardiol Cardiovasc Med*. 2022; 6(6): 550–557.

Section 3

TIPS & TRICKS IN AORTOILIAC OBSTRUCTIVE DISEASES

Toolkit A – Management of Percutaneous Access in Aortoiliac Pathology   **92**
- Tips 1 to 5B

Toolkit B – Tips & Tricks for Aortoiliac Stenoses and Occlusions   **97**
- Tips 6 to 14

Toolkit C – The CERAB Technique   **108**
- Tips 15 to 19

Toolkit D – Hybrid Procedures in the Context of Iliac–Femoral Recanalizations   **114**
- Tips 20 to 28

DOI: 10.1201/9781003567080-3

TIP #1

Lesions of the external iliac arteries should be managed through a percutaneous approach via the brachial artery or the contralateral femoral artery. This is because, in most cases, when these lesions are located at this level, they extend almost into the common femoral artery, making retrograde access from the ipsilateral side challenging. An alternative approach may be considered if the distal segment of the external iliac artery to be treated is sufficiently healthy – providing a few centimeters of usable space. In such cases, a retrograde puncture within the initial centimeters of a healthy superficial femoral artery can be performed, following the technical guidelines outlined in the first section.

TIP #2

In cases of chronic total occlusions (CTOs) of the external iliac arteries, as mentioned in the previous Tip, an anterograde approach (via the contralateral femoral artery or the brachial artery) is generally preferred. Conversely, for CTOs of the common iliac arteries, a retrograde approach from the ipsilateral femoral artery is often the first choice. In the latter scenario, if retrograde recanalization cannot be completed, attempting the procedure from the brachial artery typically allows the lesion to be crossed successfully in the vast majority of cases (Figure 3.1).

In general, brachial access provides a direct line to iliac lesions and offers superior torquability and pushability. Contralateral femoral access is usually sufficient for most external iliac CTOs. However, for common iliac CTOs, this approach does not provide adequate pushability due to the lack of an

First-choice access in iliac recanalizations

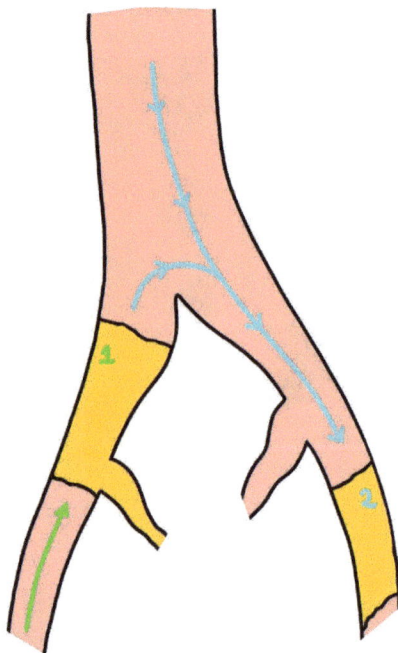

Figure 3.1 Access options for iliac recanalization procedures.

ostial zone to secure engagement with the iliac axis and provide the necessary support. In these cases, the guidewire frequently tends to jump into the aorta during the recanalization attempts.

As previously mentioned, the first-line approach for common iliac CTOs is a retrograde ipsilateral femoral access, as it is quicker and more convenient. Using this access, it is important to attempt endoluminal recanalization patiently, following the escalation strategy detailed in the earlier section. If endoluminal attempts fail (this approach is associated with a high rate of subintimal recanalization), subintimal strategies may be acceptable, but extending the dissection plane into the aorta has to be strictly avoided. In such situations, advanced recanalization techniques or re-entry devices can be beneficial.

The use of re-entry devices such as Outback or Pioneer does not appear to increase the risk of perforation complications. However, their use at the iliac level is recommended for operators already experienced with these devices in their infrainguinal applications.

It is worth noting that international statistics indicate that, in cases of long iliac CTOs (TASC D lesions), retrograde ipsilateral access is associated with the highest failure rates.

TIP #3

If recanalization of an iliac axis cannot be achieved using a single access point, a dual access strategy (ipsilateral femoral + brachial, or ipsilateral femoral + contralateral femoral) can serve as an additional tool. For instance, one possible approach might include the following steps.

- **Brachial access** with a 4 Fr sheath and ipsilateral femoral access.
- After achieving an anterograde recanalization via the brachial access, the guidewire is captured from the femoral access, enabling a **Flossing Wire Technique** to secure access to the aortic lumen from below.
- The procedure is then completed from the femoral access.

This sequence is well illustrated in Figures 3.2–3.2f.

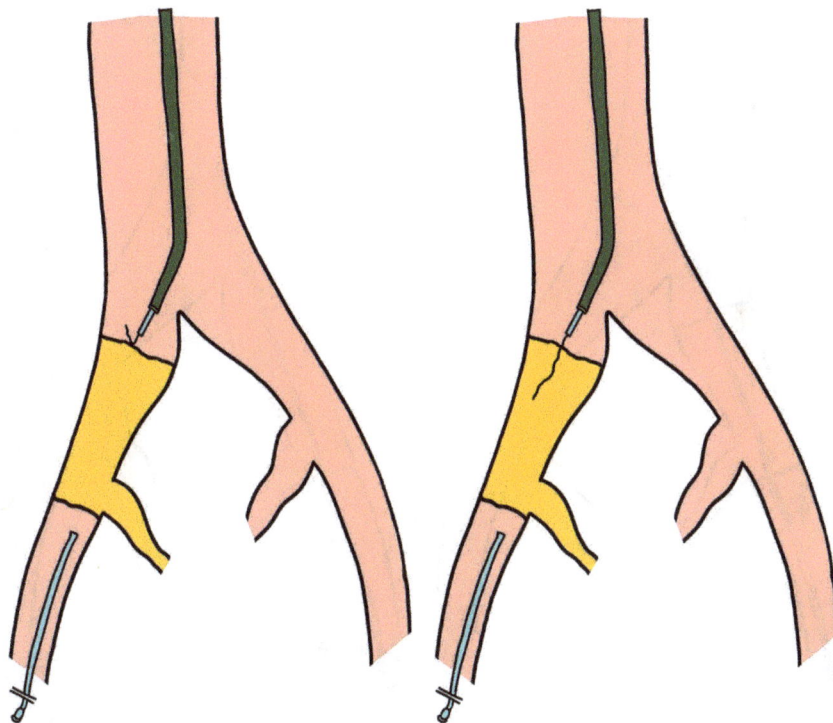

Figures 3.2–3.2a Example of dual access during an iliac recanalization.

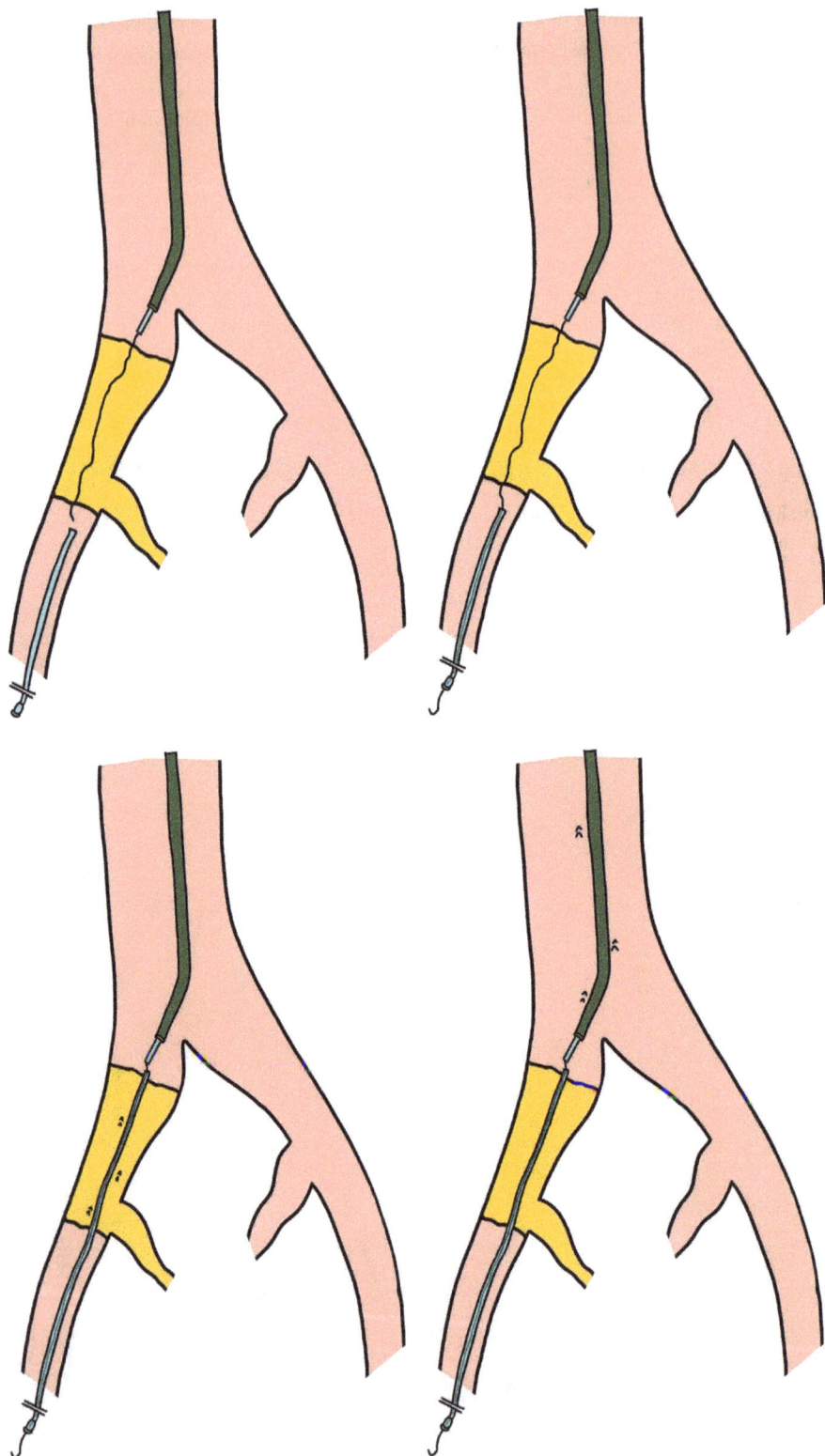

Figures 3.2b–3.2e (Continued)

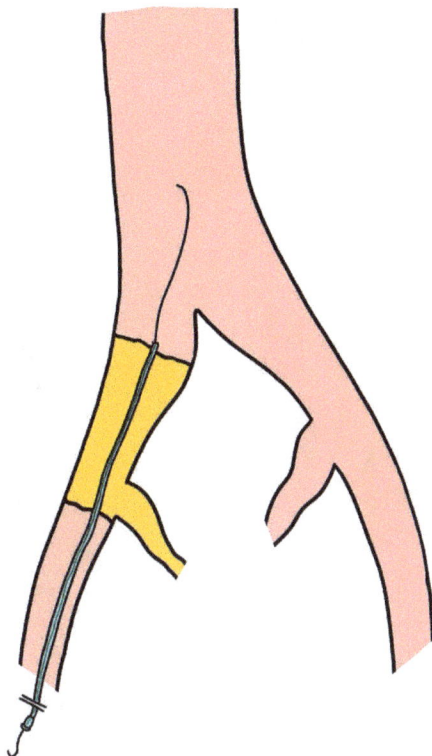

Figure 3.2f (Continued)

The necessity to perform stenting from the femoral access is largely due to the fact that balloon-expandable stents – preferable in cases of common iliac CTOs – often require a a 7 Fr platform. Such a large sheath size is associated with higher complication rates at the brachial access site, which is why many authors recommend a primary surgical approach for brachial access beyond 6 Fr.

Using dual iliac access also allows for the cautious application of all advanced subintimal techniques described in Section 2 (e.g., Crush Balloon, Parallel Wire, SAFARI, Double Balloon).

These techniques, particularly at the iliac level, should only be employed by operators with appropriate expertise and training.

TIP #4

In certain situations when both iliac axes need to be recanalized without requiring a kissing stent at the aortoiliac bifurcation, the entire procedure can be completed through a single percutaneous access point. In these cases, it is preferable to select the arterial axis with the best atherosclerotic profile and where the iliac stenosis or occlusion is located at the most proximal level. This choice facilitates better access management during the procedure and allows for the safe placement of a closure device, if necessary (Figures 3.3–3.3c).

TIP #5A

Brachial Access: Advantages

- Excellent pushability.
- Avoids aortic dissection in cases of subintimal recanalization.
- Higher success rate for endoluminal recanalization.

Distal right common iliac steno-occlusion, associated with left external iliac steno-occlusion

Step 1: *Access selection*
It is preferable to puncture on the right side, as it provides more room for maneuvering and better management of the access

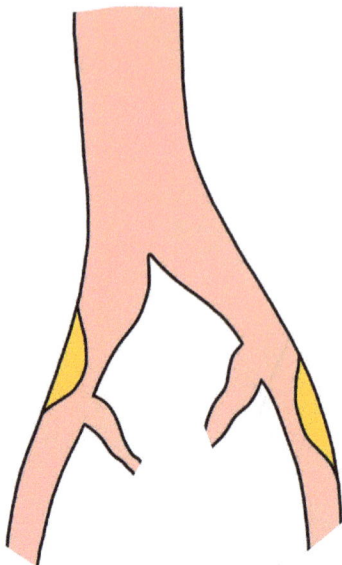

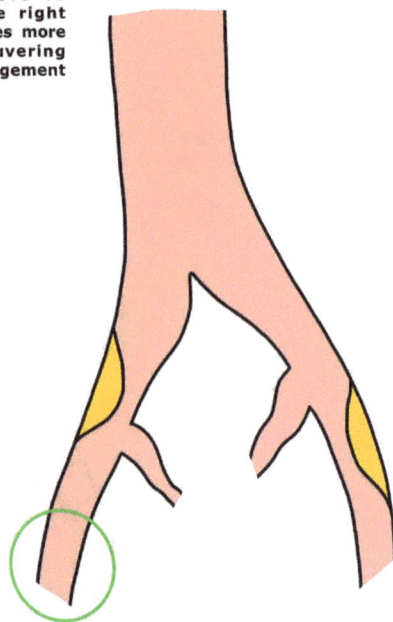

Step 2: Treat the left-sided lesion

Step 3: Upon exit, treat the right-sided lesion

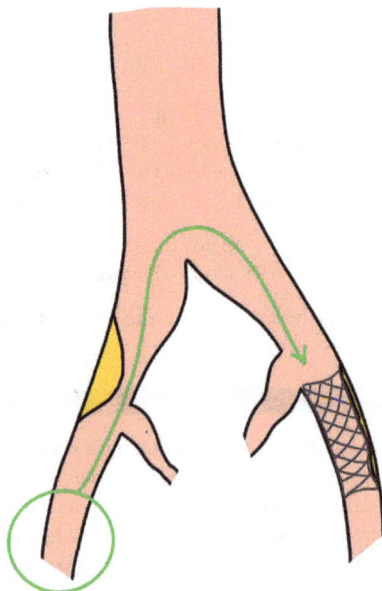

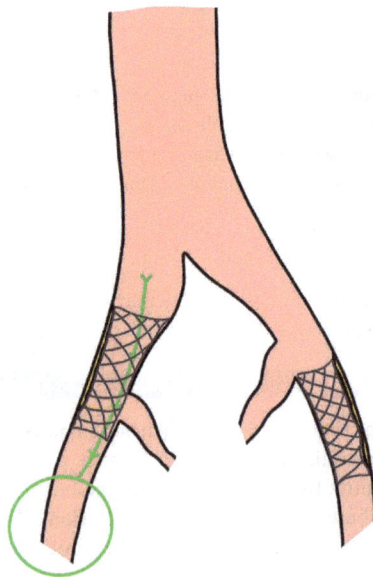

Figures 3.3–3.3c Stenting of both iliac arteries via a single femoral access.

TIP #5B

Brachial Access: Disadvantages.

- Brachial access carries a higher risk of site-related complications, such as arterial thrombosis or pseudoaneurysm. For sheath sizes exceeding 6 Fr, a small surgical access is recommended.
- Although rare, there is a potential risk of embolization into the supra-aortic trunks.

TIP #6

When it is necessary to place a balloon-expandable stent, due to the risk of its displacement from the delivery catheter (or to avoid difficulties in crossing the lesion given the high profiles of this type of stent) all pre-occlusive stenoses and iliac CTOs should be pre-dilated with a balloon, even one as small as 3 mm or 4 mm.

After pre-dilation, it is advisable to cross the stenosis with a long sheath. The stent should then be advanced within the sheath until it is positioned in the desired release zone.

Finally, the sheath is retracted, and the procedure continues with the deployment of the stent (Figures 3.4–3.4d).

Pre-occlusive lesion of the right common iliac

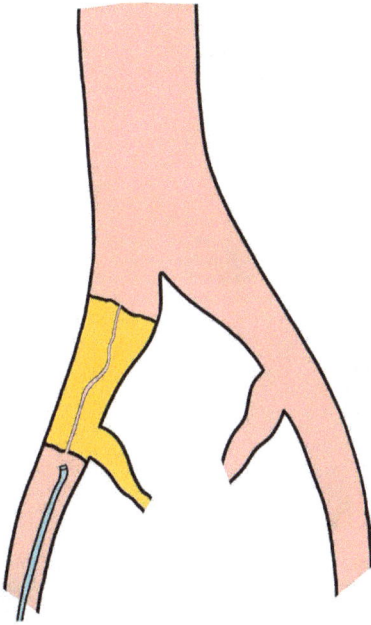

Step 1: Cross and pre-dilate the lesion

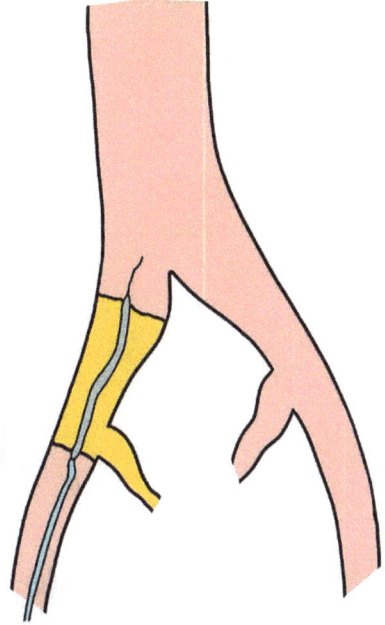

Figures 3.4–3.4a Iliac preparation prior to balloon-expandable stent deployment.

Step 2: Position a long introducer within the lesion

Step 3: Position the stent at the desired level within the introducer

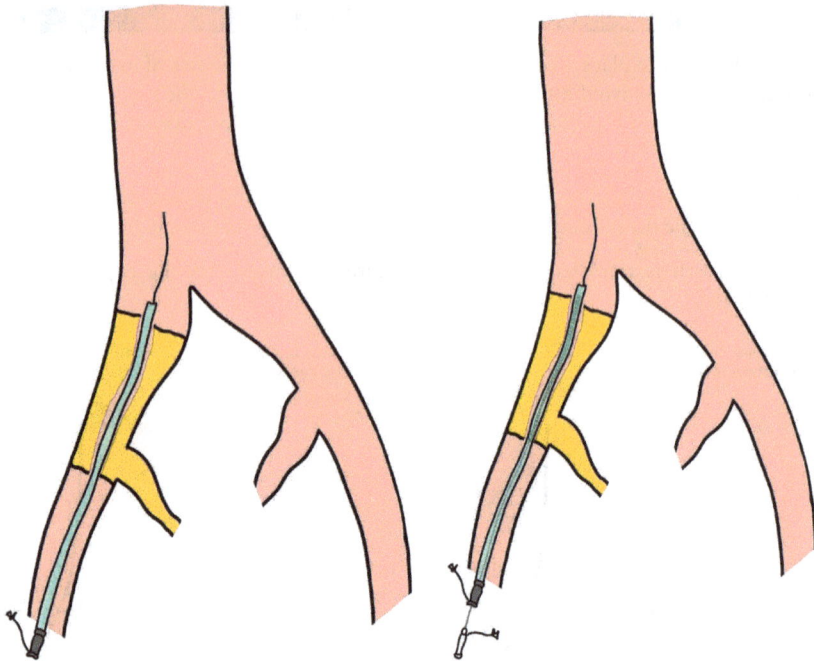

Step 4: Withdraw the introducer and deploy the stent

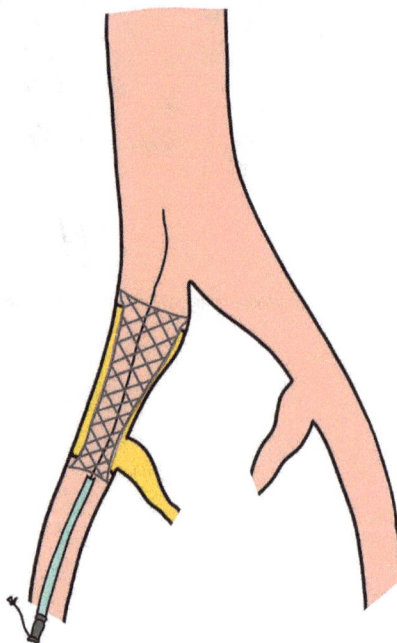

Figures 3.4b–3.4d (Continued)

TIP #7

If a critical stenosis or CTO cannot be crossed via ipsilateral femoral access, it can be helpful to advance a Bern catheter through this route to the distal zone of the lesion.

From this position, perform an angiography by forcefully injecting contrast medium. This approach allows visualization of any navigable microchannel within the lesion, which can then be engaged with a catheter and guidewire using the endoluminal handling escalation techniques previously described (Figures 3.5–3.5c).

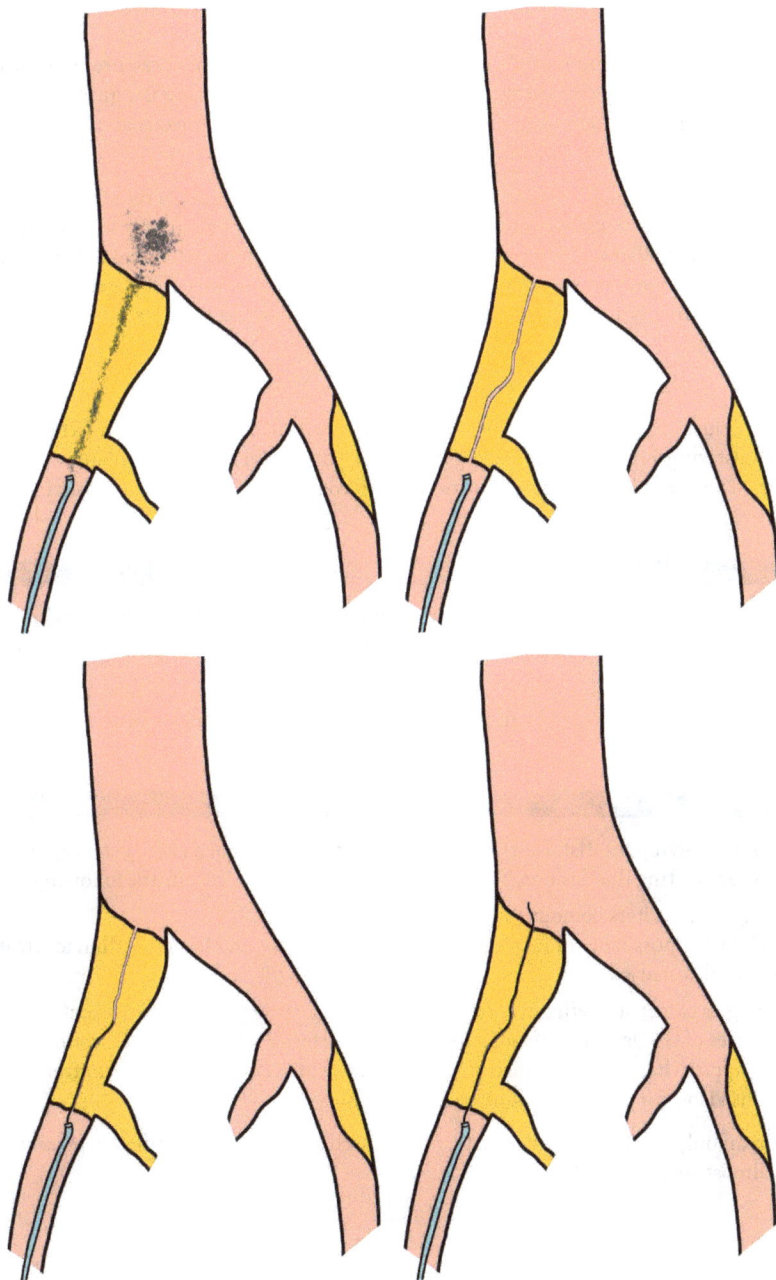

Figures 3.5–3.5c Visualization of the microchannel within an iliac CTO.

If no such microchannel is present, the CTO must be recanalized using the perforating technique or a controlled subintimal approach. Subintimal techniques in aortoiliac pathology, especially with retrograde ipsilateral access, should be employed with great caution. The goal should always be re-entry into the common iliac artery, or at most at the level of the bifurcation, to avoid extensive aortic dissections, which can sometimes lead to disastrous outcomes.

TIP #8

It may occasionally happen during iliac catheterization performed for another reason to encounter an unexpected iliac lesion. Any uncertainty about the significance of the lesion can be clarified by measuring the pressure differential.

In such cases, the pressure differential can be assessed by connecting the pressure transducer first to the catheter that has already crossed the lesion and then – after advancing the guidewire beyond the lesion and removing the catheter – to the same sheath used for percutaneous access. Pressure differences as small as 10 mmHg are considered significant.

This allows measurement of the pressure both downstream and upstream of the stenosis, regardless of the access route (ipsilateral, contralateral, or brachial), without compromising the obtained recanalization. However, the challenge lies in the fact that invasive pressure measurement through the catheter requires temporary removal of the guidewire – a maneuver that is unwise if the measurement needs to be performed proximally to the lesion (on the percutaneous access side), as this would necessitate re-crossing the lesion.

***

If there is an occlusion also of the superficial femoral artery ipsilateral to the iliac axis being evaluated, locally administering highly diluted nitroglycerin (or papaverine) can help dilate the downstream arterial bed. This prevents inadequate runoff from compromising the accuracy of the pressure evaluation.

TIP #9

For eccentric and calcified aortoiliac lesions, it is advisable to accept even a suboptimal result. Aortic ruptures pose a significant threat, which does not justify aggressive post-dilatation maneuvers for minor residual stenoses.

Balloon-expandable stents should be inflated to a maximum of **4–6 atm** in the aorta and **6–8 atm** in the iliac artery.

TIP #10A

Except in cases involving the distal aorta and the bifurcation, the use of a kissing stent approach should be avoided when treating iliac lesions. The issues with kissing stents include the following.

- Their configuration alters hemodynamics at the bifurcation.
- They preclude the possibility of future crossover femoral access, an essential option for treating a lot of infrainguinal scenarios.

Various strategies can ensure effective stenting without resorting to the Kissing Stent Technique. For instance, in cases of CTOs involving both common iliac arteries but without bifurcation involvement, a **V-stenting** approach can be used instead of a kissing stent. This ensures that contralateral femoral access remains viable for future procedures (Figure 3.6b).

Furthermore, if only one common iliac artery is diseased and a proximal stump is present, unilateral stenting is almost always feasible.

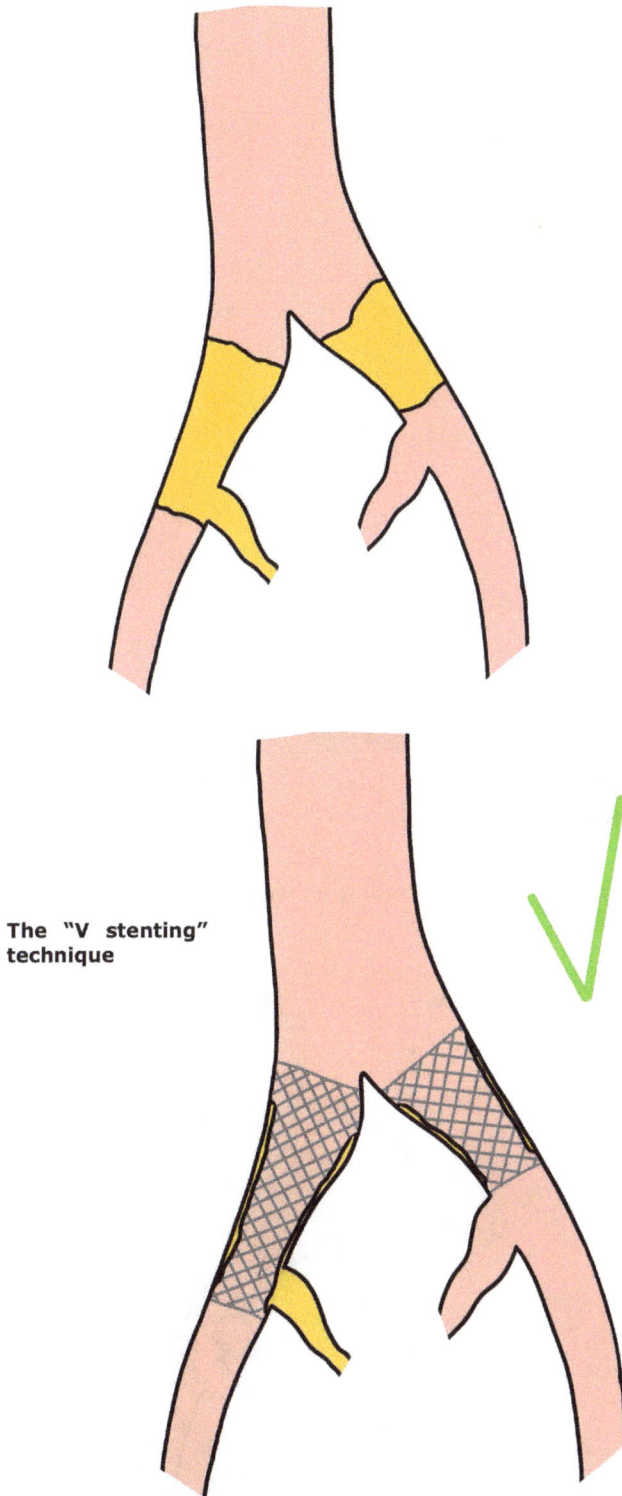

The "V stenting" technique

Figures 3.6–3.6a Comparison between V-stenting and kissing stenting.

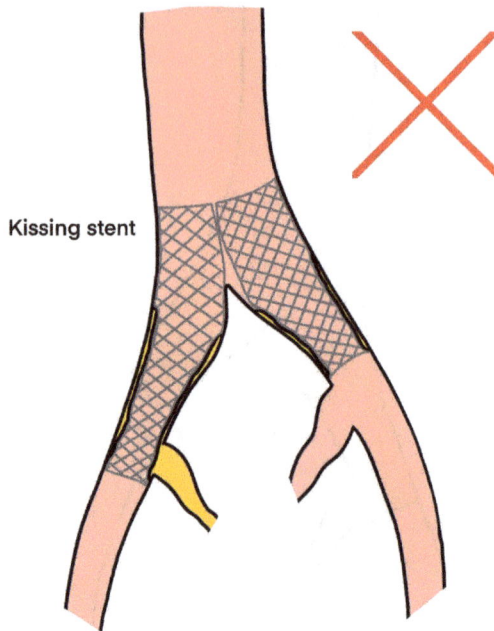

Kissing stent

Figure 3.6b (Continued)

TIP #10B

When stenting a single common iliac artery without using the Kissing Stent Technique, it is always advisable to consider protecting the contralateral iliac axis with a balloon inflated to **3–4 atm** (Figure 3.7a).

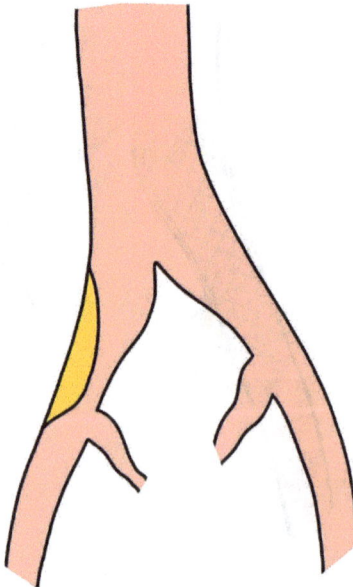

Steno-occlusion of the right
common iliac axis

Figure 3.7 Balloon protection of the iliac axis during stenting of the contralateral common iliac artery.

Stenting of the right common iliac artery
On the left, a balloon at low pressure (4 atm) is inflated, in order to protect the contralateral axis. Note that the balloon on the left terminates upstream of the hypogastric artery

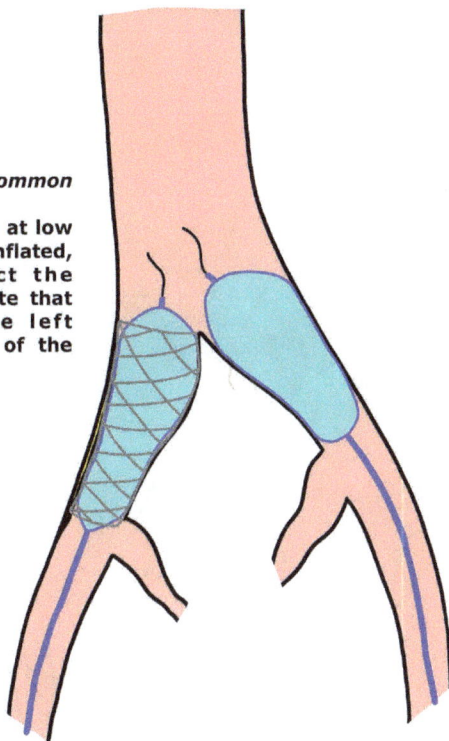

Figure 3.7a (Continued)

This precaution helps prevent the displacement of atherosclerotic plaque or dissection flaps into the contralateral iliac axis – a rare but possible complication.

TIP #11

Except for the first few centimeters of the common iliac arteries, where balloon-expandable stents are preferred – primarily for reasons of precision – the remainder of the common iliac axis and up to the distal external iliac artery is better suited for the use of self-expanding stents. This preference is due to the extreme tortuosity of these segments and the fact that, unlike at the bifurcation, precision in stent deployment is less critical at this level.

TIP #12

During an aortoiliac PTA, the patient's pain is a reliable indicator of the pressure limit to which balloon inflation should be pushed. This pain should subside once the balloon is deflated; if it persists, an aortoiliac angiography should be performed to check for potential wall ruptures or flow-limiting dissections.

TIP #13

In the case of a flush occlusion of a common iliac artery with a healthy contralateral iliac axis, if retrograde recanalization via ipsilateral femoral access fails, an alternative approach for CTO recanalization can be as follows (Figures 3.8–3.8b).

- **Contralateral femoral access** (on the healthy side) combined with **brachial access**, preferably left-sided.

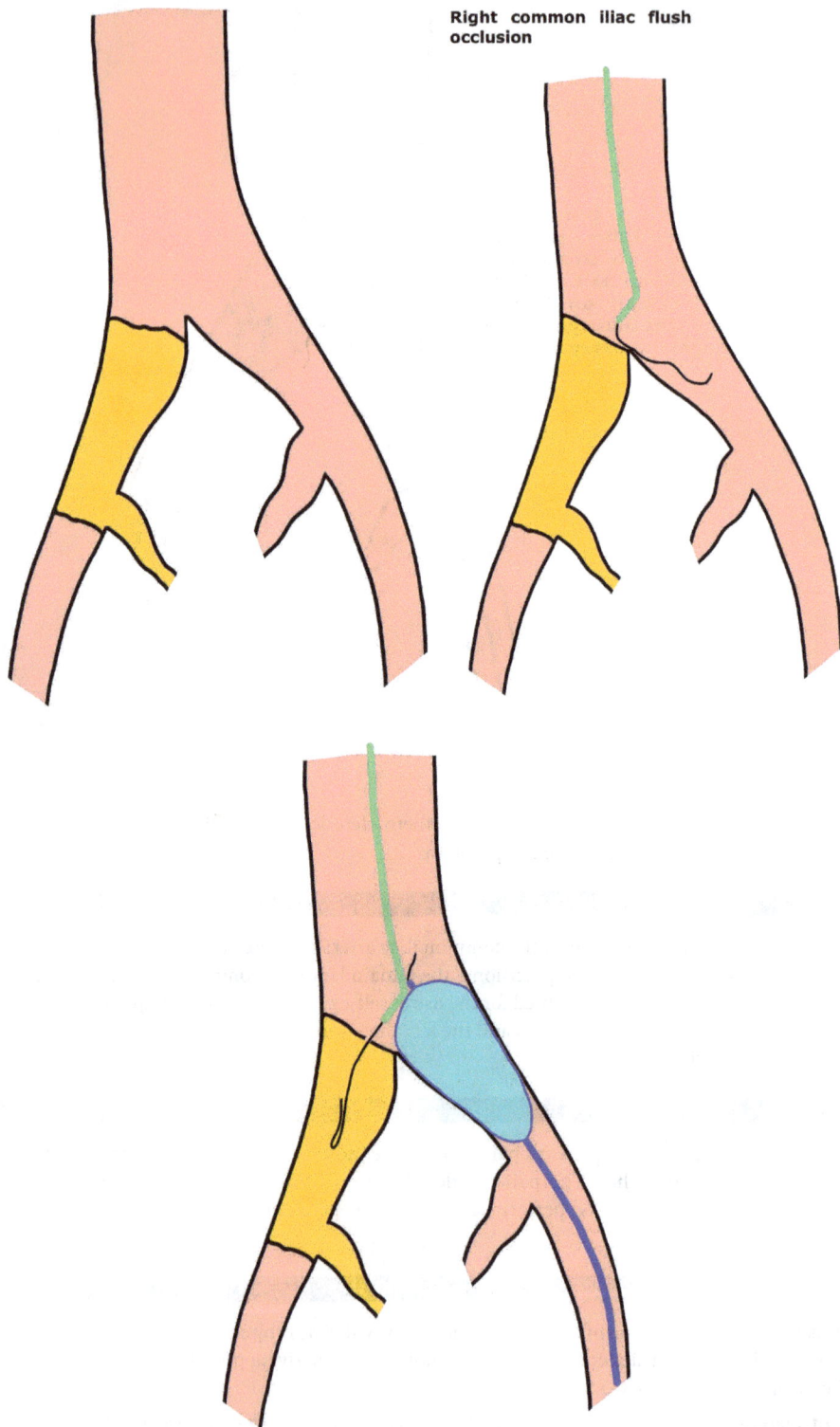

Right common iliac flush occlusion

Figures 3.8–3.8b Another example of dual access during a common iliac recanalization.

- Position and inflate a balloon at low pressure (2–4 atm) within the contralateral healthy common iliac artery. The balloon should be slightly undersized relative to the vessel diameter and should protrude approximately 1 cm into the aorta.
- Through the brachial access, position a long sheath (or guiding catheter) near the occlusion. Use the chosen guidewire and catheter to cross the CTO. The inflated balloon in the contralateral axis acts as a support for the recanalization catheter, facilitating engagement with the CTO.

This method also allows for safe subintimal recanalization, as brachial access eliminates the risk of aortic dissection.

TIP #14

The Crush Stent Technique is an endovascular tool derived from cardiology, designed to treat an iliac axis with an occluded stent that is challenging to recanalize intraluminally.

When endoluminal recanalization is deemed impossible, the procedure transitions to a subintimal recanalization strategy. This approach requires dissecting the occluded stent from the arterial wall, conducting the recanalization outside the stent.

Once re-entry is achieved, the occluded stent can be crushed by ballooning the newly gained subintimal space. A second stent is then placed in parallel to complete the crushing process.

This technique is reserved for bailout scenarios in patients who cannot be treated otherwise. However, it carries a risk of vessel rupture both during the crushing phase and afterward, due to the combined radial force of the two parallel stents. For this reason, the use of a covered stent is advisable (Figures 3.9–3.9e).

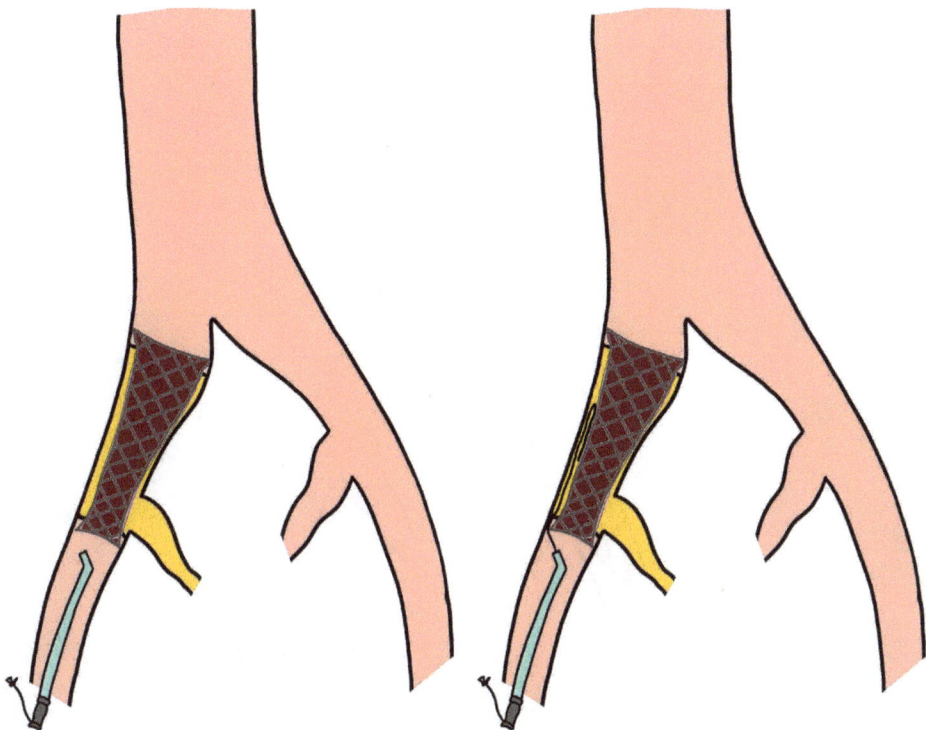

Figures 3.9–3.9a The Crush Stent Technique

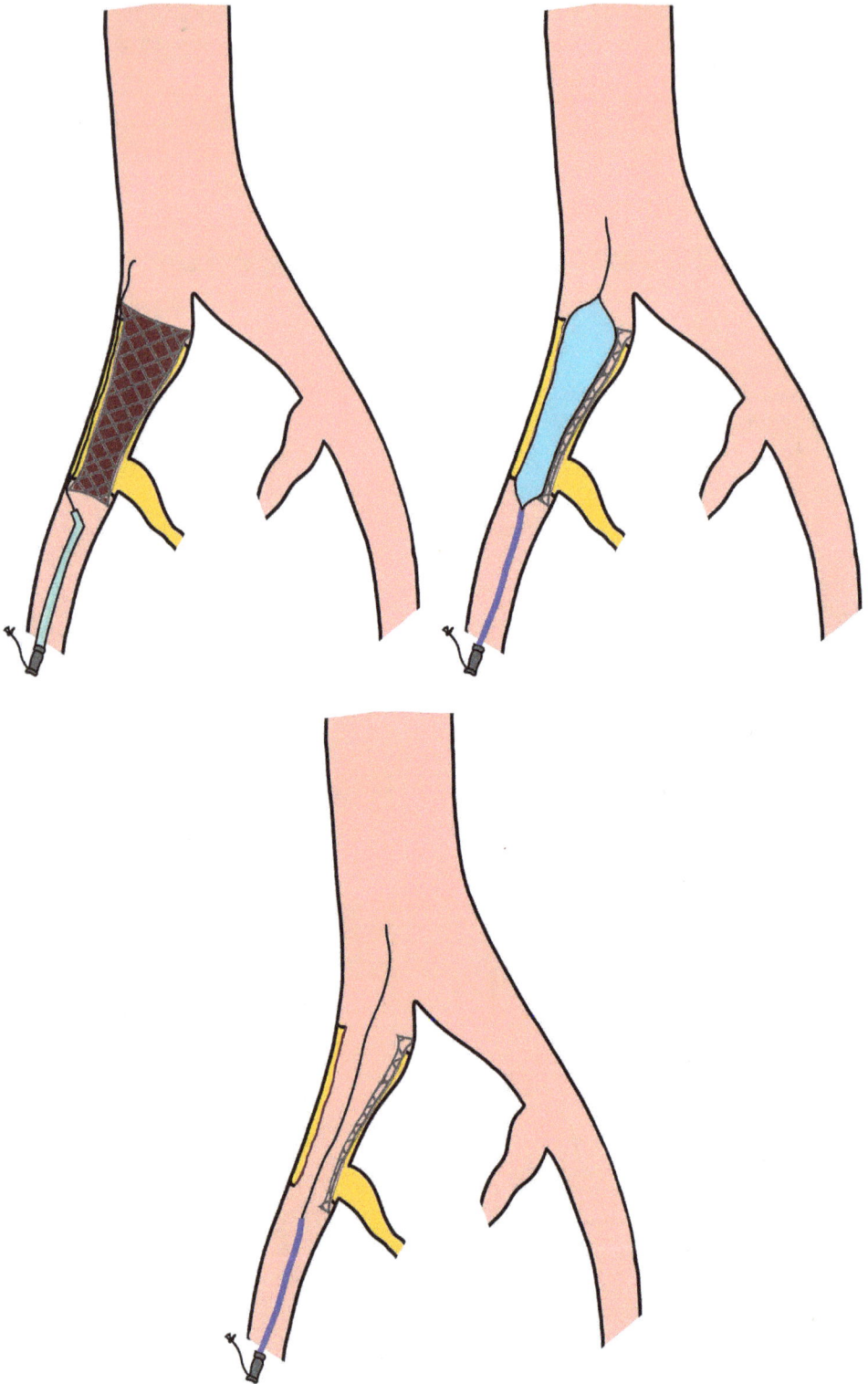

Figures 3.9b–3.9d (Continued)

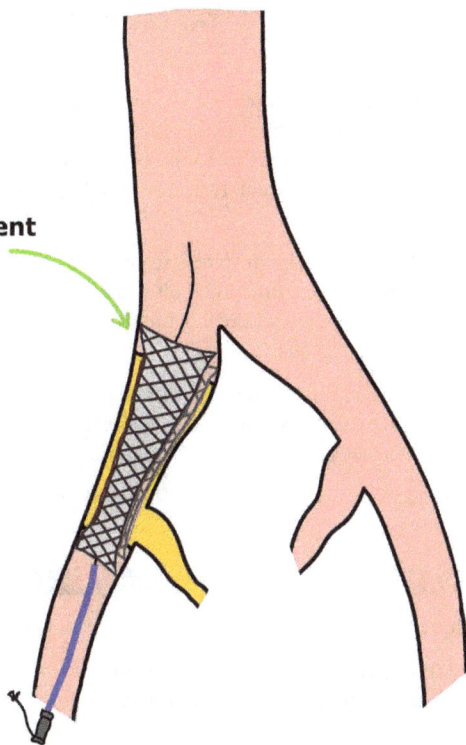

Covered stent

Figure 3.9e (Continued)

The CERAB Technique (**Covered Endovascular Reconstruction of the Aortic Bifurcation** Technique) was developed to address certain hemodynamic and anatomical limitations identified with bare-metal endovascular treatment of the aortoiliac bifurcation. There is substantial evidence suggesting that the geometry of the Kissing Stent Technique is a key factor in the development of restenosis and occlusions at this level.

The dead spaces present outside the stent struts create persistently perfused areas of native artery. At these sites, local flow dynamics are significantly altered due to the hemodynamic resistance caused by the metal structure surrounding the area outside the stent lumens. These alterations can accelerate the progression of disease in these regions.

In the space between the native bifurcation and the neobifurcation – as well as in the gutters between the stents and their metallic struts – studies have demonstrated the presence of immature mesenchymal cells, neointimal hyperplasia, and thrombotic material.

The CERAB Technique was introduced to eliminate these dead spaces and optimize local hemodynamics.

TIP #15

Procedural Technique

After achieving guidewire recanalization of the aortoiliac bifurcation, perform pre-dilation of the stenosis or occlusion using the Kissing Balloon Technique, if necessary. Subsequently, follow the following steps.

1. Advance a **9–12 Fr long sheath** (the precise size depends on the diameter of the aortic covered stent to be used) through one access route and position it in the aortic segment to be stented. Through the other access route, advance a **7 Fr long sheath** into the iliac axis (Figures 3.10–3.10b).

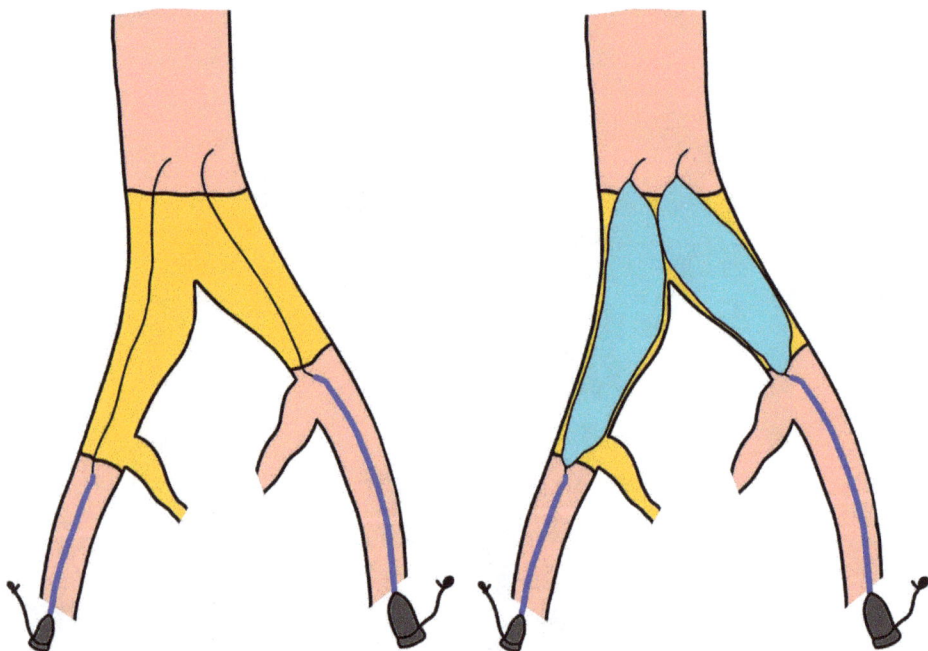

Figures 3.10–3.10a The CERAB Technique

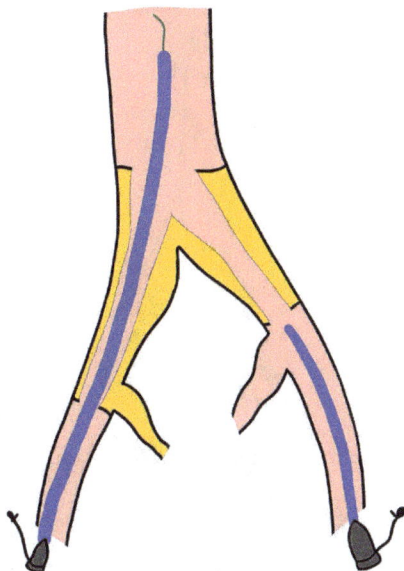

Figure 3.10b (Continued)

2. After performing a high-quality aortoiliac angiogram, insert a **12 mm diameter covered stent** of appropriate length through the sheath positioned in the aorta. This stent should be delivered over a stiff or extra-stiff guidewire, preferably Teflon-coated. Retract the sheath and expand the stent, ensuring that its distal portion ends approximately **15 mm above the native bifurcation** (Figure 3.10c).

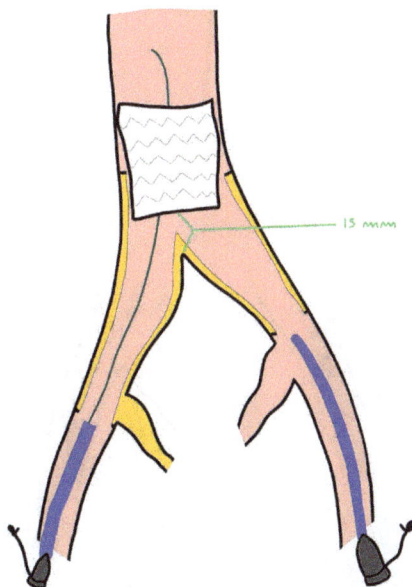

Figure 3.10c (Continued)

3. Using the same access and over the stiff guidewire, introduce a **16 mm aortic balloon** to adapt ONLY the proximal portion of the endograft to the aorta. It is critical not to balloon the distal 15–20 mm of the endograft to optimize the local anatomy and reduce radial mismatch. The distal portion of the aortic endograft should remain at **12 mm in diameter**, thereby creating a funnel-shaped configuration (Figure 3.10d).

Use a 16 mm balloon to mold the proximal portion of the stent

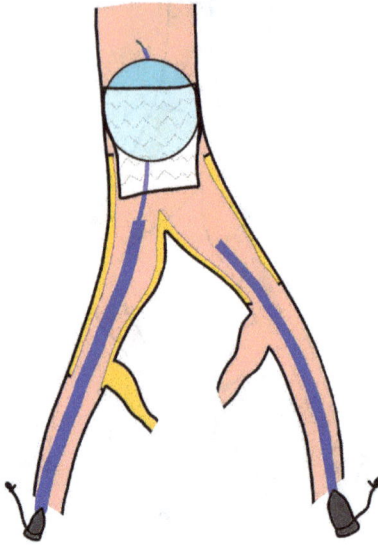

Figure 3.10d (Continued)

4. Advance both sheaths into the aortic endograft and carefully align them with the exact zone where the iliac components will be deployed (Figure 3.10e).

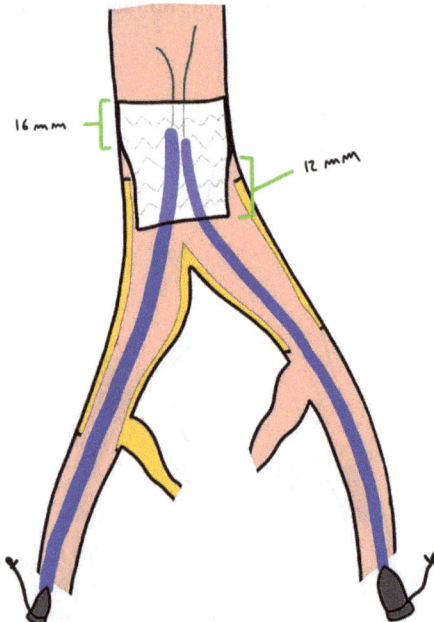

Figure 3.10e (Continued)

5. Insert **two 8 mm iliac endografts** through the sheaths, ensuring they emerge within the aortic module. The proximal edge of the iliac endografts must terminate within the distal zone of the aortic endograft, where the diameter has been deliberately maintained at 12 mm. Avoid placing the iliac endografts higher, as this would significantly increase the mismatch between the components.
6. Retract the sheaths and expand both iliac endografts (Figure 3.10f).

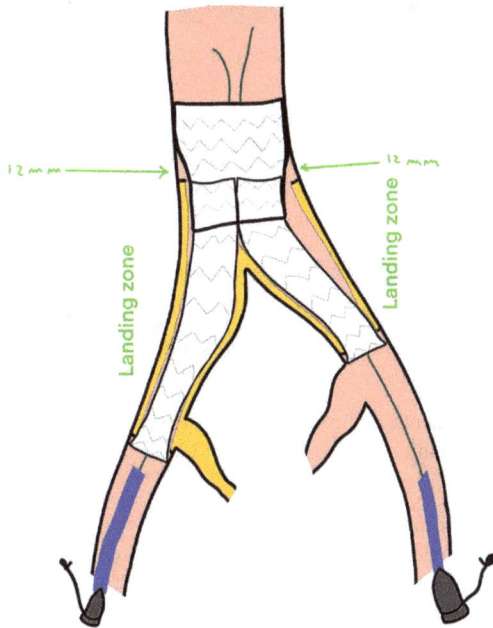

Figure 3.10f (Continued)

This configuration closely mimics the natural anatomy of the aortoiliac bifurcation, providing a more anatomically accurate solution compared to bare-metal kissing stents (Figure 3.10g).

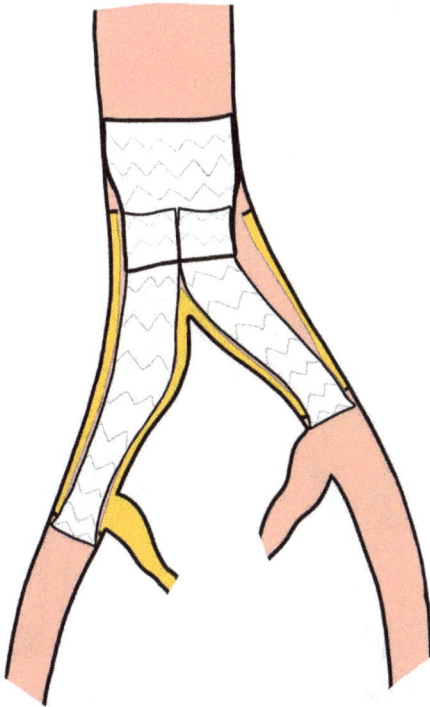

Figure 3.10g (Continued)

TIP #16

When performing a CERAB procedure, it is essential to carefully evaluate the visceral circulation during the pre-procedural CT angiography. If patent, the inferior mesenteric artery (IMA) will be covered during the procedure, as is the case with endografts.

However, unlike aneurysmal disease, the pathology in this context is obstructive. Therefore, it is critical to assess the adequacy of the superior mesenteric artery and the celiac trunk. If needed, treatment of these vessels should be planned and performed prior to the aortic reconstruction.

TIP #17

It is not the experience of the author, but cases are described in the literature in which the CERAB Technique has been performed in patients with Leriche syndrome, characterized by the classic aortoiliac occlusion with thrombosis extending up to the level of the renal arteries.

In such cases, assuming the patients are unfit for open surgery, it is important to emphasize that aortic endografts are balloon-expandable stents. When inflated, the balloon extends beyond the edges of the stent.

The potential risk in aortic thrombosis reaching the renal artery level is the displacement of thrombus into the renal arteries during endograft deployment. To mitigate this risk, it is crucial to protect the renal arteries with balloons inflated simultaneously during the procedure. Additionally, performing a Chimney Technique on these arteries (even with bare-metal stents) should be considered if the final angiographic result is suboptimal (Figure 3.11).

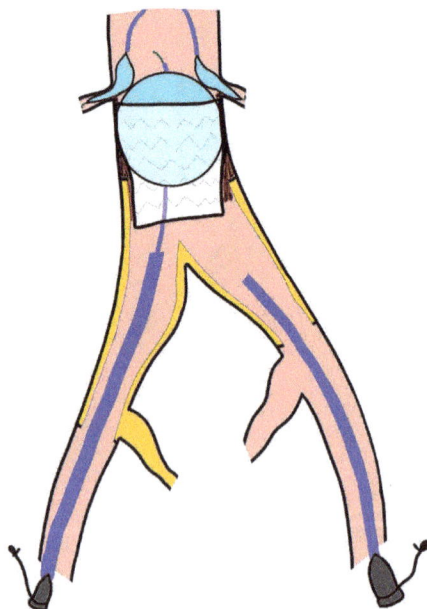

Protect the renal arteries with two balloons or perform a Chimney-CERAB if the occlusion reaches the level of the renal arteries

Figure 3.11 Protecting the renal arteries during the CERAB Technique in cases of aortic occlusion extending to the renal plane.

TIP #18

The endografts used in the CERAB Technique are balloon-expandable covered stents, as precise deployment is critical. To date, all available types have been utilized, including stainless steel, cobalt/chromium, and platinum/iridium stents, with no clear evidence of superiority among them.

TIP #19

While the CERAB Technique reduces the hemodynamic alterations typically associated with bare-metal kissing stents, it does not, in the author's opinion, address the primary anatomical disadvantage of such configurations. Specifically, as with kissing stents and most endografts used for aneurysmal aortic disease, the reconstructed bifurcation anatomy does not replicate the native bifurcation.

The main drawback – more evident in occlusive disease than in aneurysmal pathology – is that stent implantation in this configuration precludes future endovascular procedures via contralateral femoral access. This limitation is particularly significant in patients predisposed to atherosclerotic disease, where such access is frequently needed.

To address this issue, the use of the **Endologix AFX2 endograft** for aortoiliac bifurcation reconstruction has become increasingly common in recent years also in obstructive pathology. As will be discussed in the following sections, the anatomical configuration achieved by this device in the aorta enables a bifurcation reconstruction that preserves the possibility of contralateral femoral crossing in the future. This capability is invaluable in a wide range of scenarios.

Hybrid revascularization procedures can be classified into the following categories.

- Interventions whereby the endovascular component is performed **proximal** to the surgical site.
- Interventions whereby the endovascular component is performed **distal** to the surgical site.
- Interventions whereby the endovascular component is performed **both proximally and distally** to the surgical site.

These procedures are designed to avoid extensive surgical arterial reconstruction in fragile patients, who often present with complex and multilevel disease.

Hybrid procedures minimize surgical stress, reduce associated pathophysiological impacts, and lower the risk of complications typically seen with major surgeries.

TIP #20

The first and most basic piece of advice during hybrid surgery is to avoid placing your hands under the fluoroscopic beam. Pay close attention to this, as it is not always easy to keep your arms away from the radiation.

TIP #21

In hybrid surgery, the individual components – endovascular and surgical – do not differ significantly when considered separately: the procedures and maneuvers are essentially the same. The main difference – and the source of challenges in this type of procedure – lies in the phase when the two components meet each other. This includes the following.

- **Deciding how to access the surgically exposed artery** to begin the endovascular component.
- **Managing the surgical site and exposed arteries during the endovascular phase.** It is surprisingly easy, in the intensity of a complex endovascular recanalization, to overlook what is happening at the common femoral artery. Issues such as bleeding caused by a loss of tourniquet tension, laceration at the arterial access site, or rupture of the patch suture can occur – and believe me, I have experienced these myself.
- **Adhering to proper flushing techniques at the surgical site** when removing the introducer.

It is during these "transition phases" that challenges typically arise.

TIP #22

During a hybrid procedure involving iliac revascularization, the diagnostic phase achieved through contralateral femoral access is critical. For this purpose, a **5 Fr sheath** should be placed, allowing the use of a pigtail catheter connected to an injector to obtain adequate imaging. Upon removal of the contralateral sheath, it is preferable to use a closure device whenever possible, as applying a compressive bandage over the surgical wound is not only cumbersome but also more painful for the patient.

TIP #23

Do not let the convenience of ipsilateral iliac recanalization via puncture of the exposed artery dictate your approach. Instead, choose the access that is most appropriate for the type of lesion to be crossed. In this regard, all the advice provided in the chapter on percutaneous access in aortoiliac pathology applies here as well.

TIP #24

During a hybrid procedure requiring iliac stenting via access from the surgical site (e.g., femoral TEA + iliac stenting), several strategies and timing considerations come into play. In the case of an iliac CTO, an effective approach might be the following.

1. **Expose the femoral tripod** and secure the vessels with vessel loops.
2. **Puncture the femoral artery**, insert a sheath, and perform iliac axis recanalization and pre-dilation.

3. **Remove the sheath**, clamp the tripod, and perform the surgical procedure, ensuring adequate flushing of any atherosclerotic debris released during the prior ballooning.

4. Once the surgical phase is complete, resume the endovascular procedure by stenting the iliac axis using a sheath inserted through the patch.

The rationale behind this strategy is that the most technically challenging and time-consuming part of the endovascular phase – often requiring dual access – is typically the recanalization of the iliac CTO. It is not advisable to perform this phase after the patch has already been implanted, as the prolonged duration of CTO recanalization and the required maneuvers or device's manipulations could potentially damage the patch. Therefore, the sequence should follow the following logical progression.

1. **Iliac recanalization + pre-dilation**

2. **Femoral TEA + patching**

3. **Iliac axis stenting**

In contrast, for iliac stenoses rather than CTOs, the entire endovascular phase can be performed after the surgical phase, as iliac stenosis recanalization is generally quicker and less complex.

TIP #25

In the context of a hybrid procedure involving a common femoral TEA and iliac CTO recanalization, if the retrograde recanalization of the CTO from the surgical site fails, a brachial recanalization can be attempted. In this scenario, the subintimal technique can also be utilized more aggressively, with the guidewire advanced from above until it reaches the common femoral artery.

During the endarterectomy, as the plaque and intimal plane are removed with the spatula, the guidewire will "pop out" and can be easily captured. The guidewire is then externalized through the surgical site, and a sheath is placed over it to complete the endovascular phase (Figures 3.12–3.12e).

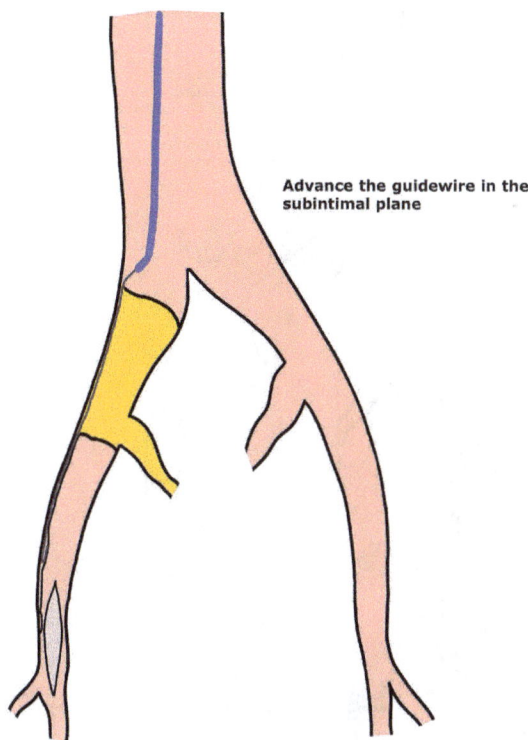

Advance the guidewire in the subintimal plane

Figure 3.12 Subintimal iliac recanalization via brachial access during a hybrid procedure.

The guidewire will emerge from the proximal edge of the endarterectomy and will be extracted from the artery

Once the introducer is inserted, using a *through-and-through technique*, a catheter is advanced along the guidewire to re-enter the aortic lumen from below

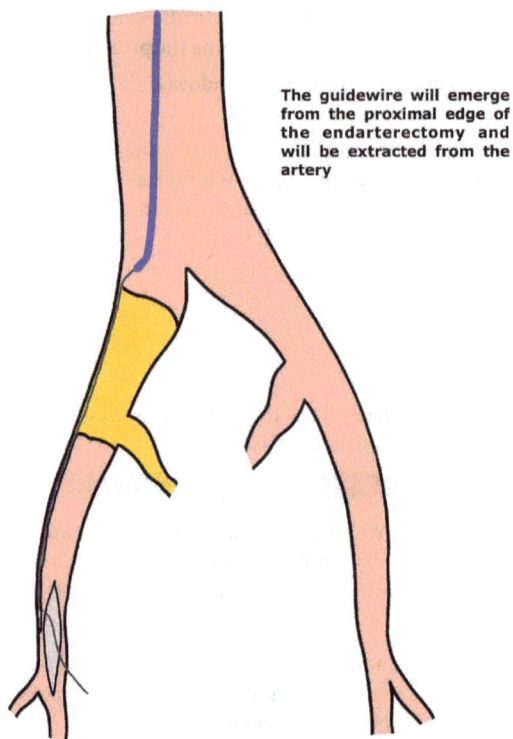

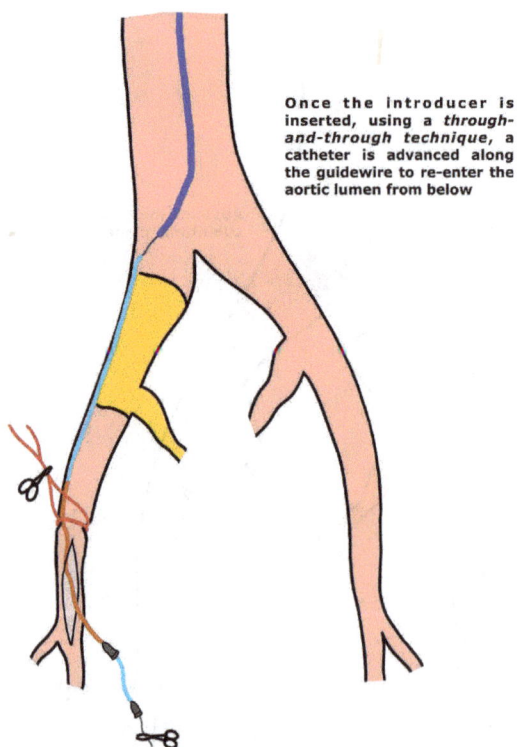

Figures 3.12a–3.12b (Continued)

The aortic lumen is reached from the femoral access

After pre-dilation, advance the stent to the chosen position

N.B. The stent should distally reach the level of the guidewire recapture plane

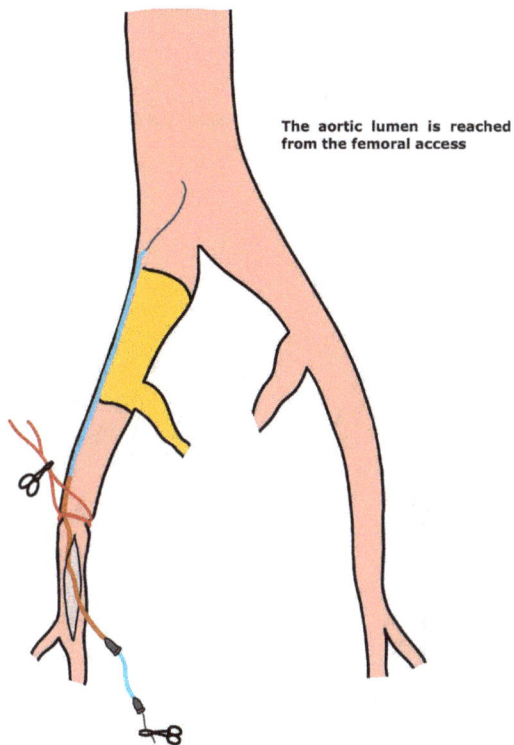

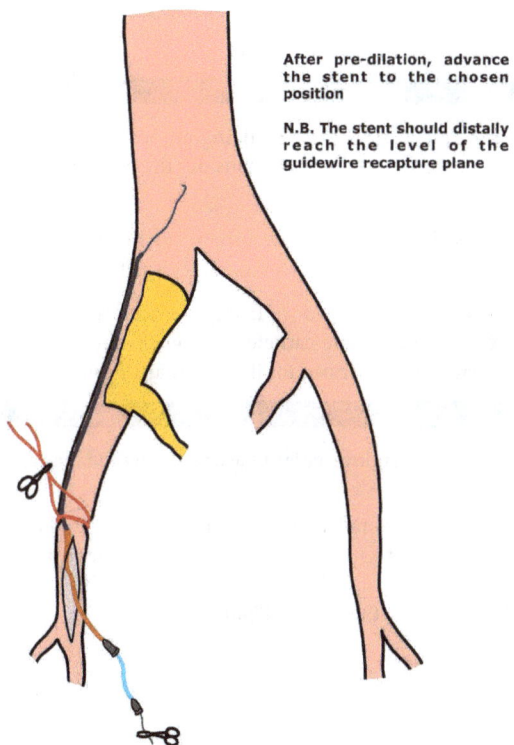

Figures 3.12c–3.12d (Continued)

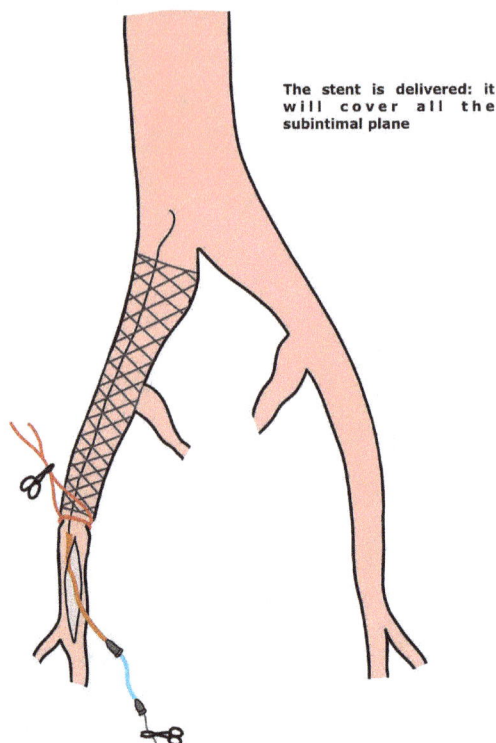

The stent is delivered: it will cover all the subintimal plane

Figure 3.12e (Continued)

TIP #26

Similarly, in cases of significant difficulty recanalizing an occluded femoropopliteal axis during a hybrid procedure with an exposed femoral tripod, consider the possibility of percutaneous retrograde access from below.

With the femoral artery exposed, the subintimal technique can be aggressively pursued from the retrograde access. The guidewire can then be easily captured through the femoral arteriotomy.

Using the captured guidewire, which is tensioned from both the femoral and retrograde access points (Flossing Wire Technique), an anterograde catheter can be advanced to complete the endovascular phase, following the same principles described for iliac recanalization.

TIP #27

If the hybrid procedure involves an endovascular phase targeting the iliac axis, access can be achieved in the following ways.

- **Via a puncture of the patch** after completing the suture (Figure 3.13). Proper management of this access is crucial to avoid blood loss. Our standard approach involves using a vessel loop to encircle both the artery and the sheath. The loop is secured by clamping its free ends with a mosquito forceps positioned immediately adjacent to the sheath (Figure 3.14).

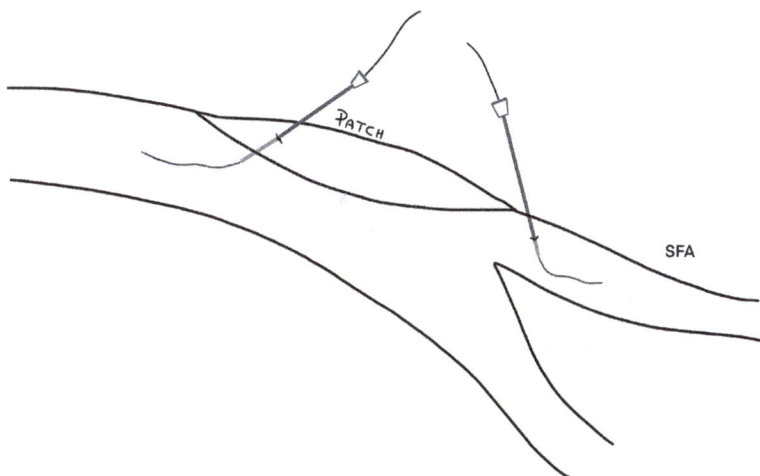

Figure 3.13 Example of puncture techniques used in hybrid procedures.

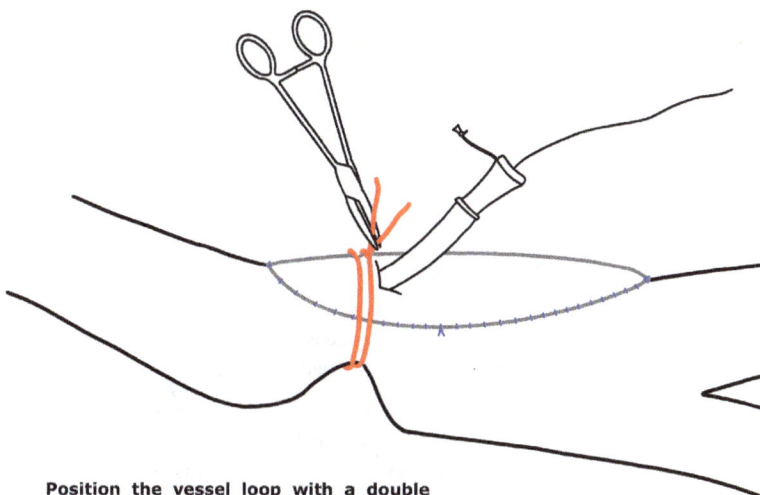

Position the vessel loop with a double pass around the artery, also looping the portion of the introducer that emerges from the access site.

Tighten the vessel loop and secure it with a mosquito clamp, right next to the artery, to achieve the desired hemostasis

Figure 3.14 Achieving hemostasis of the surgical site during a hybrid procedure (Option 1).

- **Via a service access** created through an intentionally incomplete patch suture. To prevent bleeding around the sheath, temporary hemostasis can be achieved using a tourniquet applied to the surgical suture threads. Once the endovascular phase is complete – following sheath removal and flushing maneuvers – the surgical suture is finalized as usual (Figure 3.15).

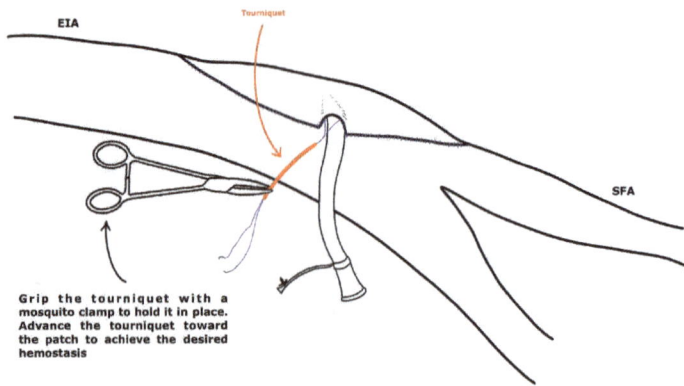

Figure 3.15 Achieving hemostasis of the surgical site during a hybrid procedure (Option 2).

In contrast, if the endovascular phase targets the femoropopliteal axis, a different approach is required. In such cases, after completing the patch, it may be useful to directly puncture the superficial femoral artery distal to the patch, provided that the first few centimeters are patent. This is a simple and safe maneuver (Figure 3.13). The surgeon's position during the endovascular phase is often uncomfortable, requiring focus on the angiographic monitor rather than the surgical field. This can lead to complications during puncture and guidewire insertion. These issues include damaging the profunda femoris artery or displacing the distal endpoint of the endarterectomy at the superficial femoral artery origin.

In our early hybrid procedures, we encountered situations in which a 0.038" guidewire appeared on the monitor to be advancing within the SFA but had actually exited through the patch suture and was traveling straight into the subcutaneous tissues. As the angiographic monitor, not the surgical site, was being observed, inserting the sheath along this misaligned guidewire tore through the entire patch suture.

TIP #28

When performing an iliac–femoral bypass (e.g., between the external iliac artery and the profunda or superficial femoral artery – or even in cases when the bypass is extended distally) combined with iliac stenting, the stent can, as a bailout maneuver if needed, be extended into the proximal segment of the bypass.

In such cases, it is crucial to ensure that the stent does not extend beyond the inguinal ligament or the upper margin of the femoral head as visualized under fluoroscopy (Figure 3.16). Proper positioning using these anatomical landmarks ensures excellent long-term patency rates.

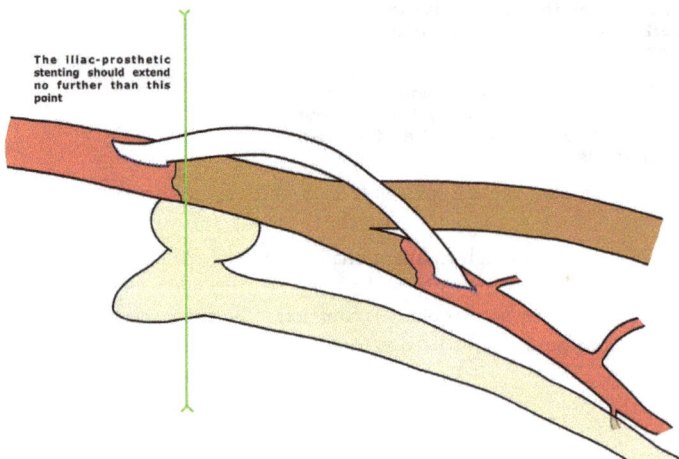

Figure 3.16 Stenting of the iliac artery extended into the proximal segment of an iliofemoral bypass.

REFERENCES

1. Zhang H, Li X, Niu L, et al. Effectiveness and long-term outcomes of different crossing strategies for the endovascular treatment of iliac artery chronic total occlusions. *BMC Cardiovasc Dis.* 2020; 20(1): 431–439.

2. Park KB, Do YS, Kim DI, et al. The trans atlantic inter society consensus (TASC) classification system in iliac arterial stent placement: Long-term patency and clinical limitations. *J Vasc Interv Radiol.* 2007; 18(2): 193–201.

3. Norgren L, Hiatt WR, Dormandy JA, et al. Inter-society consensus for the management of peripheral arterial disease (TASC II). *J Vasc Surg.* 2007; 45(Suppl S): S5–S67.

4. Dong X, Peng Z, Ren Y, et al. Endovascular treatment of aorto-iliac occlusive disease with TASC II C and D lesions: 10 years' experience of clinical technique. *BMC Cardiovasc Disord.* 2023; 23(1): 7.

5. Clair DG, Beach JM. Strategies for managing aortoiliac occlusions: Access, treatment and outcomes. *Expert Rev Cardiovasc Ther.* 2015; 13(5): 551–563.

6. Amankwah KS, Costanza MJ, Gahtan V. Percutaneous recanalization of the occluded iliac artery: Examples, techniques, and complications. *Vasc and Endovasc Surg.* 2007; 41(5): 440–447.

7. Kokkinidis DG, Alvandi B, Hossain P, et al. Midterm outcomes after endovascular intervention for occluded vs stenosed external iliac arteries. *J Endovasc Ther.* 2018; 25(2): 183–191.

8. Chen BL, Holt HR, Day JD, et al. Subintimal angioplasty of chronic total occlusion in iliac arteries: A safe and durable option. *J Vasc Surg.* 2011; 53(2): 367–373.

9. Papakostas JC, Chatzigakis PK, Peroulis M. Endovascular treatment of chronic total occlusions of the iliac arteries: Early and midterm results. *Ann Vasc Surg.* 2015; 29(8): 1508–1515.

10. Schneider PA. The infrarenal aorta, aortic bifurcation, and iliac arteries: Advice about balloon angioplasty and stent placement. In: *Endovascular Skills: Guidewire and Catheter Skills for Endovascular Surgery.* 4th ed. Boca Raton, FL: CRC Press; 2020. pp. 328–345.

11. Moore WS. Angioplasty and stenting for aortoiliac disease. In: *Vascular and Endovascular Surgery: A Comprehensive Review.* 8th ed. Philadelphia, PA: Elsevier Saunders; 2013. pp. 504–516.

12. Duc Tin L, Van Nut L, Abdalla AS. Outcomes of balloon angioplasty and stent placement for iliac artery lesions classified as TASC II A, B: A single-center study. *Front Surg.* 2024; 11: 1366338.

13. Bechara CF, Barshes NR, Lin PH, et al. Recanalization of flush iliac occlusions with the assistance of a contralateral iliac occlusive balloon. *J Vasc Surg.* 2012; 55(3): 872–874.

14. Kokkinids GD, Alvandi B, Cotter R, et al. Long-term outcomes after re-entry device use for recanalization of common iliac artery chronic total occlusions. *Cath Cardiovasc Int.* 2018: 1–7.

15. Kokkinids DG, Katsaros I, Jonnalagadda AK, et al. Use, safety and effectiveness of subintimal angioplasty and re-entry devices for the treatment of iliac artery chronic total occlusions: A systematic review of 30 studies and 1112 lesions. *Cardiovasc Revasc Med.* doi: 10.1016/j.carrev.2019.05.022.

16. Papakostas JC, Chatzigakis PK, Peroulis M, et al. Endovascular treatment of chronic total occlusions of the iliac arteries: Early and midterm results. *Ann Vasc Surg.* 2015: 1–8.

17. Suero SR, Lopez IM, Mateo MH, et al. Outcomes of the endovascular treatment of stenotic lesions versus chronic total occlusions in the iliac sector. *Ann Vasc Surg.* doi: 10.1016/j.avsg.2015.11.040.

18. Sudhakaran S, Choi JW. Coronary chronic total occlusion antegrade wire technique to successfully cross a common iliac chronic total occlusion from retrograde access. *Am J Cardiol.* doi: 10.1016/j.amjcard.2020.05.036.

19. Vuruskan E, Saracoglu E. Procedural and early outcomes of two re-entry devices for subintimal recanalization of aortoiliac and femoropopliteal chronic total occlusions. *Korean Circ J.* 2017; 47(1): 89–96.

20. Kokkinidis DG, Katsaros I, Jonnalagadda AK, et al. Use, safety and effectiveness of subintimal angioplasty and re-entry devices for the treatment of iliac artery chronic total occlusions: A systematic review of 30 studies and 1112 lesions. *Cardiovasc Revasc Med.* 2020; 21(3): 334–341.

21. Mrad MB, Hammamia MB, Emna BA, et al. Crush stent technique: A bail out technique to manage occluded iliac stent. *J Med Vasc*. 2020; 45: 18–22.

22. Reijnene MPCJ. Update on covered endovascular reconstruction of the aortic bifurcation. *Vasc.* doi: 10.1177/1708538119896197.

23. Jebbink EG, Grimme FAB, Goverde PCJM, et al. Geometrical consequences of kissing stents and the covered endovascular reconstruction of the aortic bifurcation configuration in an in vitro model for endovascular reconstruction of aortic bifurcation. *J Vasc Surg*. 2015; 61(5): 1306–1311.

24. Bontinis V, Bontinis A, Giannopoulos A. Covered stents versus bare metal stents in the treatment of aorto-iliac disease: A systematic review and individual participant data meta-analysis. *Eur J Vasc Endovasc Surg*. 2024; 68(3): 348–358.

25. Taeymans K, Goverde P, Lauwers K, et al. The CERAB technique: Tips, tricks and results. *J Cardiovasc Surg*. 2016; 57(3): 343–349.

26. Goverde PC, Grimme FA, Verbruggen PJ, et al. Covered endovascular reconstruction of aortic bifurcation (CERAB) technique: A new approach in treating extensive aortoiliac occlusive disease. *J Cardiovasc Surg*. 2013; 54(3): 383–387.

27. Semaan DB, Habib SG, Abdul-Malak OM, et al. Aortobifemoral bypass vs covered endovascular reconstruction of aortic bifurcation. *J Vasc Surg*. 2024; 80(2): 459–465.e2.

28. Bozorghadad S, Scheidt MJ, Patel PJ. Aortoiliac: Covered, uncovered, CERAB as it relates to peripheral arterial disease. *Semin Intervent Radiol*. 2023; 40(2): 151–155.

29. Reijnen MM. Update on covered endovascular reconstruction of the aortic bifurcation. *Vascular*. 2020; 28(3): 225–232.

30. Rouwenhorst KB, Abdelbaqy OMA, van der Veen D, et al. Long-term outcomes of the covered endovascular reconstruction of the aortic bifurcation (CERAB) technique in patients with aorto-iliac occlusive disease. *J Endovasc Ther*. 2023. doi: 10.1177/15266028231166539.

31. Kruszyna Ł, Strauss E, Tomczak J. Outcomes of covered endovascular reconstruction of the aortic bifurcation (CERAB) procedure for the treatment of extensive aortoiliac occlusive disease using the BeGraft balloon-expandable covered stent: A multicenter observational study. *J Endovasc Ther*. 2023. doi: 10.1177/15266028231180350.

32. Huffman J, Nicjols WK, Bath J. Current hybrid interventions in vascular surgery: Merging past and present. *Mo Med*. 2021; 118(4): 381–386.

33. Kinlay S. Management of critical limb ischemia. *Circ Cardiovasc Interv*. 2016; 9(2): e001946.

34. Chen TW, Huang CY, Chen PL. Endovascular and hybrid revascularization for complicated aorto-iliac occlusive disease: Short-term results in single institute experience. *Acta Cardiol Sin*. 2018; 34(4): 313–320.

35. Dabas AK, Dhillan R, Gambhir RPS. Journey of hybrid procedures in peripheral vascular diseases. *J Vasc Surg*. 2017; 66(1): 323–325.

36. Murakami A. Hybrid operations in patients with peripheral arterial disease. *Ann Vasc Dis*. 2018; 11(1): 57–65.

37. Serna Santos J, Laukontaus S, Laine M, et al. Hybrid revascularization for extensive iliofemoral occlusive disease. *Ann Vasc Surg*. 2023; 88: 90–99.

38. Taurino M, Persiani F, Fantozzi C, et al. Trans-atlantic inter-society consensus II C and D iliac lesions can be treated by endovascular and hybrid approach: A single-center experience. *Vasc Endovascular Surg*. 2014; 48(2): 123–128.

39. Soares TR, Manuel V, Amorim P, et al. Hybrid surgery in lower limb revascularization: A real-world experience from a single center. *Ann Vasc Surg*. 2019; 60: 355–363.

40. Georgakarakos E, Dimitriadis K, Parisidis S, et al. Tips and tricks to facilitate the combined iliofemoral endarterectomy with stenting for heavily calcified common femoral artery atherosclerosis with involvement of the external iliac artery. *Vasc Endovascular Surg*. 2024; 58(5): 571–576.

Section 4

TIPS & TRICKS IN ABDOMINAL AORTIC ANEURYSMS

Toolkit A – **Tips & Tricks in Infrarenal AAAs**   **124**
- Tips 1 to 21

Toolkit B – **Tips & Tricks for Challenging Necks in AAA**   **141**
- Tips 22 to 37

Toolkit C – **Tips & Tricks in the Choice of Infrarenal Endograft**   **154**
- Tips 38 to 47

DOI: 10.1201/9781003567080-4

TIP #1

The risk associated with an iliac extension released beyond the point of minimal overlap is that it may disconnect from the main body. This occurrence, not uncommon, can develop over time due to the natural remodeling mechanisms of the endograft (Figures 4.1–4.1a). The Type III endoleak that results from this disconnection can, in some cases, be difficult (or impossible) to resolve endovascularly. This challenge arises from the way the iliac extension positions itself within the aneurysmal sac, as follows.

- If the disconnection is only partial, performing a relining of the endograft axis will suffice to resolve the situation (Figure 4.2).
- If, however, the disconnection is complete, the severity of the morphological scenario will depend directly on the direction in which the proximal neck of the iliac extension migrates. If it migrates distally, there remains a possibility of relining through the simple interposition of an additional endograft (Figure 4.2a). The main difficulty in this case lies in the cannulation of the lost gate. Conversely, if the neck of the iliac endograft migrates proximally, beyond the level of the lost gate, engaging the main body will become virtually impossible, and concurrent occlusion of the iliac extension is not uncommon. In such cases, open or hybrid surgery will be the only viable solution (Figure 4.2b).

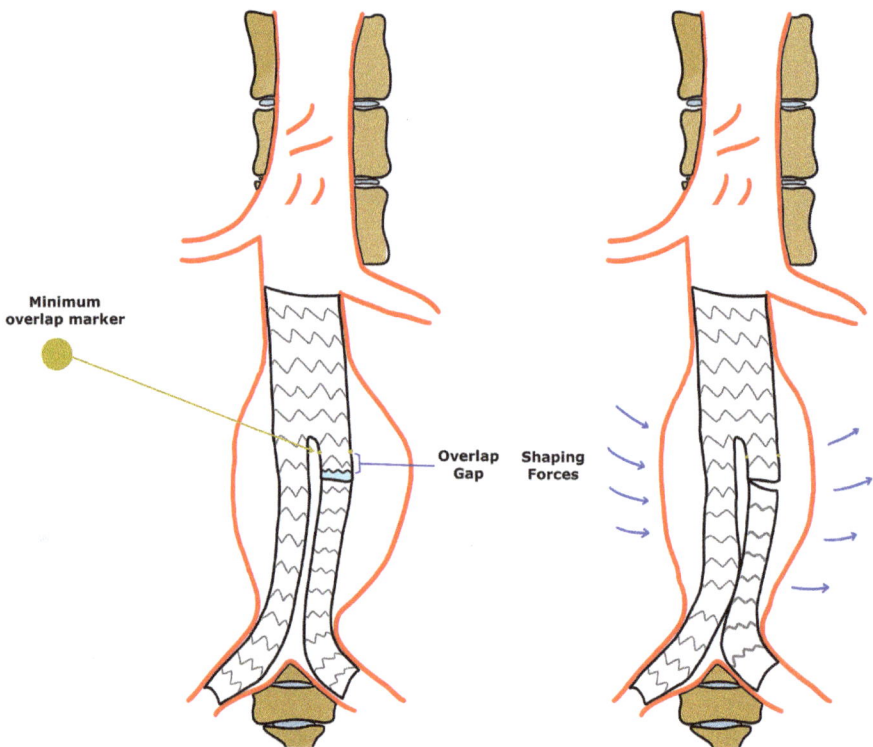

Figures 4.1–4.1a An iliac extension released beyond the point of minimal overlap may disconnect from the main body.

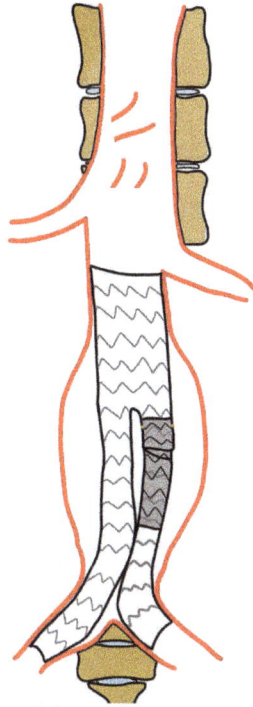

Figure 4.2 In case of partial disconnection of the iliac module, a simple relining can be performed.

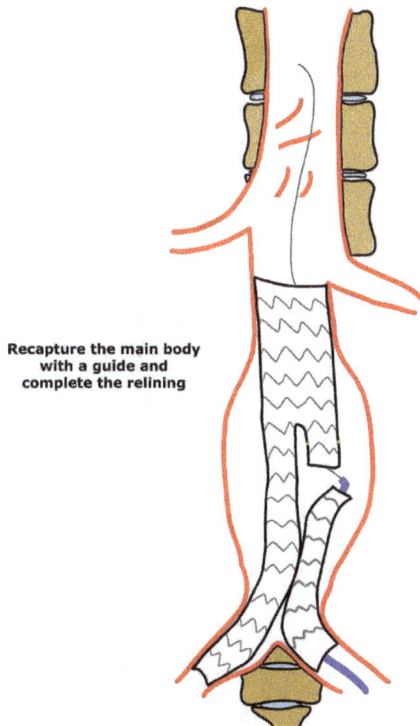

Recapture the main body
with a guide and
complete the relining

Figure 4.2a In case of total disconnection and distal migration of iliac module, the relining can still be performed.

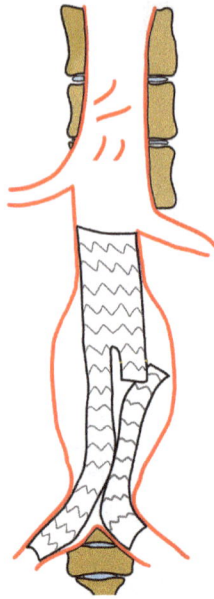

Figure 4.2b In case of total disconnection and proximal migration of iliac module, an endovascular repair is almost impossible.

TIP #2

In the case of a trimodular endograft, the ipsilateral and contralateral iliac extensions should always be implanted at the same proximal overlap level.

If one of the two is released above the other or beyond the point of maximal overlap for any reason, it is crucial to seriously consider the option of performing a kissing stent placement at the level of the flow divider, because there is a significant risk of subsequent occlusion of the contralateral limb (Figures 4.3–4.3b).

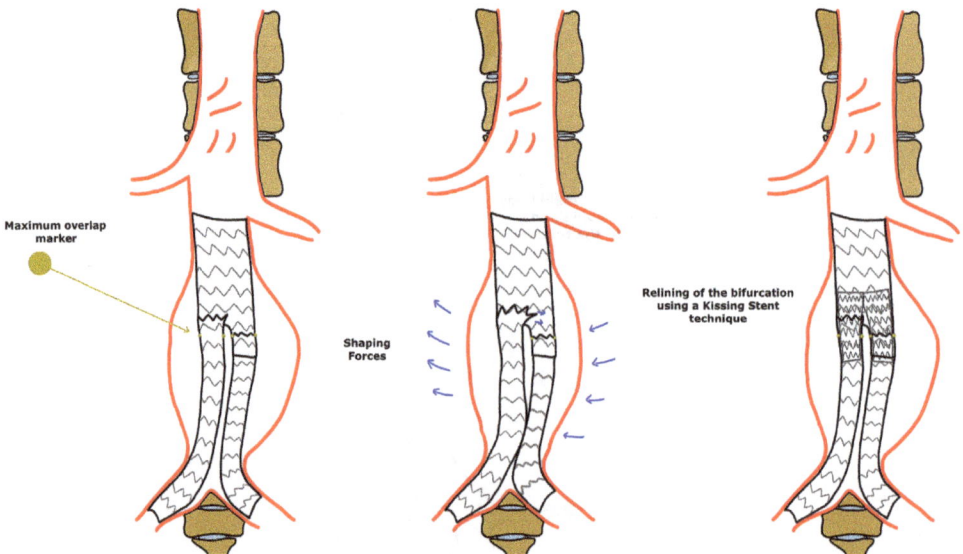

Figures 4.3–4.3b In case of iliac module released above the other or beyond the point of maximum overlap, the risk is the occlusion of the contralateral gate for the competition occurring between the iliac limbs. If this occurs, take into consideration a kissing stent at the flow divider.

TIP #3

If the iliac extension proves to be longer than anticipated during the intraoperative phase, thereby covering the hypogastric artery ostium, the following maneuver can be used to correct the issue.

- Begin by deploying the iliac extension until the first 3–4 cm are released, ensuring it is securely anchored to the main body (Figure 4.4).
- At this point, push the extension forward toward the main body until it is distally aligned with the hypogastric artery, which has been angiographically marked. This maneuver causes the limb to invaginate on itself (Figure 4.4a).
- Complete the deployment of the extension (Figure 4.4b).

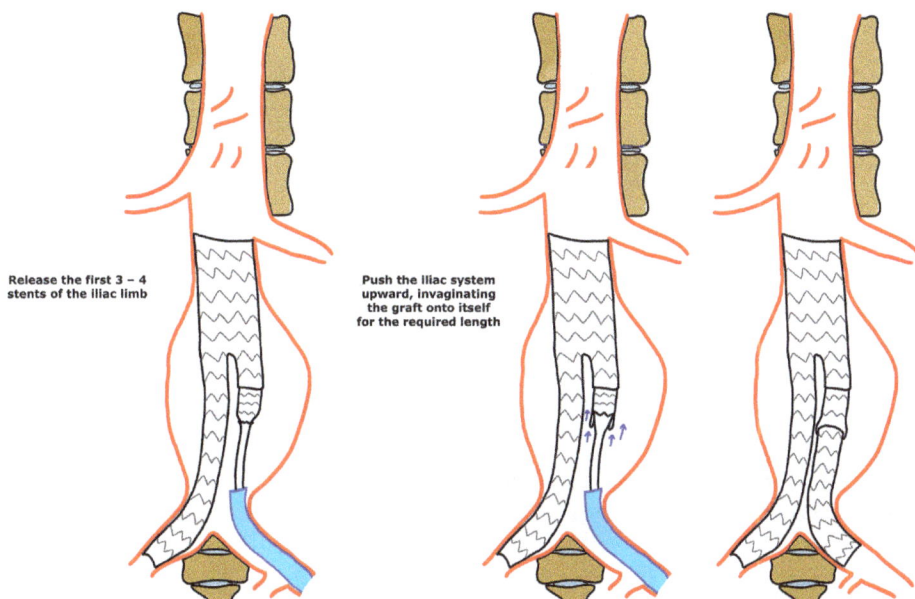

Figures 4.4–4.4b How to fix an iliac extension longer than preoperatively anticipated.

TIP #4

If, during an EVAR procedure, it becomes necessary to perform a retrograde angiography through the large-caliber sheath (or using the delivery systems of Cook Zenith or Bolton Treo, which function as large-caliber sheaths once the endograft is deployed), the manual technique for performing such angiography – required, for example, to map the hypogastric artery – should be as follows.

- Gently inject contrast medium into the sheath system using a 20 mL syringe.
- Subsequently, inject saline solution forcefully while simultaneously performing the angiography.
- Due to the differing densities of the two fluids, this maneuver allows the saline solution to push out the contrast medium with sufficient force to achieve the desired angiographic examination.

TIP #5

In the case of a residual stenosis >30% in an iliac limb post-EVAR, the placement of an uncovered self-expanding stent is mandatory, especially if the stenosis is located at the distal end of the iliac extension (Figures 4.5–4.5a). This simple measure ensures a relining of the transition segment between the endograft and the native iliac artery, effectively preventing potential future occlusions of the prosthetic limb.

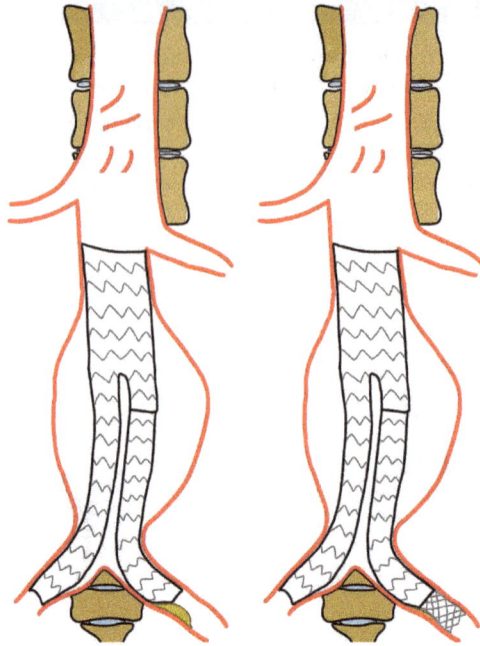

Figures 4.5–4.5a In case of stenosis along the iliac artery covered by endograft, its treatment is strongly advised.

TIP #6

If advancing the main body to the desired position proves particularly challenging due to iliac tortuosity or excessive angulation of the aortic aneurysm (Figure 4.6), the following Flossing Technique with brachial access can be a valid solution.

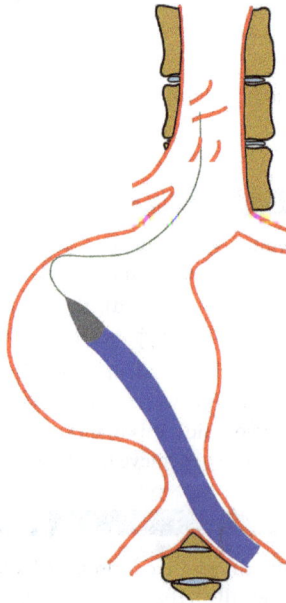

Figure 4.6 The Flossing Technique from brachial access, in case of difficult in advancing the endograft to its final location.

- Obtain a second access via the left brachial artery and insert a snare from this entry point (Figure 4.6a).
- Capture the guidewire, ideally at the level of the descending thoracic aorta (Figure 4.6b), and retrieve it through the brachial access. It is essential to protect the brachial artery from potential dissections by using a catheter or a long introducer extending into the descending thoracic aorta.
- Slightly retract the endograft to move it away from areas of the aneurysmal sac where it might have become stuck.
- While applying gentle manual tension externally on both ends of the guidewire, push the main body into the desired position (Figure 4.6c).

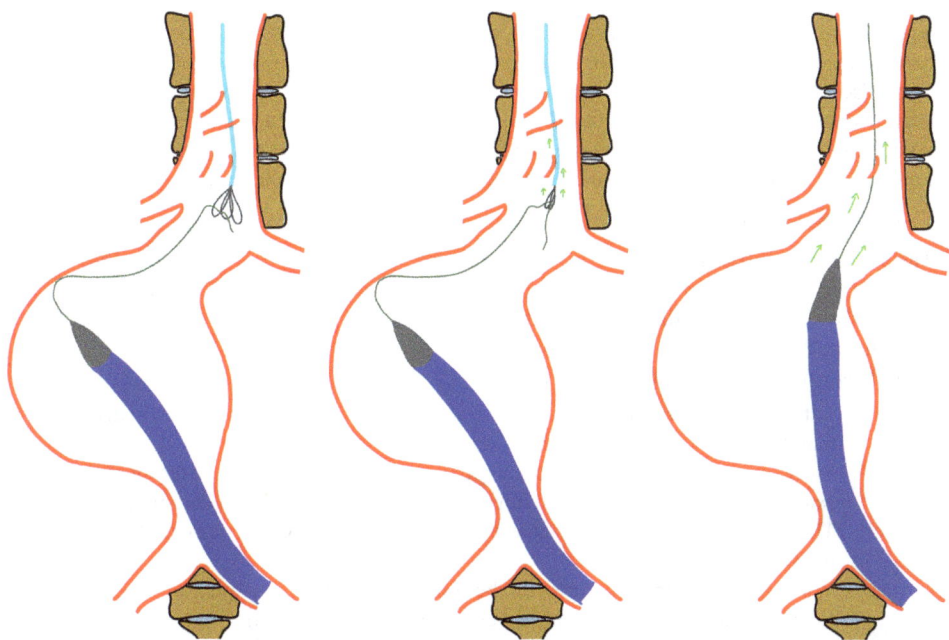

Figures 4.6a–4.6c (Continued)

TIP #7

If a critical stenosis or occlusion of the superior mesenteric artery (SMA) is present and the inferior mesenteric artery (IMA) serves as a key collateral branch, the SMA lesion should be treated as a priority before proceeding with EVAR for an abdominal aortic aneurysm (AAA). This is because excluding the IMA after endograft placement could result in visceral ischemia.

TIP #8

Accessory renal arteries are generally covered by the endograft. They should be preserved through targeted fenestration if their diameter exceeds 4 mm.

HOW TO MANAGE COMPLEX ILIAC ARTERIES

Proper management of the iliac arteries is critical during the endovascular treatment of abdominal aortic aneurysms. Accurate planning of how to approach these arteries is one of the most critical steps in preparing for an endovascular procedure, essential to preventing significant complications at this level (which, moreover, are among the most common during EVAR).

To this end, the following four categories of challenges may be encountered.

1. Stenosis
2. Calcifications
3. Vessel tortuosity
4. Iliac occlusion

For each category, we will attempt to analyze the essential technical tips to ensure the success of the procedure.

TIP #9

Iliac Stenosis

The presence of stenosis along the iliac arteries – which can vary in number and severity – is a common occurrence, particularly when addressing purely atherosclerotic aortic aneurysms. These stenoses can compromise the procedure due to the obstruction they pose to the passage of devices. Additionally, there is a significant risk of intra-procedural iliac thrombosis caused by the prolonged presence of large-caliber, often fully occlusive, sheaths. Finally, untreated iliac stenoses can lead to reduced long-term patency of the endograft. For all these reasons, managing iliac stenoses requires a vigilant and resolute approach.

The available technical solutions, in order of increasing complexity, are as follows.

- **The use of low-profile endografts** is strongly recommended. Additionally, hydrophilic sheaths such as Gore DrySeal significantly facilitate navigation through stenotic or calcified iliac arteries.
- **Progressive dilation** using dilators or sheaths of increasing caliber, advancing gradually until reaching the diameter required for the procedure.
- **PTA:** This procedure should follow these steps.
    a) Initially perform pre-dilation with a semi-compliant balloon of a diameter smaller than the nominal diameter of the iliac artery.
    b) Proceed with POBA, using balloons approximately 6–8 mm in diameter for the external iliac artery and/or 8–10 mm in diameter for the common iliac artery.
    c) These balloon sizes generally achieve an adequate lumen for the passage of commonly used devices.
    d) When necessary, the procedure can be completed with the implantation of stents (self-expanding or balloon-expandable, depending on the situation).
- **Open Conduit Technique:** This method is reserved for severely diseased iliac arteries. It involves using a prosthesis, typically 10 mm in diameter, anastomosed to the iliac artery in an end-to-side fashion (Figure 4.7). The surgical access is performed retroperitoneally through an oblique incision a few centimeters above the inguinal crease. At the end of the procedure, the prosthesis is sutured and transected flush with the anastomosis to the iliac artery (Figure 4.7a). Alternatively, as will be discussed later, the prosthesis may be used to perform an iliofemoral bypass if it is also necessary to treat the pathological iliac segment.
- **Endoconduit Technique:** This is an endovascular evolution of the Open Conduit Technique, eliminating the need for open surgical access. The procedure involves the placement of covered stents (self-expanding or balloon-expandable) of adequate length to treat the entire stenotic segment (Figures 4.8 and 4.8a). Multiple covered stents in a tandem configuration may be used, provided they are appropriately overlapped. The stent diameter is generally 10 mm. After stent placement, dilation is performed using the **Paving & Cracking Technique**, employing high-pressure non-compliant balloons to achieve the desired diameter (approximately 9–10 mm for the external iliac artery and 10–12 mm for the common iliac artery), creating a controlled fracture of the iliac artery (Figure 4.8b). Covered stents ensure the necessary protection against hemorrhagic complications. A critical aspect of the endoconduit procedure is the management of the hypogastric artery. If the artery is patent and of adequate caliber, and if the endoconduit must cover its ostium – a frequent occurrence given that controlled rupture during the Paving & Cracking phase typically occurs at this level – there is a risk of an endoleak that could feed retroperitoneal bleeding through the

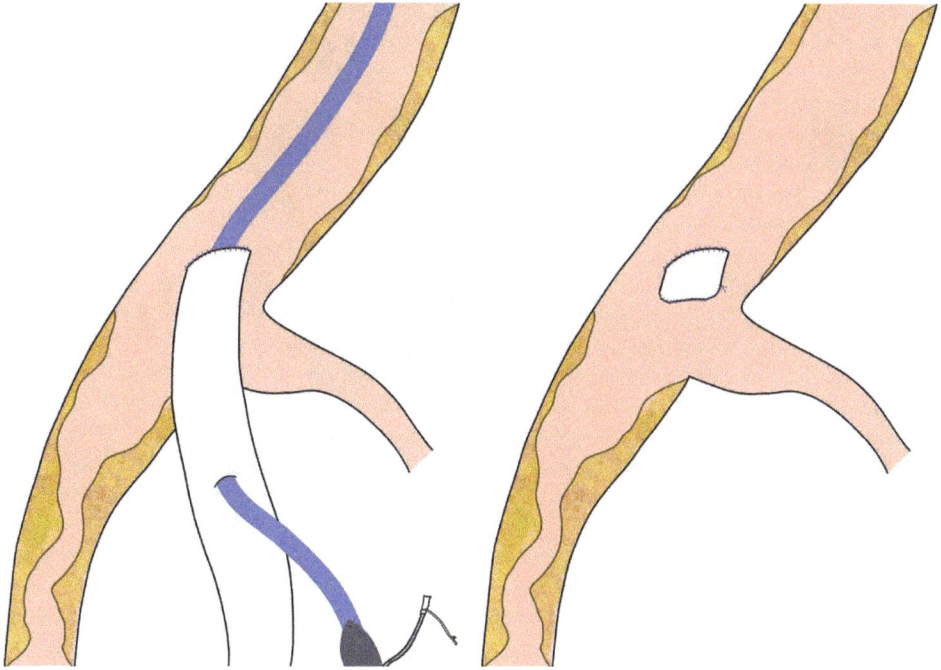

Figures 4.7–4.7a The Open Conduit Technique

The iliac artery is recanalized

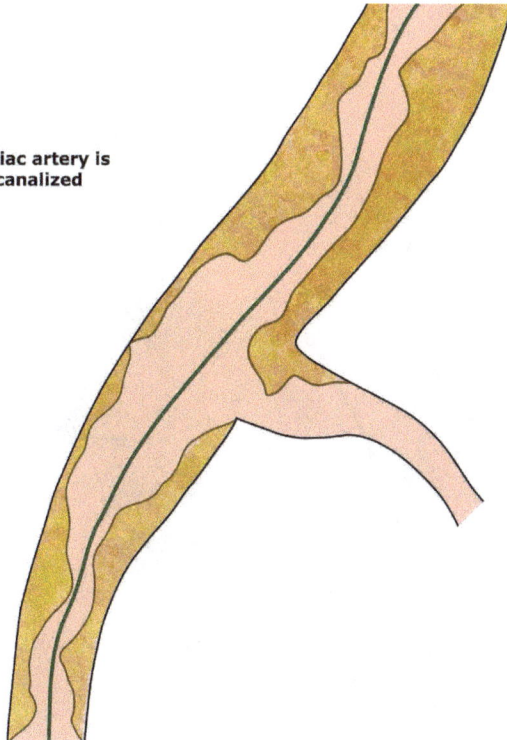

Figure 4.8 The Endoconduit Technique

The covered stent is deployed

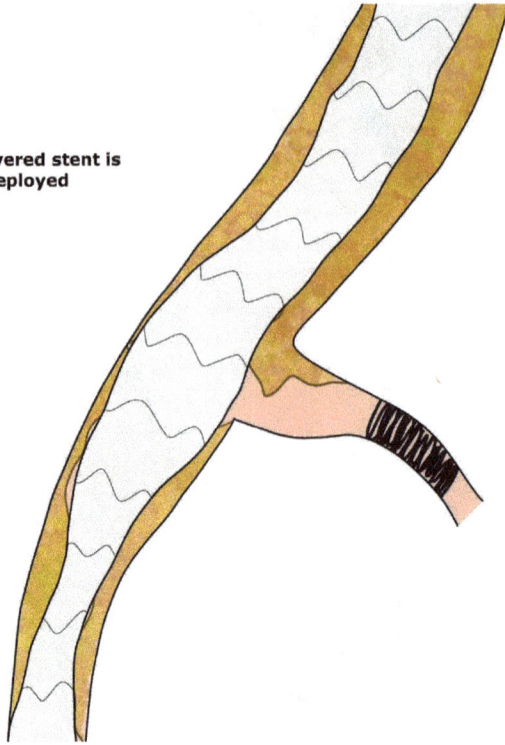

Microrupture of the vessel

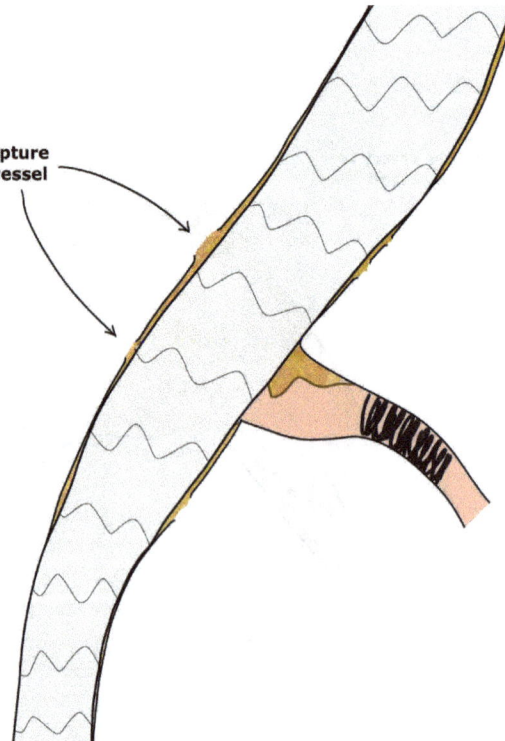

Figures 4.8a–4.8b (Continued)

fractured iliac segment. Although the literature is not unanimous, **preventive embolization of the hypogastric artery** is recommended in such cases.

TIP #10

Calcifications

The presence of calcifications along the iliac arteries can create challenges in device navigation due to the high friction generated against the vascular wall. Severe calcifications can also compromise the long-term patency of devices due to the progression of atherosclerotic disease. An especially concerning risk during the procedure is the potential avulsion of the iliac artery caused by the forced passage of devices through heavily calcified segments.

In cases of heavily calcified iliac arteries, the technical strategies include the following.

- As in previous cases, the use of low-profile endografts and hydrophilic sheaths.
- **PTA or PTA with stenting**.
- A recently introduced and appealing option is **vessel preparation** of the iliac arteries using **Shockwave balloons** for intravascular lithotripsy (see the chapter on vessel preparation in the previous section). The calcium fragmentation they induce enhances the efficacy of PTA or PTA/ stenting techniques.
- **Endoconduit Technique:** In cases of severely calcified iliac arteries, the Endoconduit Technique is preferable to the Open Conduit Technique. Surgical manipulation of calcified arteries and the creation of anastomoses on such walls often pose a technically prohibitive challenge.

TIP # 11

Tortuosities

The presence of varying degrees of tortuosity along the iliac arteries severely compromises device navigability and deployability, in addition to being a risk factor for reduced long-term patency of the endograft.

A frequent risk is the potential occlusion of the iliac artery caused by arterial twisting due to the straightening effect induced by the passage of extra-stiff guidewires and devices through the vessel. If not promptly recognized, deploying the endograft in a twisted artery can solidify this anatomy, leading to vessel occlusion during the procedure or shortly thereafter.

- The technical approach first requires meticulous attention to preventing arterial twisting during the advancement of super-stiff/extra-stiff guidewires or endograft devices. A simple maneuver involves continuous manual monitoring of the femoral pulse, which is typically lost when the artery twists upon itself. If this occurs, a guidewire de-escalation is necessary, switching to progressively less stiff wires until the appropriate stiffness is reached, ensuring adequate system support without causing twisting of the vessel.
- If the chosen guidewire does not provide sufficient support for advancing the system through the iliac tortuosity, buddy wiring can be used to straighten the vessel and enhance support.
- If advancing the device remains problematic, the flossing wire technique via brachial or axillary access, as previously described in *Tip #6* (Figures 4.6–4.6c), can be employed. In such cases, it is critical to protect the axillosubclavian artery with a long sheath to prevent vessel wall trauma caused by the guidewire.

TIP #12

Occlusions

Iliac occlusion associated with aneurysmal disease represents a not uncommon technical challenge. Strategies to optimize iliac access in these cases include the following.

- **Endovascular recanalization** followed by PTA, potentially completed with stenting. Brachial access is particularly useful in such procedures, especially if subintimal recanalization is anticipated, as it allows the extension of the subintimal plane toward the femoral axis rather than the aorta.

- **Recanalization with PTA** followed by the **Endoconduit Technique** as an alternative to conventional stenting.
- **Open repair**, which is the gold standard in these cases. Alternatively, an aortouniiliac endograft with a femoro–femoral crossover bypass may be employed.
- **Iliac Open Conduit Technique:** At the end of the procedure, the conduit can be tunneled beneath the inguinal ligament and anastomosed to the iliofemoral axis (Figures 4.9–4.9a). In this way, it is converted into an iliofemoral bypass, restoring direct blood flow to the lower limb.

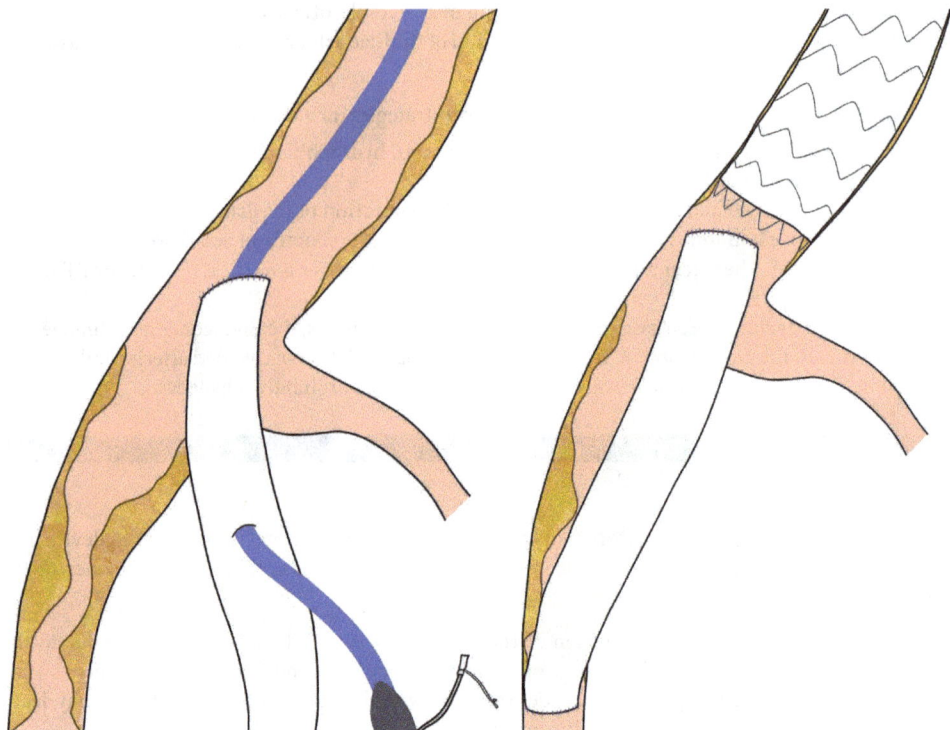

Figures 4.9–4.9a At the end of the procedure, the open conduit can be used to perform an iliofemoral bypass, if needed.

AORTIC ENDOCLAMPING

TIP #13

Endoclamping is an extremely useful maneuver for the hemodynamic stabilization of patients with ruptured aortic aneurysms (Figure 4.10). Its utility is not limited to endovascular treatment but is also an invaluable resource for unstable patients undergoing traditional surgical management.

It allows hemorrhage control and restoration of stable hemodynamics. Endoclamping can be performed via femoral or brachial access. The steps, considering femoral access, are as follows.

- A **0.035" stiff guidewire** (e.g., Lunderquist, Amplatz Super-Stiff) is placed in the aortic arch (Figure 4.10a).
- The standard sheath is replaced with a **12–14 Fr, 45 cm long one** whose distal tip is positioned at the level of the celiac aorta (Figure 4.10b).
- An **aortic balloon** (if using a molding balloon without an occlusive component a three-way stopcock should be connected to its inflation port) is advanced through the sheath and deployed just distal to it, at the level of the diaphragmatic aorta. It is inflated to occlude the aorta using a 1:1 mixture of saline and contrast medium (Figure 4.10c).

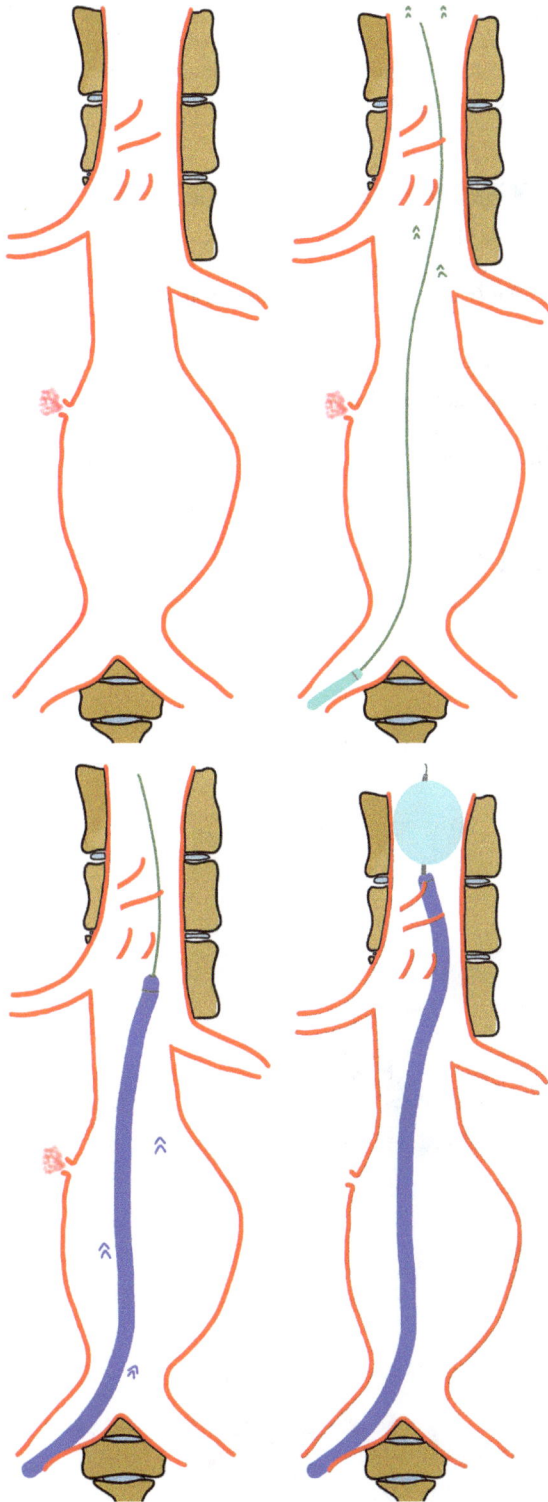

Figures 4.10–4.10c Aortic endoclamping.

- The sheath, left in place just below the balloon, serves to prevent distal migration of the endoclamp due to pressurization forces, which can occur as soon as adequate hemodynamics are restored.
- The balloon should be deflated as soon as possible and should not remain inflated for more than 10–15 minutes, as the risk of renal and mesenteric ischemic damage increases exponentially beyond this timeframe.

TIP #14

If endoclamping is performed via brachial access, it can be combined – though this is rarely necessary – with simultaneous iliac endoclamping. This maneuver is useful in cases of extreme ruptured abdominal aortic aneurysms (rAAA), particularly when an associated iliac arteriovenous fistula (AVF) or aorto-caval fistula is present.

Additionally, it may be beneficial if aortic endoclamping alone fails to restore adequate hemodynamics. Through bilateral femoral access, a balloon is inserted and inflated at the level of each common iliac artery, enabling distal hemostasis (Figure 4.11). This is achieved by halting retrograde inflow into the aneurysmal sac, which is supported by collateral circulation through the hypogastric, circumflex, and epigastric arteries.

CONTRALATERAL GATE CANNULATION

Cannulation of the contralateral gate is almost always the most time-consuming step for operators during an EVAR procedure.

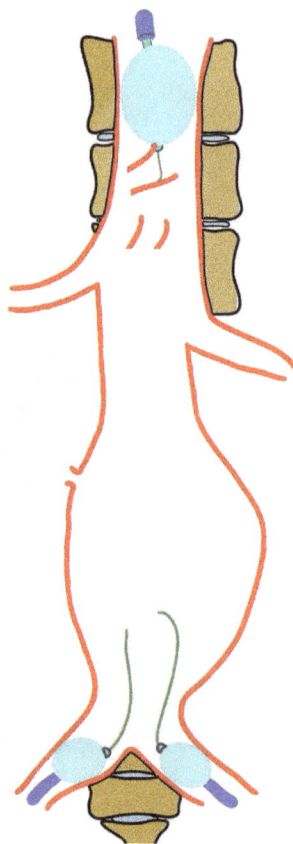

Figure 4.11 Aortoiliac endoclamping.

Significant prolongation of procedural times during this phase has become increasingly common due to the constant evolution of the endograft portfolio, which now allows the treatment of even the most complex anatomies. Extended procedural times also lead to the following.

- An exponential increase in radiological exposure.
- Greater discomfort for both the patient and the operators.
- Increased risk of thrombotic or embolic complications caused by guidewire and catheter manipulation within the aneurysmal sac, which almost always contains parietal thrombotic deposits.
- Prolonged anesthesia times and higher costs.

It is therefore essential to adopt a series of technical and strategic measures to optimize and accelerate this phase of the endovascular procedure. Doing so minimizes or eliminates the aforementioned issues while improving the overall efficiency of the intervention.

TIP #15

The engagement of the contralateral gate begins with the analysis of the preoperative CT angiography. It is crucial to plan and anticipate where the gate will open or where it should be made to open. The distance between the lowest renal artery and the aortic bifurcation must be assessed to select a main body whose gate is not positioned too far from the aortic carrefour. This prevents the gate from opening in the widest area of the aneurysmal sac, where the maneuver would be more challenging (Figures 4.12–4.12a).

Additionally, a longer main body provides greater columnar strength to the system, making the gate more stable and less susceptible to movements caused by blood flow.

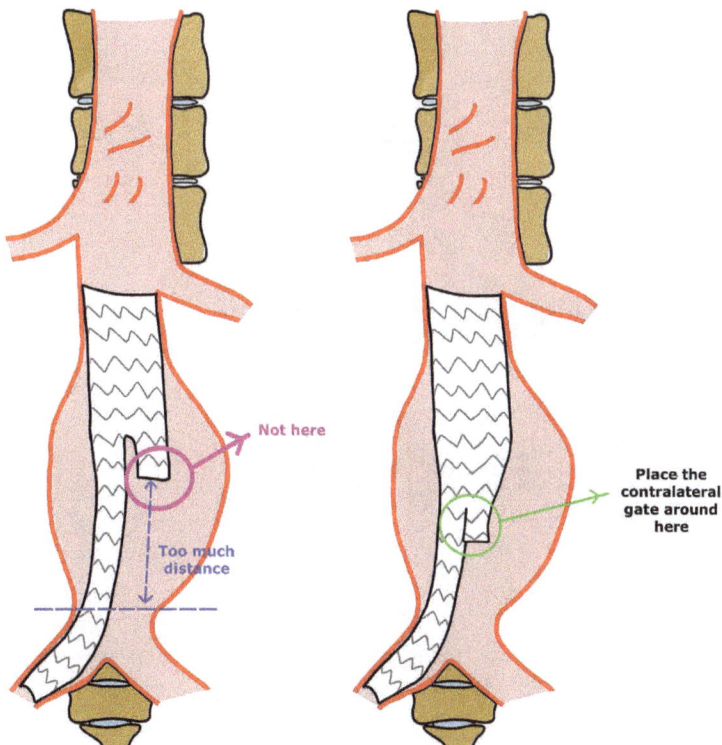

Figures 4.12–4.12a Tips & Tricks to engage the contralateral gate.

TIP #16

The first and most important advice is to remain patient and avoid persistently using a single catheter. Additionally, the following should be kept in mind.

- Many operators often insist on using the **Pigtail catheter**, which is already in place for aortography. Personally, I typically start this maneuver with a **Bern catheter**, whose angled and upward-oriented tip allows for 360° guidewire orientation toward the gate.
- Depending on how the catheter positions itself within the sac, I may switch to a catheter with a different shape (e.g., a Cobra or a Bern with a different tip angle).
- The catheter tip should be kept close to the gate (within 1–2 cm), as being too far from the gate makes precise guidewire orientation much more challenging (Figure 4.12b).
- Guidewire manipulations should be very slow. Additionally, attention should be paid to how the tip of the guidewire moves during maneuvers. Occasionally – once advanced beyond the gate – retracting the guidewire causes it to contact the endograft wall and spontaneously "jump" into the gate. Pay attention to this jump.
- Do not hesitate to use a 0.035 torque device, which allows precise control and direction of the guidewire.
- Be mindful of optical illusions caused by parallax effects. For example, in a frontal projection, it may appear that the catheter is correctly oriented toward the gate, but a steep lateral projection could reveal that it is completely off course. For this reason, during a challenging cannulation, frequent adjustments to the fluoroscopic projection are necessary. (My personal rule of thumb is to change the projection approximately every 2 minutes.)

TIP #17

An anteromedial orientation of 30–45° of the gate – obtained by rotating the main body – facilitates cannulation. This positioning aligns the gate approximately along the natural path of the guidewire (Figures 4.12c–4.12d).

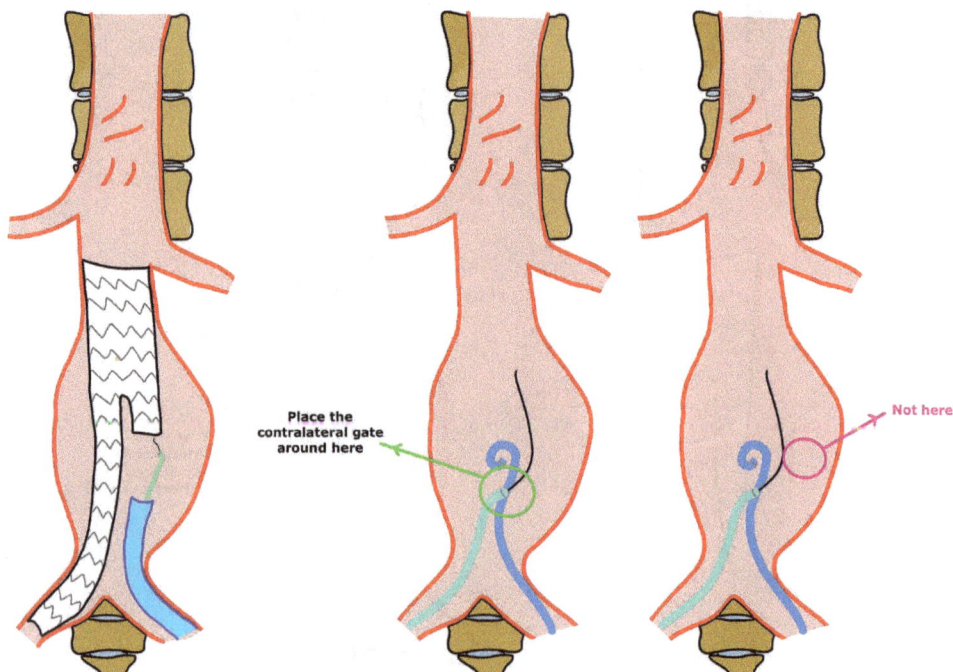

Figures 4.12b–4.12d (Continued)

TIP #18

Consider the possibility of a "ballerina" deployment. This technique can facilitate gate engagement in cases of highly angulated necks or severely tortuous iliac arteries when the curve is unfavorable relative to the main body axis (Figures 4.12e–4.12f).

Place the
contralateral gate
around here

Not here

Ideal route
of the GW

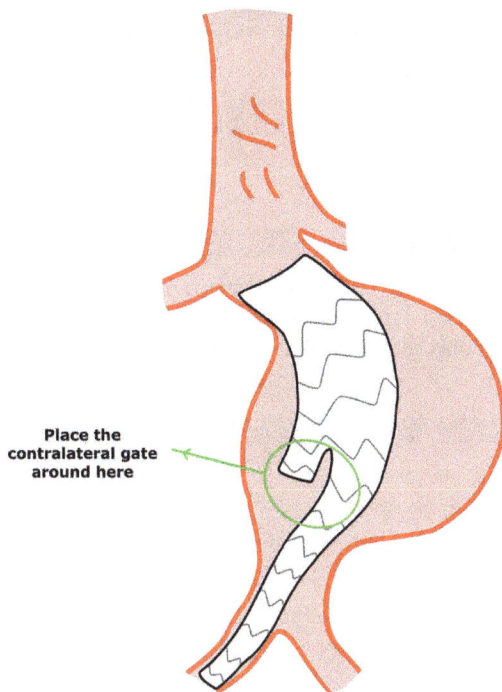

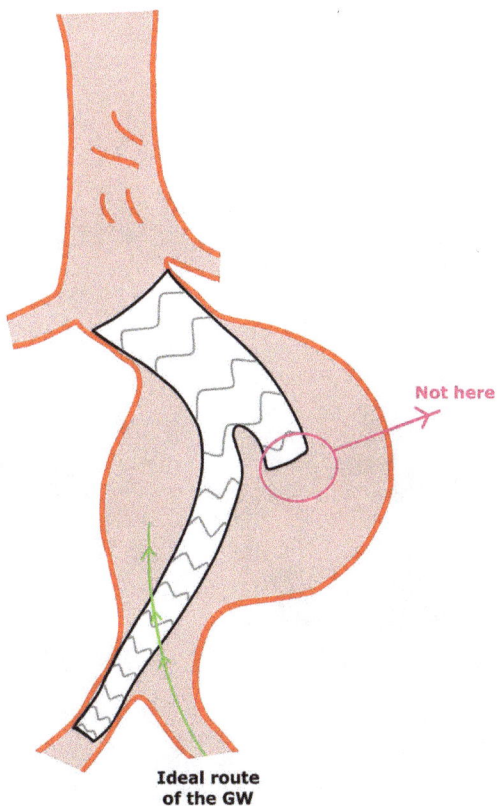

Figures 4.12e–4.12f (Continued)

TIP #19

During a difficult cannulation, if the tip of the guidewire exhibits a ticking motion synchronized with systole, it indicates that the guidewire is very close to the gate (as, at this stage of the procedure, the sac is pressurized only through the gate itself). At this point, very slow movements should be combined with attempts to engage the gate during diastole, as this phase of the cardiac cycle offers less resistance to the guidewire's advancement into the ostium to be engaged.

TIP #20

If preoperative CT angiography reveals a highly tortuous aortic anatomy and a difficult cannulation is anticipated, consider the implantation of an **Anaconda endograft**, provided it is within the IFU. This device features a magnetic mechanism for guided gate cannulation, significantly simplifying and accelerating the maneuver.

TIP #21

As a last resort, I would like to emphasize that in cases of genuine difficulty, opting for the use of a **snare** inserted via brachial access can be a wise choice. It is simple, quick, and safe.

These represent approximately 20–30% of all infrarenal aneurysms. Challenging necks in AAA are defined by the following criteria.

- A neck < 10 mm in length.
- A neck angulation > 60°.
- A conical neck (i.e., a distal neck diameter > 10% larger than the diameter immediately below the renal plane).
- A neck diameter > 28–30 mm.
- A neck with calcifications involving more than 50% of the circumference.

There is still no unanimous consensus on considering the presence of mural thrombus as a criterion of complexity.

The concept of a challenging neck has emerged over the years alongside the establishment of EVAR as the standard therapy for AAA. Despite the phenomenal technological advancements in endograft design, a challenging neck remains a critical factor of complexity in the standard endovascular treatment of infrarenal aneurysms. A challenging neck significantly reduces the proximal sealing and fixation capabilities of the endograft, exponentially increasing the risk of developing a **Type IA endoleak** or distal migration of the device.

Currently, it is the leading contraindication for standard endovascular treatment of infrarenal aneurysms. Additionally, the presence of a challenging neck greatly increases the following.

- Operative times.
- The incidence of perioperative and postoperative complications.
- Procedure costs.
- The technical skill requirements for operators.
- Radiation exposure for both patients and operators.

Aneurysms with challenging necks are typically treated with open surgery – when the patient is eligible – or with **FEVAR/BEVAR techniques**.

Here, I propose a series of strategies to enable adequate infrarenal treatment even in these cases. It is important to emphasize that these should not be the go-to solutions for elective procedures but can be invaluable in **bailout situations** or emergencies, where other technical or technological solutions are unavailable or impractical. Finally, these are technical gems that may provoke skepticism among proponents of suprarenal treatments but are nevertheless worth having in your toolbox.

TIP #22

How to Calculate the Neck Angle: Using a DICOM file management software package (freeware options include Osirix for Macintosh or Radiant DICOM Viewer for PC), the neck angle should be measured as shown in Figure 4.13.

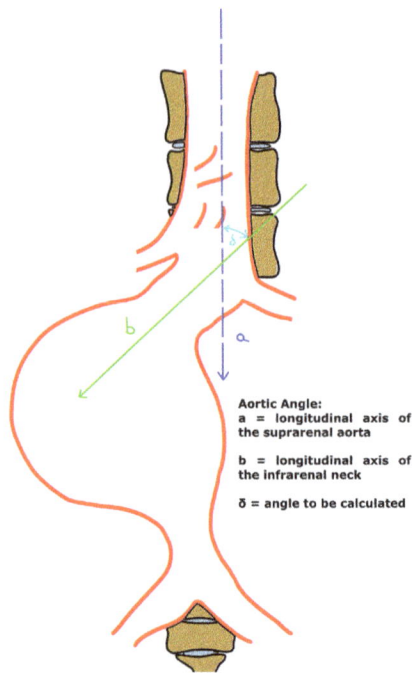

Aortic Angle:
a = longitudinal axis of the suprarenal aorta

b = longitudinal axis of the infrarenal neck

δ = angle to be calculated

Figure 4.13 How to calculate the neck angle.

TIP #23

Here is a fact: Each millimeter of proximal neck length reduces the 2.5-year risk of distal endograft migration by 5.8%, thereby lowering the risk of late Type IA endoleak.

TIP #24

In highly angulated necks or significantly tortuous aortic anatomies, it is advisable to insert the main endograft body from the side opposite to the angulation. This approach facilitates navigation through the neck and simplifies endograft deployment (Figure 4.14).

Indeed, when the main system is inserted through the other side, the sheath tip may press against the aortic wall (Figure 4.14a), making advancement toward the desired location particularly challenging.

TIP #25

Endografts tend to "fall" toward the side of the contralateral gate during deployment. To achieve better sealing in highly angulated necks, the system can be rotated so that the contralateral gate aligns with the lesser curvature of the aneurysm (Figures 4.15–4.15a).

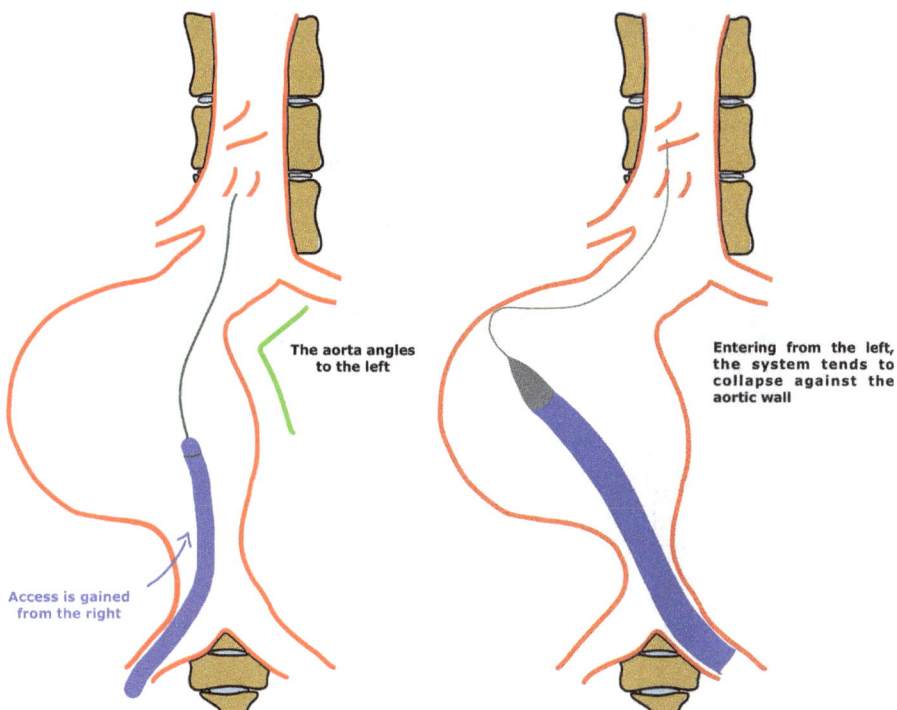

The aorta angles
to the left

Entering from the left,
the system tends to
collapse against the
aortic wall

Access is gained
from the right

Figures 4.14–4.14a In highly angulated necks or tortuous anatomies, insert the main endograft body from the side opposite to the angulation.

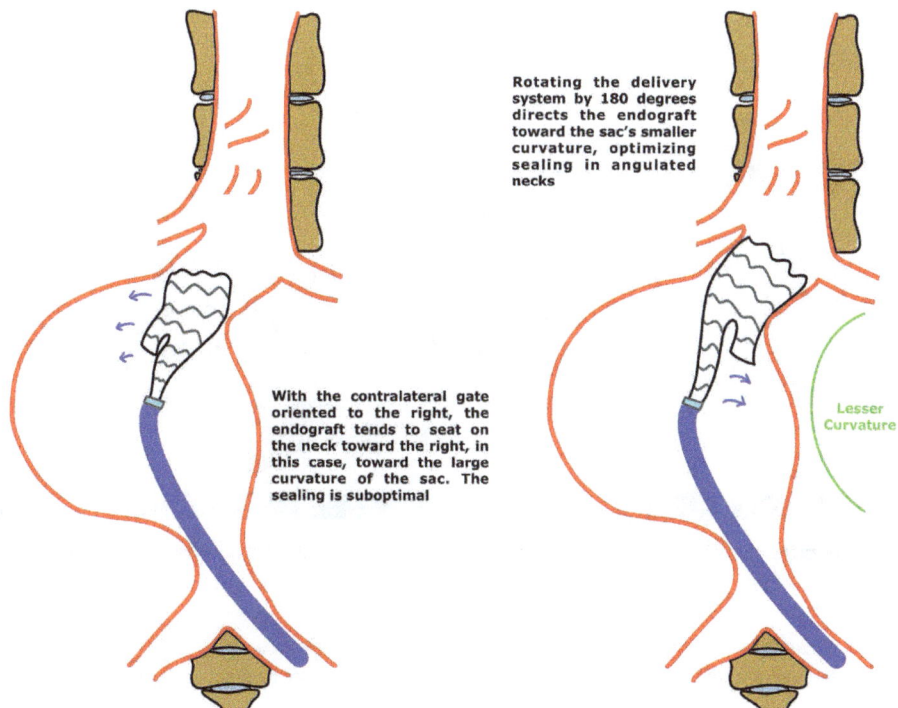

Rotating the delivery
system by 180 degrees
directs the endograft
toward the sac's smaller
curvature, optimizing
sealing in angulated
necks

With the contralateral gate
oriented to the right, the
endograft tends to seat on
the neck toward the right, in
this case, toward the large
curvature of the sac. The
sealing is suboptimal

Lesser
Curvature

Figures 4.15–4.15a Align the contralateral gate with the lesser curvature of the aneurysm to achieve better sealing in highly angulated necks.

TIP #26

In necks that are borderline in terms of length, and when no other options are available aside from a traditional implantation, the following maneuver can help ensure precise endograft deployment and maximize every millimeter of the neck.

- Position an **18 Fr sheath** just below the emergence of the contralateral gate.
- Deploy the endograft up to the contralateral gate (Figure 4.16).
- Engage the contralateral gate and advance an **aortic balloon** over a super-stiff/extra-stiff guidewire into the gate. Inflate the balloon at the infrarenal portion of the endograft, so sealing it to the neck (Figure 4.16a).
- Complete the deployment of the endograft with the balloon inflated in its proximal portion. This anchors the endograft firmly to the neck, preventing distal migration or malposition during implantation (Figure 4.16b).

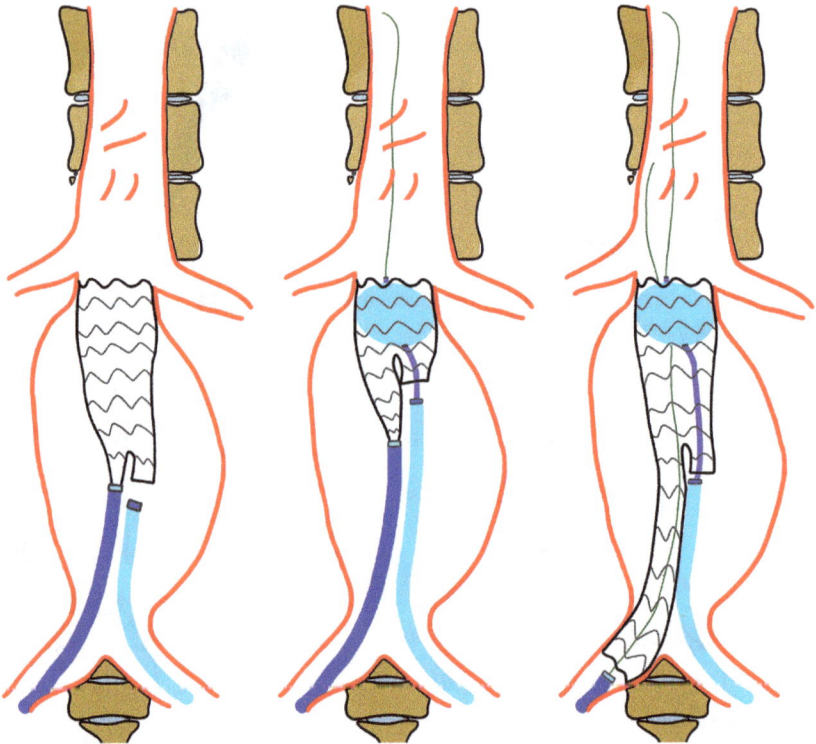

Figures 4.16–4.16b How to maximize every millimeter of a short neck with contemporary endograft molding ballooning and releasing.

TIP #27

After endograft deployment, when the guidewire is removed and the aorta returns to its natural conformation, it is possible – having deployed the endograft over an extra-stiff guidewire, which unnaturally straightens the anatomy – that the following may happen.

- The endograft may migrate distally, resulting in a **Type IA endoleak**.
- The endograft may shift upward, increasing the risk of covering the lowest renal artery.

A useful maneuver in these cases is to pre-bend the extra-stiff guidewire to match the curvature of the aorta as visualized on the preoperative CT angiography (Figure 4.17). This allows for a more anatomically accurate endograft deployment.

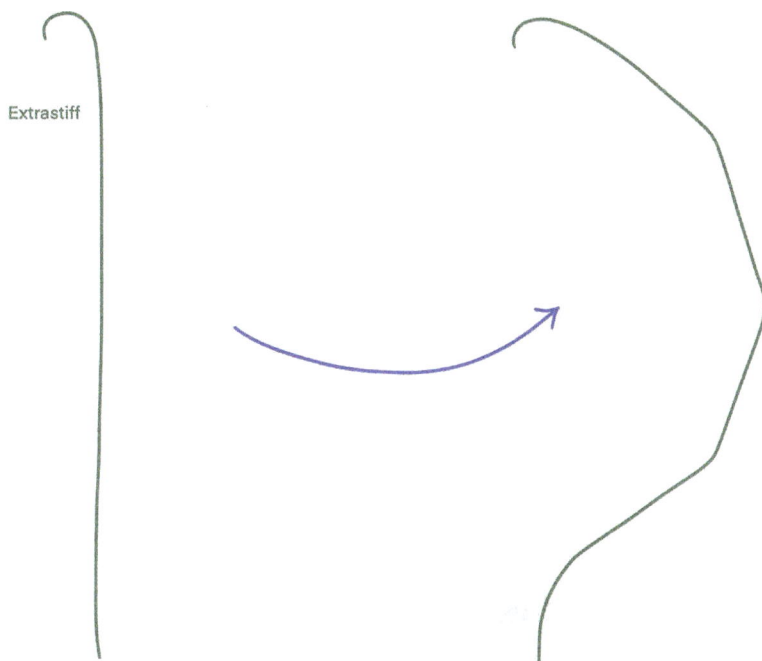

Extrastiff

Figure 4.17 Pre-bend the extra-stiff guidewire for an anatomical endograft deployment.

TIP #28

The Gore Excluder in its standard version (a subrenal fixation endograft) features an edging, a sort of **"microscalloping"** of 4 mm along the entire circumference of the proximal border (Figure 4.18). This scalloping is present on all diameters except for the 31 mm and 35 mm sizes.

The rationale behind this design, according to the manufacturer, is that this configuration creates an asymmetry in the distribution of the radial forces the endograft exerts against the aortic neck. This phenomenon optimizes sealing, reducing the risk of a **Type IA endoleak**, while also minimizing the likelihood of future aortic wall dilation.

For borderline necks, the **Endowedge Technique** can leverage this feature, as follows.

- Deploy the first 2–3 cm of the endograft.
- Using single or dual brachial access, cannulate one or both renal arteries with atraumatic Teflon-coated guidewires. (The Abbott Supracore is a good choice.) If one renal artery originates slightly lower than the contralateral, you may choose to cannulate only the lower artery.
- Advance a 0.035" balloon into each renal artery and inflate (Figure 4.18a).
- The proximal part of the endograft is constricted and gently pushed upward toward the renal arteries (Figure 4.18b). This allows the microscalloping at the proximal edge to wedge against the balloons, gaining precious millimeters (Figure 4.18c). Complete the endograft deployment.
- Perform post-implantation angiography and carefully check the renal arteries' condition before removing the guidewires.

Microscalloping

4 mm

Infrarenal space to be gained

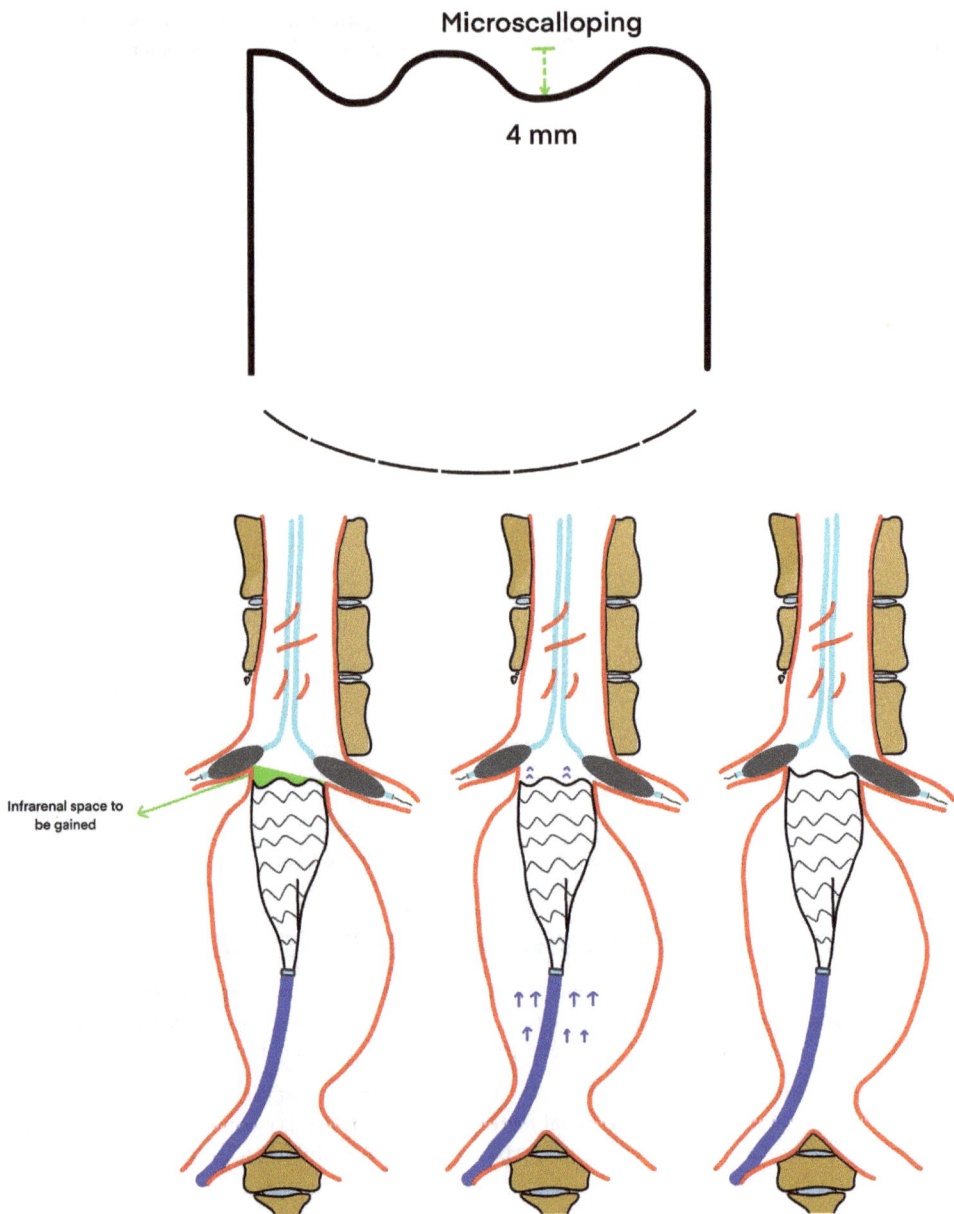

Figures 4.18–4.18c The Endowedge Technique

Alternatively, due to the endograft's repositionability (up to two times, according to the manufacturer), the following maneuver can be performed using only femoral access, avoiding brachial artery access.

- The endograft is positioned in place and deployed, up to the emergence of the contralateral gate.
- The contralateral gate is cannulated using previously described techniques. Through this access, one or both renal arteries are accessed with guidewires, as outlined earlier, and balloons are positioned in the renal arteries. Since access to the renal arteries is now from below, excessive angulation may create stability issues. In this case, a guiding catheter or a long introducer shaped to the renal artery anatomy can be helpful.
- Inflate the renal balloons; then the endograft is reconstrained in its delivery system and gently pushed against the balloons to utilize the microscalloping.
- Redeploy the endograft, continuing with the standard technique.

This maneuver is undoubtedly aggressive and should be reserved for bailout scenarios and selected cases. However, its benefits in terms of sealing are noteworthy. Consider a scenario with an 11 mm neck, where the Excluder appears to be the best-suited endograft (or the only one available in an emergency). Utilizing the 4 mm microscalloping extends the neck length to 15 mm, aligning with the manufacturer's IFU. This represents an approximately 36% increase in neck length compared to the original neck.

TIP #29

In anatomies with highly angulated aortas (Figure 4.19), a technique known as the **Kilt Technique** can be employed to correct the angle, optimize endograft positioning, and prevent future endoleaks or distal migrations.

The steps are as follows.

- Cross the renal artery plane and perform the pre-procedural angiography.
- Advance an extra-stiff guidewire (e.g., Boston BackUp Meier or Cook Lunderquist) into the thoracic aorta. The guidewire serves here not only to provide the necessary support during endograft deployment but also to straighten the aortic angle (Figure 4.19a). If a single guidewire is insufficient, a second extra-stiff guidewire or a long sheath through which the endograft can travel may be required for additional support.
- Once the native anatomy is corrected, advance an appropriately sized aortic cuff to the renal artery plane and deploy it approximately 5 mm below the inferior margin of the lowest renal artery. The aortic cuff stabilizes the newly corrected anatomy (Figure 4.19b).
- Complete the procedure using the standard technique by implanting an aortobiiliac endograft through the cuff. This endograft should be deployed flush with the renal arteries (slightly above the level where the cuff was placed). For greater system stability, it is preferable to use a device with suprarenal free flow and, if possible, infrarenal barbs. The presence of the cuff, positioned outside the bifurcated body, ensures the necessary stability for the entire system.

One (or more)
extra-stiff GWs
straighten the
anatomy

An aortic cuff will
stabilize the neck

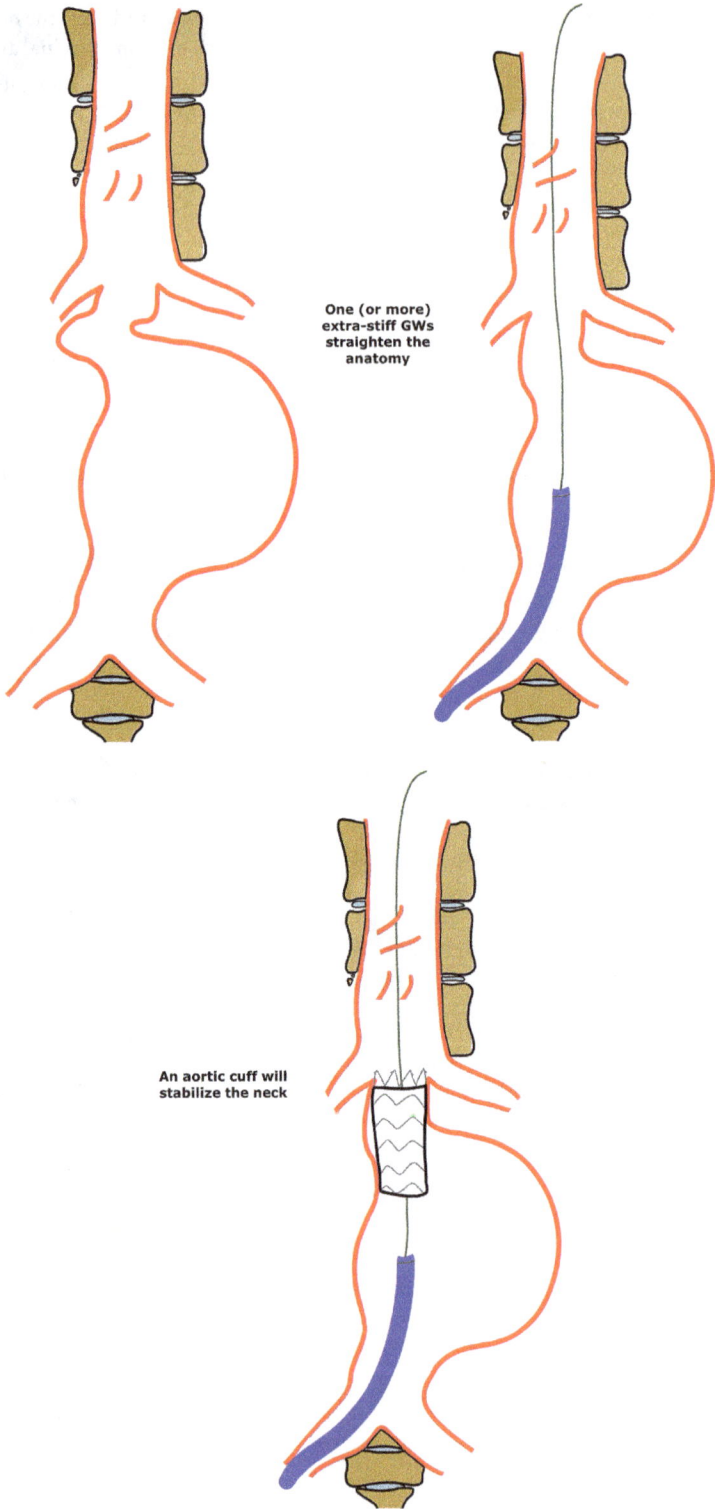

Figures 4.19–4.19b The Kilt Technique in a highly angulated aorta.

The **Kilt Technique** is also helpful in cases of a **"Dumbbell Aorta"** (Figure 4.20 – aorta with tandem dilations, the first located at the level of the infrarenal neck). In such cases, the indication for a Kilt Technique depends on the presence of proximal and distal sealing zones, with a dilated neck segment in between (Figure 4.20a).

For this type of anatomy, the technique is as follows.

• Deploy an aortic cuff in a way that connects the proximal and distal sealing zones. (Ideally, the cuff should be located approximately 10–15 mm below the proximal landing zone of the bifurcated endograft to be implanted.) The cuff will cover the dilated portion of the neck, extending to the junction between the two dilations (the distal sealing zone, Figure 4.20b).
• Deploy a bifurcated endograft (preferably a device equipped with proximal barbs as well as a free flow section) inside the cuff, flush with the renal arteries (Figure 4.20c).

This technique provides the following two key advantages in such situations.

1. It increases the usable length of the infrarenal neck for sealing, as the cuff acts as a distal extension of the infrarenal neck (Figure 4.20d).
2. In the event of distal migration of the bifurcated endograft, its barbs will anchor to the cuff (Figure 4.20c).

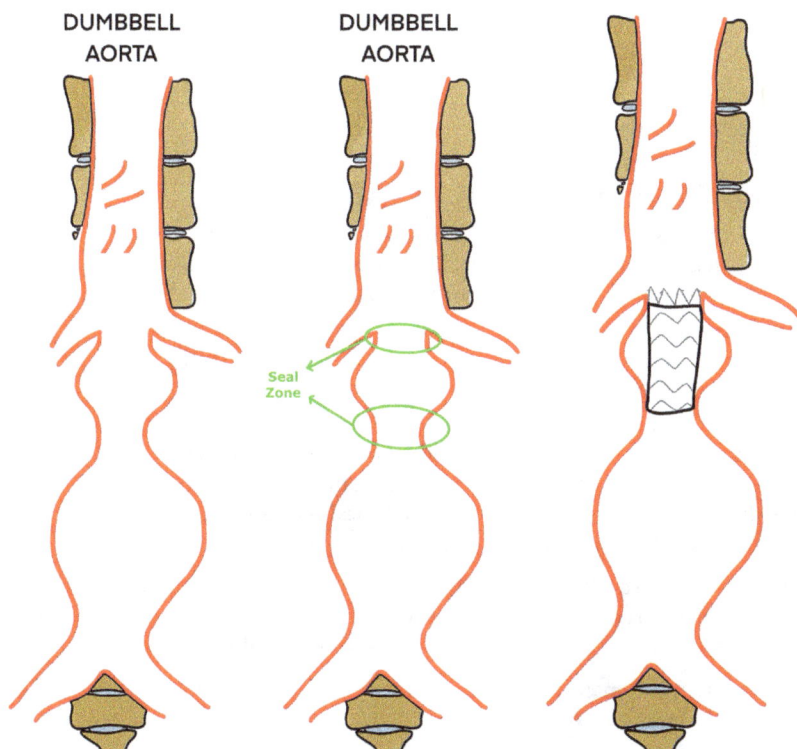

Figures 4.20–4.20b The Kilt Technique in a dumbbell aorta.

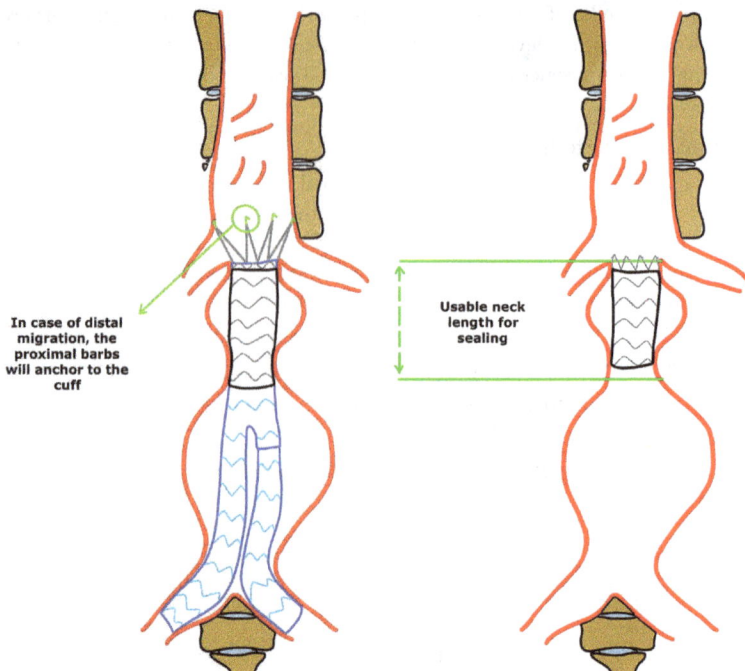

Figures 4.20c–4.20d (Continued)

THE CHIMNEY TECHNIQUE (ChEVAR)

The **Chimney Technique (ChEVAR)** was originally developed for the salvage of visceral branches acciden-tally covered during endovascular treatment (EVAR) of complex infrarenal aortic pathologies. First described in the literature by the late and brilliant Greenberg, its current indications include the following.

- Emergency scenarios.
- Situations when other endovascular options are unavailable or impractical, and the patient is not a candidate for open surgery.
- As a salvage (bailout) procedure to ensure the patency of one or more visceral branches.

In summary, the technique involves positioning one or more covered stents (rarely uncovered stents) parallel to the main endograft. This approach allows for the extension of the proximal sealing zone in cases where the aortic neck is inadequate or pathological – thus unsuitable for standard infrarenal treatment – while simultaneously maintaining the patency of the involved visceral vessels.

The primary risk associated with this procedure is the formation of so-called **gutters**, residual spaces where the stents, the main endograft, and the aortic wall fail to adhere completely. These gutters allow persistent flow into the aneurysmal sac, leading to **Type IA endoleaks**.

However, most gutters are small and tend to thrombose spontaneously. In the literature, the reported incidence of Type IA endoleak ranges from 6% to 7%.

TIP #30

Strategies to minimize the risk of complications include the following.

- Oversizing of the main body by 20–30%.
- Oversizing of the covered stents by 1–2 mm compared to the diameter of the target visceral vessel.
- The presence of an infrarenal neck, even minimal, for sealing.
- An expected sealing zone of at least 15–20 mm, once the Chimney is completed.
- The use of no more than two Chimney grafts, limiting the technique to the preservation of two visceral vessels.

TIP #31

Preoperative Planning

Preoperative planning requires a detailed CT angiography study to determine the appropriate length of the covered stent to be used. This should consider the following.

1. The length of parallel overlap between the main body and the stent.
2. The proximal protrusion of the covered stent beyond the proximal edge of the main endograft (which should be at least 5 mm).
3. The length of the covered stent required for anchoring in the visceral vessel (at least 15–20 mm).
4. The need to ensure an adequate sealing zone, which should be at least 15 mm (preferably 20 mm).

Proper preoperative planning that accounts for these factors will, in most cases, allow for the use of a single covered stent per target vessel, thereby avoiding the need for a second stent in overlap. This reduces the risk of their disconnection, malpositioning, or long-term thrombosis.

TIP #32

Access Strategy

The Chimney Technique can involve, in addition to femoral access, the use of one or more access points (percutaneous or surgical) from the upper limbs, which may include the following.

1. **Left brachial or axillary access:** This is generally preferred to reduce the risk of cerebral embolization associated with passing through the brachiocephalic trunk or aortic arch when using the right upper limb.
2. **Both brachial or both axillary accesses** in particularly complex cases.

TIP #33

Technical Procedure

The steps are as follows.

- Cannulate the visceral branches to be stented via arm access and position a stiff guidewire within them. Over this guidewire, advance a 6–8 Fr sheath, 70–90 cm in length, in each aortic branch to be stented (Figure 4.21). In case of difficulties with cannulation or system instability (e.g., if it tends to "jump" into the aorta), an aortic molding balloon inflated at the infrarenal neck can be used to provide the necessary support and stabilization.
- A covered stent is then advanced through each sheath. As previously emphasized, this stent should be oversized by 1–2 mm relative to the target vessel (Figure 4.21a). Its length must ensure at least 15–20 mm of anchorage within the vessel and a proximal protrusion of at least 5 mm into the aorta, beyond the upper edge of the main body.
- Position the aortic main body at the chosen location and slowly deploy it, maintaining a clear view of its proximal edge in relation to the covered stents (Figure 4.21b).
- Verify the correct positioning of the covered stents and withdraw the sheath into the aorta to expose the stents. During the withdrawal maneuver, the sheaths should first be advanced by a few millimeters and then retracted to minimize the rare risk of it catching on the proximal barbs of the aortic endograft.
- Deploy the covered stents (Figure 4.21c). After deployment, perform an angiographic check to confirm the correct positioning of the stents and the patency of the stented visceral branch.
- Perform simultaneous ballooning of the aortic endograft and the covered stents (Kissing Balloon Technique, Figure 4.21d). This step is critical to optimize conformability and ensure adequate sealing between the devices and the aortic wall, minimizing gutters as much as possible.
- Conduct a control angiography.
- Remove the guidewires from the stented visceral branches only at the end of the procedure, after the correct positioning of the iliac modules.

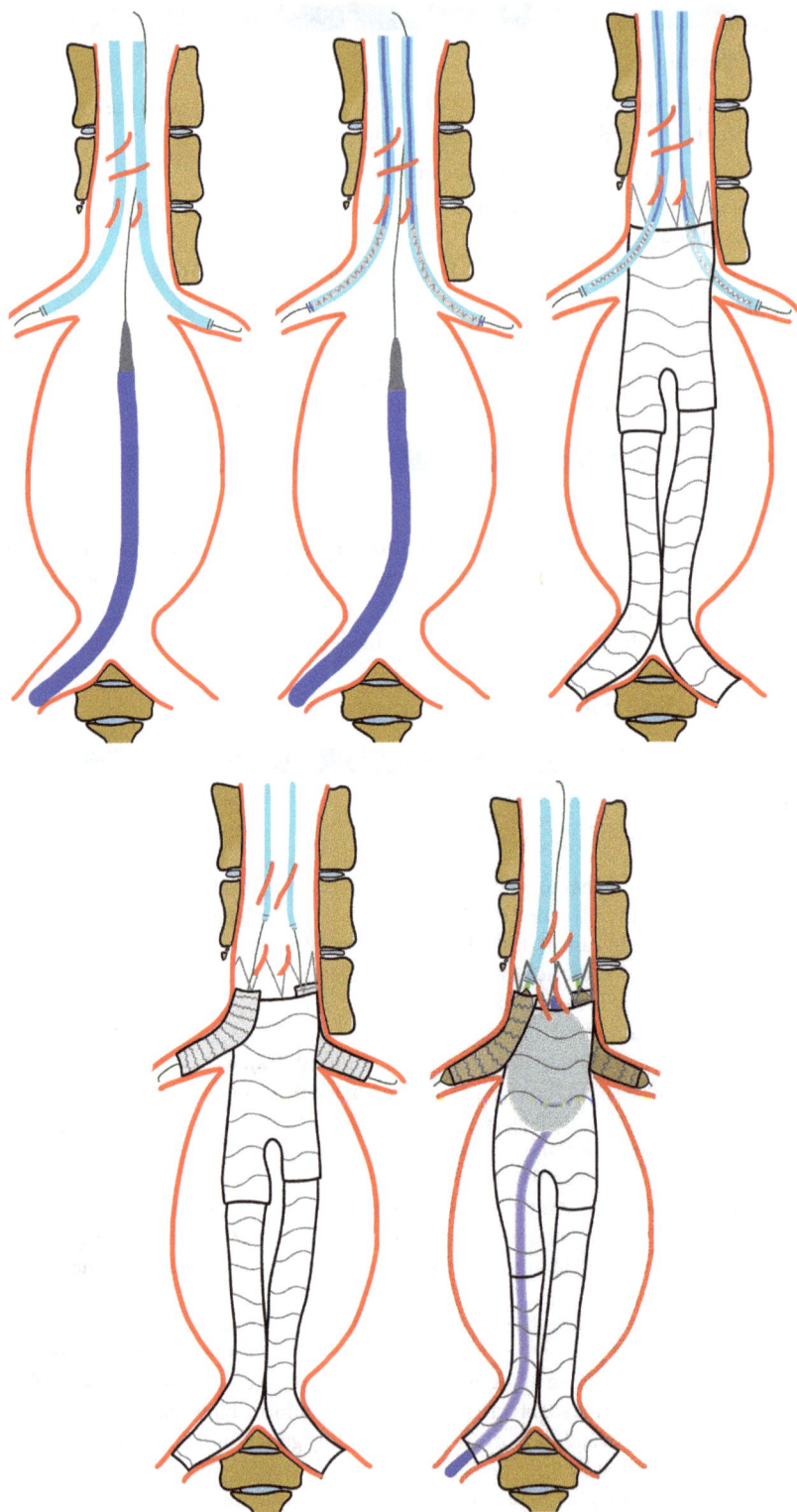

Figures 4.21–4.21d The Chimney Technique

TIP #34

Types of Stents

The stents used in the Chimney Technique can include the following.

- **Balloon-expandable covered stents:** These stents have high radial force and offer exceptional deployment precision.
- **Self-expanding stents:** These provide greater flexibility, high resistance to kinking, and superior conformability. However, they have lower radial force compared to balloon-expandable stents.

The most commonly used type is the balloon-expandable stent, but self-expanding stents may be preferable in highly angulated anatomies. However, no study has demonstrated a clear superiority of one type over the other in medium- and long-term follow-up.

TIP #35

As previously mentioned, based on the current literature, **ChEVAR** cannot be considered an elective option and should be reserved for emergencies and bailout situations.

A specific case when the Chimney Technique may be a practical choice is a pararenal aortic PAU (a rare condition). In such cases, the anatomy – due to smaller diameters compared to aneurysmal aortas – is generally unsuitable for the currently available off-the-shelf fenestrated endografts. Furthermore, since this condition falls under the category of Acute Aortic Syndromes, waiting the 8–12 weeks required for the production of a custom-made endograft is not advisable.

TIP #36

Contraindications to ChEVAR, due to extremely small diameters in these cases, include aortic dissection with a markedly reduced true lumen and aortic stenoses.

TIP #37

If the guidewire causes perforation of a distal branch of the renal artery during Chimney stenting, the following steps should be taken.

- Inflate a balloon within the stent to stop the bleeding and perform angiography of the distal arterial segment through it.
- Perform superselective catheterization of the bleeding branch with a microcatheter and embolize it with coils.

If the perforation is located in the renal artery just distal to the stent, it can be treated simply by deploying a second covered stent to extend further distally. If the guidewire causes vessel dissection, the solution is to deploy an uncovered self-expanding stent.

To avoid such complications, the best guidewires for bridging stents are the **Abbott Supracore** or the **Boston Scientific Rosen**. During the procedure, maintain a fluoroscopic view that ensures visibility of the guidewire tip at all times.

The endovascular treatment of infrarenal aortic aneurysms is one of the most common procedures in vascular surgery. Despite significant technological advances in recent decades and the availability of increasingly sophisticated devices, selecting the most appropriate endograft for each individual case remains a challenge for the vascular surgeon.

The difficulties in making this choice are manifold. First, the extreme anatomical variability of infrarenal aneurysms demands highly customized solutions. In addition, the lack of robust comparative studies between the various devices available on the market makes it difficult to determine the superiority of one endograft over another in specific anatomical situations. Furthermore, the rapid technological evolution in the field, with the continuous introduction of new devices and modifications to existing ones, adds further complexity to the decision-making process.

The consequences of a suboptimal endograft selection can be significant. Complications such as endoleaks, device migration, branch occlusions, and iliac module detachment not only jeopardize the technical success of the procedure but may also require secondary interventions, leading to increased morbidity and costs associated with the condition. It is therefore essential to develop a systematic approach to endograft selection that maximizes the chances of treatment success. Unfortunately, the literature provides little guidance in this regard. To date, the only reviews (see Duffy et al., 2013, 2015) that have attempted to establish whether objective criteria could guide this choice have concluded that no such evidence exists.

In this chapter, we aim to provide practical guidance to inform the selection of the appropriate endograft based on patients' anatomical and clinical characteristics. We will begin by detailing the various devices currently available on the market.

Note: The following material refers to European IFUs that were available to the author at the time of writing. The recommendations may vary in other countries.

ENDOGRAFTS WITH INFRARENAL FIXATION

TIP #38

Gore Excluder (Figure 4.22)

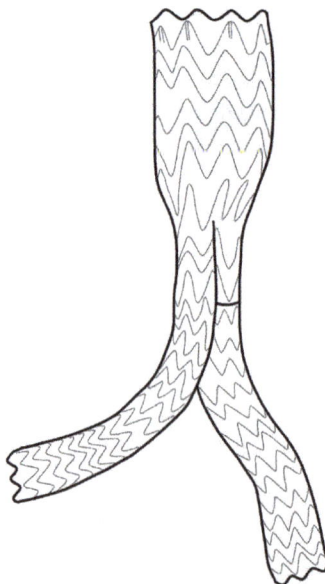

Figure 4.22 The Gore Excluder

- It is available in two versions. The ***standard version*** is indicated for necks up to 15 mm in length. While excellent in its performance, it is suited to standard anatomical scenarios. The ***conformable version***, on the other hand, allows adjustment of the angulation of its proximal portion and is thus indicated for highly angulated necks – up to 90°, according to the manufacturer. Despite lacking the suprarenal free flow (whose harmlessness to the renal arteries has never been clearly demonstrated), it is indicated for necks as short as 10 mm.
- It should be noted that the conformable version lacks the 4 mm microscalloping discussed earlier; thus, optimizing the neck with the Endowedge Technique is not possible.
- The Excluder is an endograft that, according to the manufacturer, can be repositioned up to two times.
- Its deployment is simple, precise, and rapid, closely resembling the deployment mechanism of a Viabahn.
- As mentioned, the proximal portion of the conformable version can be angled up to 90° via a wheel mechanism to better conform to highly angulated aortic necks (indicated for necks with angles up to 90°). However, it should be noted that for extreme neck angles, specifically between 60° and 90°, the minimum required neck length is 15 mm and not 10 mm.
- Due to the tendency of extra-stiff guidewires to straighten the angulation of the proximal aortic neck, a key tip to keep in mind during the deployment of the conformable version in highly angulated anatomies is to withdraw the stiff guidewire from the proximal aorta during the conforming of the device's proximal portion, keeping it within the main body of the endograft. This allows the proximal neck to recover its natural anatomy, thereby optimizing the device's conformability.
- The Gore endograft portfolio also includes a system for iliac branch treatment.
- Its features, despite the absence of suprarenal fixation, allow it to adapt to most anatomies, including challenging necks and configurations requiring preservation of at least one hypogastric artery. A small gem from the trusted and time-tested Gore lineup.

TIP #39

Terumo Anaconda (Figure 4.23)

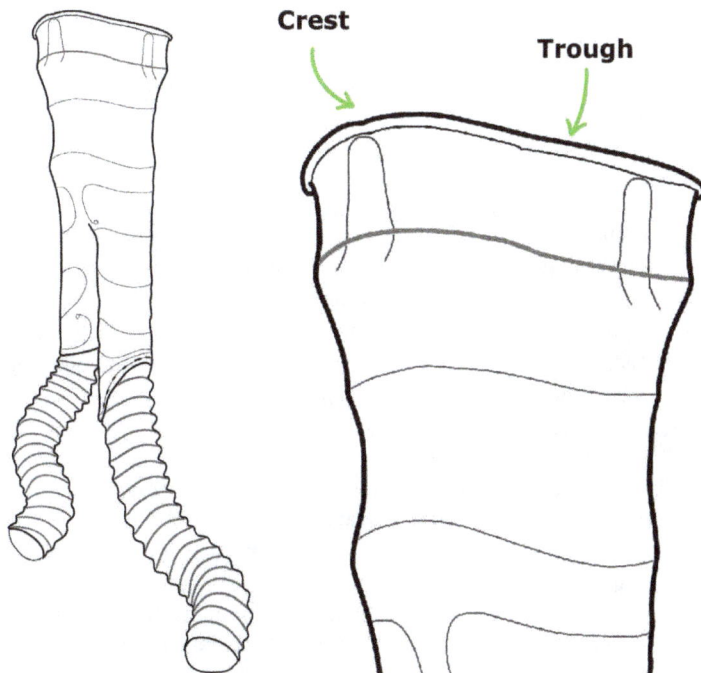

Figures 4.23–4.23a The Terumo Vascultek Anaconda and the saddle-shaped configuration of its proximal edge.

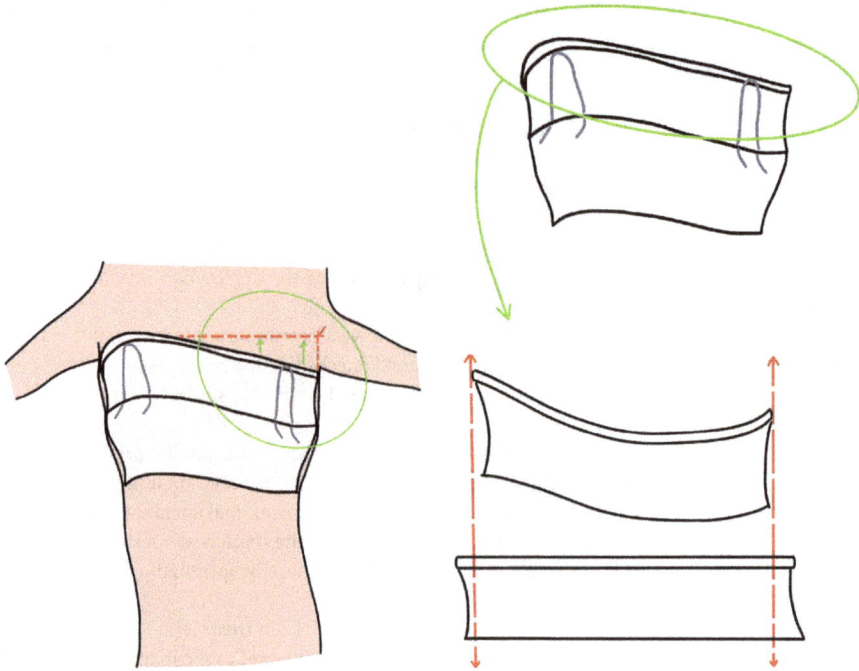

Figures 4.23b–4.23c (Continued)

- Indicated for necks up to 15 mm in length.
- A fully repositionable endograft, with no limit on the number of repositioning attempts.
- Features a magnetic mechanism that facilitates fast gate cannulation, enabling a rapid and assisted maneuver thanks to the presence of a magnet.
- Exceptionally flexible, it adapts to highly tortuous anatomies (hence its name) and necks with angles up to 90°, made possible by its independent ring stent configuration, which provides great adaptability.
- Its assisted cannulation, repositionability, and high conformability make it ideal for angulated and tortuous anatomies, provided the proximal neck is at least 15 mm long.
- Due to its circumferential stent design, this endograft typically does not require post-implant ballooning – a maneuver generally necessary for endografts with Z-, W-, or M-shaped stent designs.
- The Anaconda endograft is characterized by its unique stent design, which, as noted, has a circular orientation. Specifically, at its proximal edge, it features a distinctive horseshoe saddle shape, with two lateral depressions and two curvilinear peaks, one anterior and one posterior (Figure 4.23a). The lateral depressions are typically positioned below the renal arteries.

Over time following implantation, this saddle configuration may be lost, with the stents – and consequently the proximal edge of the endograft – flattening out. This change has the following implications.

1. It is important to use the peaks of the proximal edge as reference points relative to the lower margin of the renal arteries, not the depressions. If the endograft is positioned with the lateral depressions flush with the lower margin of the renal arteries, subsequent flattening of the proximal edge could cause the lateral segments to rise, overlapping the ostia of the renal arteries and potentially leading to occlusion of one or both arteries (Figure 4.23b).

2. The saddle-shaped proximal configuration also necessitates a precise oversizing of no more than 10% of the aortic diameter. Excessive oversizing can – due to the aforementioned flattening – increase the device's radial forces, which over time may promote dilation of the proximal aortic neck. This occurs because the flattening of the proximal edge increases its diameter (Figure 4.23c).

This phenomenon, reported in international case series with an incidence of up to **5%**, can lead to the development of a **Type IA endoleak** or caudal migration of the endograft.

ENDOGRAFTS WITH SUPRARENAL FIXATION

TIP #40

Terumo Bolton Treo (Figure 4.24)

- Indicated for necks as short as 10 mm. It is not repositionable.
- A trimodular endograft with a wide range of solutions and sizes available.
- The delivery system features an integrated and detachable sheath. This allows the sheath to remain in place even after the endograft is deployed, eliminating the need to replace it with a large-caliber one during the final stages of the procedure.
- The IFU permits its use even in more complex neck anatomies.
- It features a double row of hooks, with both suprarenal and infrarenal barbs (Figure 4.24a). The infrarenal barbs are particularly important in angulated necks, where the aortic angulation exposes them, providing greater fixation stability.
- The inner face of the penultimate stent of the iliac gates of the main body contains a row of hooks (lock-stent technology) that anchor the iliac limbs, minimizing the risk of branch disconnections.
- Due to its characteristics, this endograft is highly versatile and suitable for a variety of anatomical scenarios. In our experience, it is one of the best on the market.

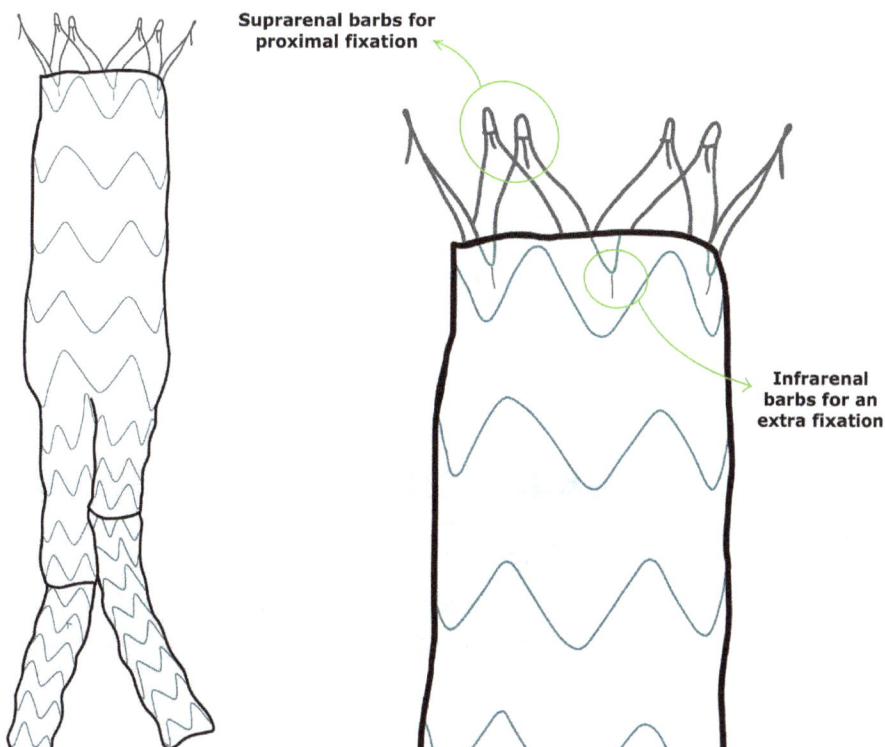

Suprarenal barbs for proximal fixation

Infrarenal barbs for an extra fixation

Figures 4.24–4.24a The Terumo Bolton Treo

TIP #41

Medtronic Endurant II

- Indicated for necks as short as 10 mm and is not repositionable.
- It offers a broad range of solutions, available in both bimodular and trimodular configurations, accommodating a wide variety of infrarenal anatomies.

- Its IFU includes indications for use in the Chimney Technique, as well as its application in more complex neck anatomies. This is particularly notable, considering that the Chimney Technique has historically been regarded as an off-label procedure.
- Additionally, when paired with the Heli-Fx EndoAnchor system, the IFU allows its use for necks as short as 4 mm.
- This endograft is well established and historically highly versatile. Even today, it remains the most widely used – Medtronic reports a global utilization rate of up to 50% of all implanted endografts.

TIP #42

Cook Zenith

- Indicated for necks up to 15 mm and is not repositionable.
- One of the standout features of this endograft is that the prostheses come preloaded within the sheaths, eliminating the need to use additional sheaths beyond those provided with the device. For example, if three components need to be implanted, only the three sheaths provided with the endografts will be used, one of which will be inserted coaxially into the one of the main body.
- The main body is longer compared to other endografts, providing greater column strength comparable to that of the native aorta. However, this may make it unsuitable for certain anatomies.
- At the suprarenal fixation level, the hooks are staggered rather than aligned at the same level. This design reduces the tangential force exerted on the aortic wall.
- Its product portfolio also includes a system for iliac branch treatment.

TIP #43

Cordis Incraft

- Indicated for necks as short as 10 mm.
- It is an ultra-low-profile endograft, featuring the lowest profile currently available on the market (14 Fr for the main body). This makes it ideal for anatomies with particularly narrow aortic bifurcations, tortuous, atherosclerotic, calcified, and small-caliber iliac arteries. It can also be used in patients with small-caliber femoral access arteries, down to 5 mm in diameter, according to the manufacturer.
- On the downside, the contralateral gate measures only 11 mm in diameter, which may make cannulation challenging.
- The delivery system for the bifurcated body includes an integrated introducer, eliminating the need for an additional introducer to deploy the ipsilateral iliac limb.

TIP #44

Endologix AFX2 (Figure 4.25)

- Indicated for necks up to 15 mm.
- This is a conceptually distinct endograft, characterized by the following two modules.
    1. A **distal bifurcated module**, designed to anatomically reconstruct the aortoiliac bifurcation without the need for contralateral gate cannulation. Essentially, the graft "sits" on the bifurcation (Figure 4.25a).
    2. A **proximal tubular module** (referred to as **VELA**) that is inserted into the distal module. Once deployed, the proximal sealing zone of this module adopts a "trunk-like" configuration (Figure 4.25a).
- Unlike traditional endografts, where both proximal sealing and fixation are achieved at the proximal neck of the aneurysm, the AFX2 operates differently, as follows.
    1. **Proximal sealing** occurs at the neck (Figure 4.25a).
    2. **Fixation**, referred to as anatomical fixation, occurs at both the proximal neck and the aortic bifurcation, where the endograft sits in its final configuration.

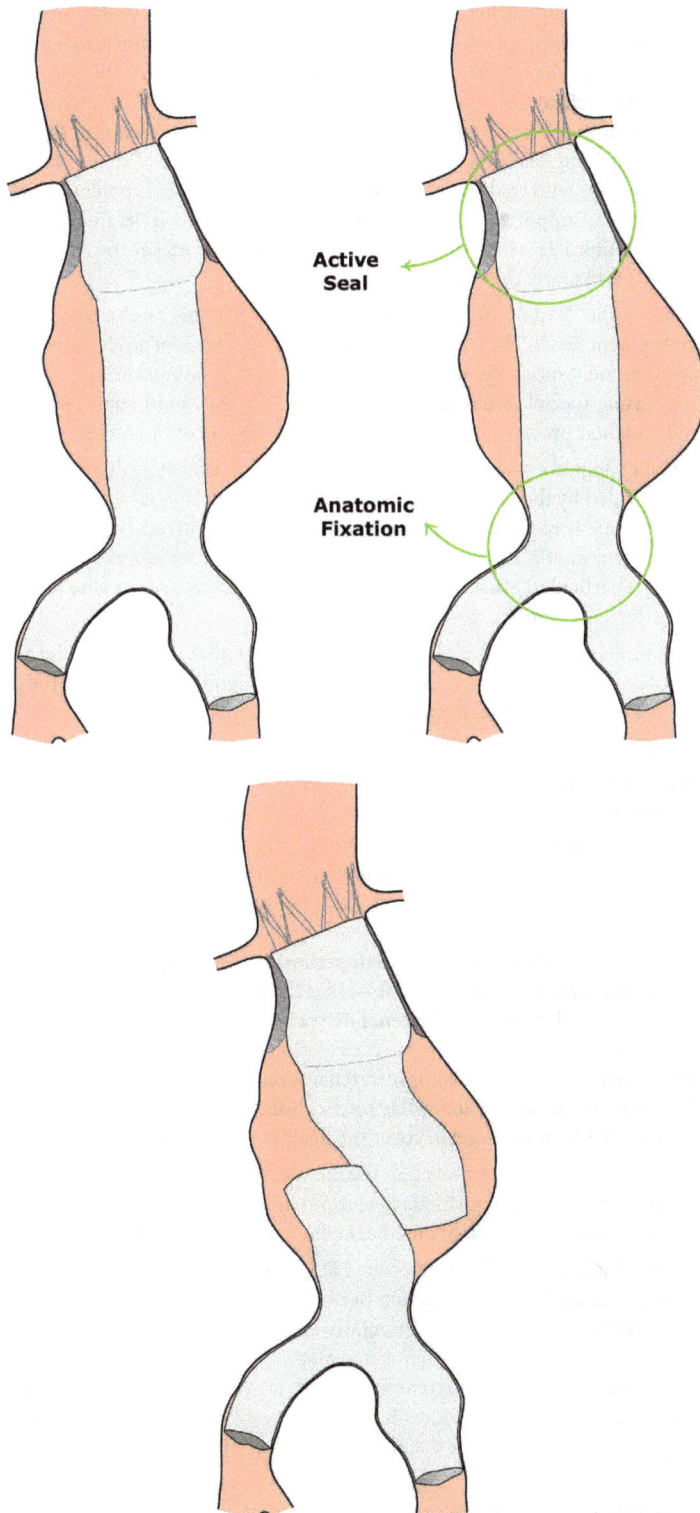

Active Seal

Anatomic Fixation

Figures 4.25–4.25b The Endologix AFX2 with its active seal and anatomic fixation characteristics.

- The endograft's covering fabric is located on the outside of the stents, the latter forming an endoskeleton supporting the graft. The PTFE material, known as *Duraply*, is independent of the stents in the proximal and distal portions of the endoskeleton. This allows the material, through a mechanism called **ActiveSeal**, to "expand" (producing the "VELA effect") and separate from the stent mesh, enabling it to conform to the neck. In this way, the PTFE adheres to the inner surface of the aortic wall, providing sealing without relying on the radial force of stents pressing against the aortic neck, as is the case with traditional endografts. This feature avoids potential long-term aortic dilative degeneration, as supported by significant scientific literature. In its final configuration, the endograft forms a "trunk-like" shape at the aortic neck. ActiveSeal makes the AFX2 feasible even in challenging necks, particularly the reversed-tapered ones.

- One disadvantage of the "VELA effect" is that in the areas where this mechanism occurs, the PTFE separates from the stent mesh. This separation may increase the risk of guidewires and catheters slipping between the stent mesh and the Duraply, instead of navigating within the true endograft lumen. For this reason, special care is needed when using this endograft, especially during subsequent endovascular procedures, to ensure proper navigation of instruments within the graft.

- Unlike traditional endografts where the main body bifurcates with a flow divider, the anatomical reconstruction provided by the AFX2 allows for subsequent contralateral access for peripheral procedures. This feature is particularly advantageous in patients with atherosclerosis, as it is not uncommon to perform multiple and repeated crossover femoral procedures over time. For this reason, the AFX2 is particularly suitable for patients with aortic aneurysms who also have an occlusive atherosclerotic component.

- Because the iliac limbs of the AFX2 are located anatomically rather than within the aortic lumen, there is no risk of competition between the iliac limbs. This significantly reduces the risk of iliac limb occlusion in cases of narrow anatomies.

- Due to these features, the AFX2 is particularly indicated for the following anatomical conditions.
  1. **Narrow aortic bifurcations** (D < 18 mm).
  2. As previously mentioned, in aneurysms associated with **obstructive disease**. The anatomical reconstruction of the aortoiliac axis ensures the possibility of contralateral access if needed. Furthermore, for addressing obstructive aortoiliac disease, the use of the AFX2 may be a more advantageous solution than the CERAB Technique described in earlier sections.
  3. **Aneurysms associated with focal aortic stenosis.** The endograft will treat also this focal pathology, once again without the risk of iliac limb occlusion.
  4. **Aneurysms associated with infrarenal dissection,** as dissections can result in narrow anatomies or make contralateral gate cannulation challenging.
  5. **Pararenal aortic ulcers (PAUs)** or infrarenal saccular aneurysms.
  6. **Isolated aneurysms of the aortoiliac bifurcation**, whereby the distal bifurcated body alone can be used, without the need to cover the healthy proximal aorta with the VELA module.

- One disadvantage of the AFX2, as reported in the literature, is the rigidity of the system, which becomes particularly significant in tortuous iliac anatomies, whereby it may struggle to conform adequately. This can increase the risk of bird-beak phenomena at the level of the distal sealing zone.

- This endograft has been subjected to numerous FDA reviews and inspections due to a high risk of Type III endoleak caused by disconnection between the two modules, observed in the follow-ups of earlier versions. This risk is particularly concerning because the disconnection occurs between the two aortic "tubes" (rather than between the gates and iliac limbs, as in standard endografts), making subsequent relining extremely difficult (Figure 4.25b). This complication is likely caused by post-implant sac remodeling, which in some cases leads to a gradual deformation of the endograft body until the two modules disconnect, in a manner akin to "uncorking" a champagne bottle.

In a standard endograft, such an endoleak could be resolved, if relining is impossible, by excluding the disconnected segment from circulation using a plug in the contralateral gate of the main body and performing a crossover femoro–femoral bypass. However, this bailout strategy is not feasible for the type of Type III endoleak observed with the AFX. Additionally, this type of endoleak results in severe pressurization of the sac, requiring urgent intervention.

To address this issue, Endologix, with the current version of the AFX2 (the only version available), has attempted to mitigate the problem by lengthening the aortic bodies of both modules, thereby increasing the overlap surface. However, data from the scientific literature – most of which are based on small patient cohorts – remain inconclusive and warrant further evaluation.

As of the time of this edition's publication, the implantation of this endograft is subject to strict health monitoring and stringent follow-ups. Furthermore, the use of this device remains tied to solid clinical indications.

TIP #45

Endologix ALTO (Figure 4.26)

- An ultra-low-profile, trimodular endograft, representing the latest version of the Ovation, which is no longer on the market.
- Its IFU indicates suitability for necks as short as 7 mm, currently the most inclusive criterion available on the market.
- The proximal sealing mechanism is achieved not through stent apposition but via a system called Custom Seal, which provides what can be described as dynamic sealing, adaptable to the anatomy (adaptive sealing). Specifically, the proximal portion of the main body features a series of rings that are filled during the procedure with a low-viscosity radiopaque polymer. The first two circumferential rings, located along the upper edge of the graft, expand with the polymer to create a sealing tailored to the neck anatomy (Figure 4.26a). Neither the stents nor the graft body make contact with the aortic wall – only the rings do. According to the manufacturer, this mechanism avoids potential neck degeneration caused by the radial force of stents against the aortic wall.

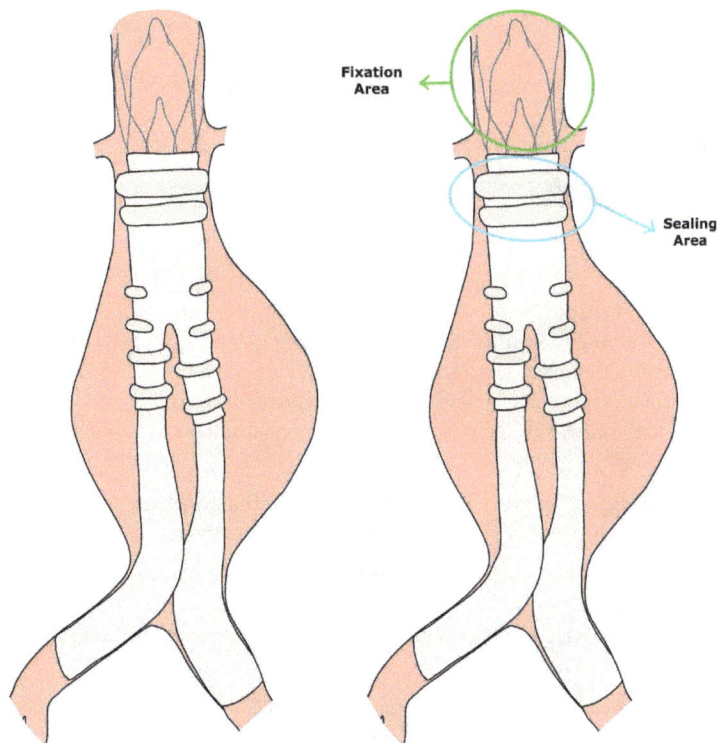

Figures 4.26–4.26a The Endologix ALTO with its Custom Seal characteristic.

- The concept of adaptive sealing, introduced for the first time with the Ovation, represents a paradigm shift in the endovascular management of infraneal aneurysms. The ability of the rings to dynamically adapt to irregularities in the aortic neck allows for precise and individualized sealing, enabling treatment in short, angulated, conical, or reverse-tapered necks while simultaneously reducing the risk of Type Ia endoleak.
- The introducer system includes an integrated compliant balloon for shaping the graft body, which accelerates the procedure.
- Thanks to these features, this endograft is indicated for challenging necks, short necks, and tortuous, narrow, or atherosclerotic anatomies.
- The iliac limbs, inherited from the previous Ovation, are composed of sinusoidal nitinol stents encapsulated in low-permeability PTFE fabric.
- This is a highly promising but relatively new endograft, requiring further studies to validate its efficacy.

TIP #46

Jotec E-Tegra

- A repositionable endograft, available in bimodular or trimodular configurations, indicated for necks up to 15 mm.
- The manufacturer's product portfolio addresses the full range of aortic surgery needs, and this system includes also a module for iliac branch treatment.
- The stent mesh design is distinctive and can be divided into the following three zones.
  1. **Proximal Zone (Sealing Zone):** Features a W-shaped stent configuration designed to optimize proximal sealing and ensure proper alignment with neck angulations up to **75°**.
  2. **Intermediate Zone (Flexibility Zone):** The stent design is asymmetric, enhancing flexibility and adaptability to various anatomies.
  3. **Distal Zone (Patency Zone):** At the level of the flow divider, the stent configuration is ovoid (the apex of each stent is rounded rather than pointed). This design increases resistance to external stresses and improves long-term patency, even in cases where there is asymmetry in the overlap levels of the iliac limbs (see *Tip #2*).
- The deployment mechanism is highly intuitive and simple, featuring a control similar to a bicycle brake lever.
- This is a relatively recent endograft, with limited studies conducted to date.

TIP #47

Endologix Nellix – This tip has primarily historical value, as the Nellix is no longer on the market at the time of writing.

It is worth discussing because Endologix, with this endograft, introduced a truly innovative concept: **Endovascular Aneurysm Sealing (EVAS)**. This endograft consists of two separate tubular grafts, placed in parallel within the aorta starting at the infrarenal neck (Figure 4.27). Each endograft anchors distally into its respective iliac artery and remains independent from the other one along its entire course. Surrounding the outer surface of each module is a polyurethane endobag (essentially, an empty sac).

Once the EVAS procedure is completed, these endobags are filled with a polymer (Figures 4.27 and 4.27a); this maneuver obliterates the aneurysm sac and eliminates the risk of Type II endoleaks.

The Nellix has undergone numerous revisions, criticisms, and evaluations due to its association with high rates of Type I endoleaks, graft migration, and sac expansion. A particular type of Type I endoleak associated with this system arises not between the endograft and the neck but in the space that inevitably exists between the two endobags.

Another significant limitation of this system is that, in cases of failure and the need for reintervention, its design makes it impossible to resolve the issue with a traditional EVAR or relining. Instead, the operator must extend the repair above the level of the renal arteries using FEVAR, BEVAR, or ChEVAR techniques.

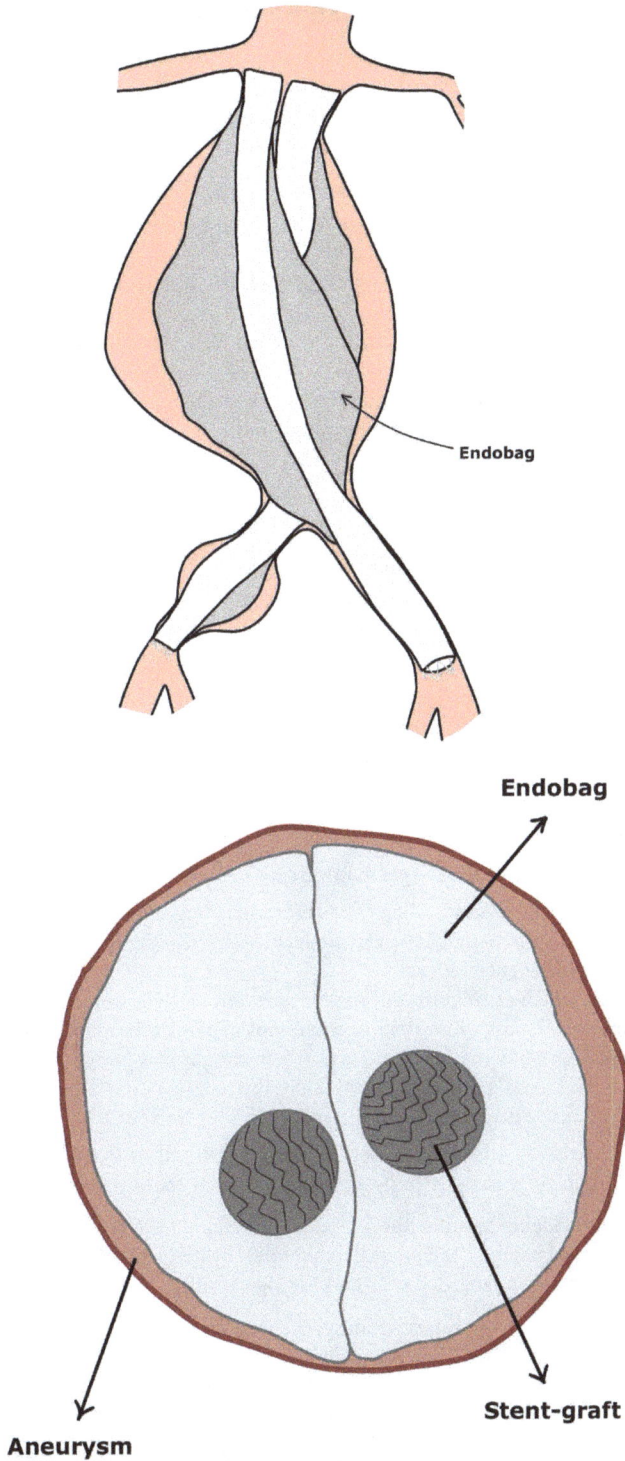

Figures 4.27–4.27a The Endologix Nellix

ALGORITHM FOR SELECTING INFRARENAL ENDOGRAFTS

The difficulty encountered in attempting to systematize the process of selecting the appropriate endograft arises primarily from the fact that, at present, there is no perfect endograft for every anatomical scenario. To generalize the discussion, it can be stated that, as of now, the concept of what might constitute a perfect endograft is likely still missing.

What characteristics should such an endograft (an ideal endograft) possess?

- Such a device should evidently ensure effective sealing, both proximally and distally, to prevent type IA and type IB endoleaks.
- It should be atraumatic to the aortic wall to prevent potential degenerative changes, whether dilatative or stenotic-occlusive.
- Conformability to native anatomy is another fundamental requirement, allowing the device to adapt to tortuous anatomies, particularly at the iliac axes.
- The material composing it must be inert, durable, and resistant.
- Finally, the endograft must be stable over time, maintaining its shape to prevent branch disconnections or proximal and distal migrations.

It is clear that, as of today, relying solely on a single type of endograft – or on a limited number of those available – does not allow for the achievement of the results that a hypothetical ideal endograft could provide.

The most functional and intelligent solution, therefore, seems to be to consider the entire range of endografts currently available on the market as a single comprehensive portfolio of options. Following this approach, and based on the technical and technological features unique to each endograft, every device should be evaluated as the best choice for the anatomical niche for which it was designed.

Such an approach enables the identification of the most appropriate and effective endograft for each clinical and anatomical scenario, maximizing the benefits for the patient by leveraging the technical and technological advantages of the selected device.

Within the process of selecting an endograft, the decision regarding the most suitable option for a specific case should be grounded in an analysis of the potential challenges present in the aneurysm to be treated.

The most commonly encountered challenges in infrarenal aneurysmal pathology include the following.

- The presence of a challenging neck, which often results in suboptimal proximal sealing and consequently leads to the development of Type IA endoleaks.
- The presence of a highly angulated neck.
- Tortuous anatomies, which can significantly complicate device navigation along the native vessels and, over time, may lead to disconnections or occlusions of part or the entirety of the endograft.
- The presence of occlusive atherosclerotic disease, which complicates device passage due to the reduced caliber of the arterial pathways. Additionally, the progression of atherosclerotic disease may result in stenotic occlusive degeneration of the endograft over time.

The evaluation of these critical factors is essential to identifying the most suitable endograft for the specific anatomical scenario, ensuring the best possible outcome for the treatment.

In the absence of clear evidence to guide the operator's selection of the most appropriate endograft for a given case – and to avoid having the choice dictated solely by market logic – there arises the question of what constitutes the most suitable decision-making algorithm.

Although it may seem obvious upon first reading, the most rational and functional approach, in the author's opinion, is to consider the IFU of each endograft as the guiding principle for this decision. More specifically, attention should be focused on the particular part of the IFU that specifies the anatomical niche most suited to the device being considered.

An algorithm that takes into account the technical and technological characteristics of each device – identifying its suitability for specific anatomical conditions and thereby the niche in which it ideally performs best – remains, to date, the most evident criterion available to us.

By reviewing the IFUs of the analyzed endografts (Figure 4.28) and considering the anatomical niche each one addresses, it is possible to simplify the decision-making process, as illustrated in Figure 4.29.

INFRARENAL ENDOGRAFT IFUs

	Gore Excluder	Terumo Anaconda LoPro	Bolton Treo	Medtronic Endurant II	Cordis Incraft	Cook Zenith	Endologix AFX2	Endologix Alto	Jotec E-tegra
Suprarenal fixation	No	No	Yes	Yes	Yes	Yes	Yes	Yes	Yes
Neck length (mm)	≥ 15 (10 in Conformable version)	≥ 15	≥ 10	≥ 10 ≥ 4 (if implanted with Endoanchors)	≥ 10	≥ 15	≥ 15	≥ 7	≥ 15
Neck diameter (mm)	16 - 32	17.5 - 31	17 - 32 (with neck lenght ≥ 10) 16 - 30 (with neck lenght ≥ 15)	19 - 32	17 - 31	18 - 32	18 - 32	16 - 30	19 - 32
Neck angulation (°)	≤ 60 (90 in Conformable version)	≤ 90	≤ 60 (if neck lenght 10 - 14) ≤ 75 (if neck lenght ≥ 15)	≤ 60 (if neck lenght 10 - 14) < 75 (if neck lenght > 15)	≤ 60	≤ 60 (relative to aneurysm) ≤ 45 (relative to suprarenal aorta)	≤ 60	≤ 60	≤ 75
Distal fixation length (mm)	≥ 10	≥ 20	≥ 10 (with diameter 8 - 13) ≥ 15 (with diameter 14 - 20)	≥ 15	≥ 15	≥ 10	≥ 15	≥ 10	≥ 15
Iliac diameters (mm)	10 - 25	8.5 - 21	8 - 13 (if iliac lenght ≥ 10) 14 - 20 (if iliac lenght ≥ 15)	8 - 25	7 - 22	8 - 20	10 - 23	8 - 25	8 - 25
Main body sheath size (Fr)	16 - 18	20 - 22	18 - 19	18 - 20	14	16 - 17	19	15	18 - 20
Limb sheath size (Fr)	12 - 15	18	13 - 14	14 - 16	12	12 - 14	9	10 - 15	16
Repositionability	Yes (until 2 times)	Yes	No	No	Yes	No	No	No	Yes

Figure 4.28 Indications for use (IFUs) of the infrarenal endografts.

This algorithm may be bypassed in standard situations where the aforementioned anatomical complexities are absent and where any endograft can theoretically be used with the expectation of similar outcomes (while bearing in mind the strengths and limitations of each).

However, when faced with a case presenting one or more of the anatomical challenges highlighted earlier, the algorithm depicted in Figure 4.29 proves invaluable in determining the optimal endograft choice.

This approach offers several advantages, making it particularly useful and functional for managing the anatomical complexities of infrarenal aneurysms. Among its key strengths is its flexibility, enabling the selection of an endograft tailored to the specific needs of each patient without being limited to a single device or a narrow set of options. This ability to customize treatment translates into improved clinical efficacy.

Another benefit lies in its independence from market dynamics. By considering the full spectrum of available endografts, the algorithm minimizes the influence of commercial constraints or brand preferences, prioritizing the clinical needs of the patient in the decision-making process. Furthermore, it enhances the surgeon's role by emphasizing their expertise and decision-making abilities. Finally, it serves as a valuable educational tool for less experienced operators, offering a logical framework for selecting endografts.

Nonetheless, there are certain limitations. First, the algorithm lacks scientific validation supported by robust evidence. Another critical issue is the requirement for the operator to have access to, theoretical knowledge of, and practical familiarity with all the endografts available on the market. This technical expertise demands continuous learning and experience, which not all surgeons possess, potentially limiting the algorithm's applicability in less advanced settings or among less experienced operators.

These limitations can, however, be mitigated by ensuring availability and familiarity with at least one endograft for each anatomical niche. Relying solely on a single endograft for all situations, in principle, is a flawed approach.

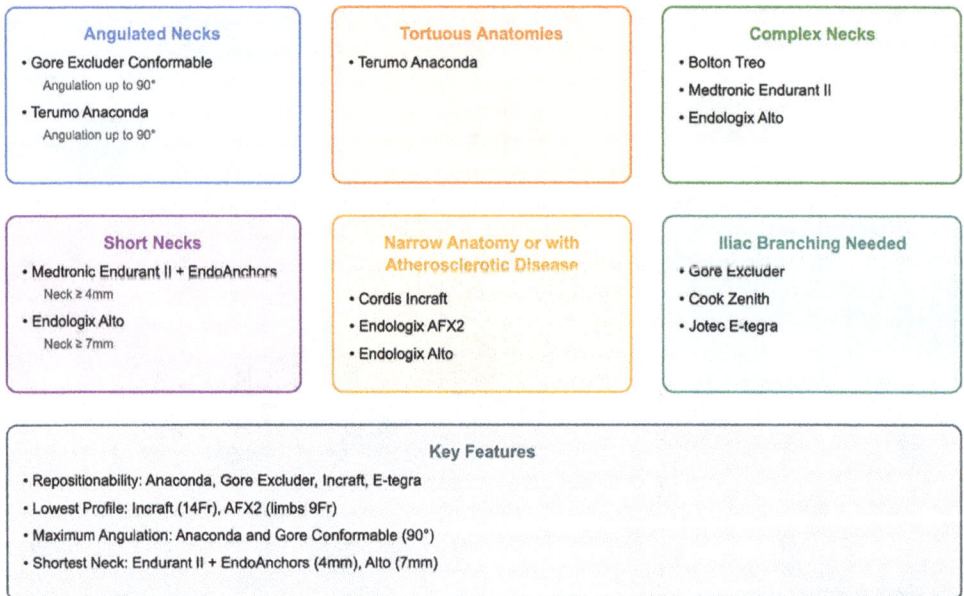

Angulated Necks
- Gore Excluder Conformable
  Angulation up to 90°
- Terumo Anaconda
  Angulation up to 90°

Tortuous Anatomies
- Terumo Anaconda

Complex Necks
- Bolton Treo
- Medtronic Endurant II
- Endologix Alto

Short Necks
- Medtronic Endurant II + EndoAnchors
  Neck ≥ 4mm
- Endologix Alto
  Neck ≥ 7mm

Narrow Anatomy or with Atherosclerotic Disease
- Cordis Incraft
- Endologix AFX2
- Endologix Alto

Iliac Branching Needed
- Gore Excluder
- Cook Zenith
- Jotec E-tegra

Key Features
- Repositionability: Anaconda, Gore Excluder, Incraft, E-tegra
- Lowest Profile: Incraft (14Fr), AFX2 (limbs 9Fr)
- Maximum Angulation: Anaconda and Gore Conformable (90°)
- Shortest Neck: Endurant II + EndoAnchors (4mm), Alto (7mm)

Figure 4.29 Algorithm for infrarenal endograft selection.

REFERENCES

1. Nano G, Gargiulo M. Endovascular treatment of aortic aneurysms durable solutions. *Pavia, Medea*. 2018; 3: 11–16.

2. Hans SS, Shepard AD, Weaver MR, et al. *Endovascular and Open Vascular Reconstruction. A Practical Approach*. London: Taylor & Francis; 2018. Vol. 12, pp. 75–85.

3. van Bogerijen GHW, Williams DM, Eliason JL, et al. Alternative access techniques with thoracic endovascular aortic repair, open iliac conduit versus endoconduit technique. *J Vasc Surg*. 2014; 60(5): 1168–1176.

4. Asciutto G, Aronici M, Resch T, et al. Endoconduits with "pave and crack" technique avoid open ilio-femoral conduits with sustainable mid-term results. *Eur J Vasc Endovasc Surg*. 2017; 54(4): 472–479.

5. Hinchliffe RJ, Ivancev K, Sonesson B. "Paving and cracking": An endovascular technique to facilitate the introduction of aortic stent-grafts through stenosed iliac arteries. *J Endovasc Ther*. 2007; 14(5): 630–633.

6. Giannopoulos S, Malgor RD, Sobreira ML, et al. Iliac conduits for endovascular treatment of aortic pathologies: A systematic review and meta-analysis. *J Endovasc Ther*. 2021; 28(4): 499–509.

7. Spath P, Campana F, Gallitto E, et al. Impact of iliac access in elective and non-elective endovascular repair of abdominal aortic aneurysm. *J Cardiovasc Surg*, 2024; 65(2): 85–98.

8. Berland TL, Veith FJ, Cayne NS, et al. Technique of supraceliac balloon control of the aorta during endovascular repair of ruptured abdominal aortic aneurysms. *J Vasc Surg*. 2013; 57(1): 272–275.

9. Nakayama H, Toma M, Kobayashi T, et al. Ruptured abdominal aortic aneurysm treated by double-balloon technique and endovascular strategy: Case series. *Ann Thorac Cardiovasc Surg*. 2019; 25(4): 211–214.

10. Wongwanit C, Mutirangura P, Chinsakchai K, et al. Transfemoral temporary aortic balloon occlusion assisting open repair for ruptured abdominal aortic aneurysms. *J Med Assoc Thai*. 2013; 96(6): 742–748.

11. Karkos CD, Papadimitriou CT, Chatzivasileiadis TN. The impact of aortic occlusion balloon on mortality after endovascular repair of ruptured abdominal aortic aneurysms: A meta-analysis and meta-regression analysis. *Cardiovasc Intervent Radiol*. 2015; 38(6): 1425–1437.

12. Hallett RL, Ullery BW, et al. Abdominal aortic aneurysm: Pre- and post- procedural imaging. *Abdominal Radiology*. doi: 10.1007/s00261-018-1520-5.

13. Minion DJ, Xenos ES. The femoral-based endowedge technique to increase juxtarenal seal and correct graft tilt. *J Vasc Surg*. 2012; 55(5): 1522–1525.

14. Igari K, Kudo T, Uchiyama H, et al. Early experience with the endowedge technique and snorkel technique for endovascular aneurysm repair with challenging neck anatomy. *Ann Vasc Dis*. 2014; 7(1): 46–51.

15. Kim TH, Jang HJ, Choi YJ, et al. Kilt technique as an angle modification method for endovascular repair of abdominal aortic aneurysm with severe neck angle. *Ann Thorac Cardiovasc Surg*. 2017; 23(2): 96–103.

16. Jeon YS, Cho YK, Song MG, et al. Clinical outcomes of endovascular aneurysm repair with the Kilt technique for abdominal aortic aneurysms with hostile aneurysm neck anatomy: A Korean multicenter retrospective study. *Cardiovasc Intervent Radiol*. 2018; 41(4): 554–563.

17. Jimenez JC, Quinones-Baldrich WJ. Technical modifications for endovascular infrarenal AAA repair for the angulated and dumbbell-shaped neck: The precuff Kilt technique. *Ann Vasc Surg*. 2011; 25(3): 423–430.

18. Greenberg RK, Clair D, Srivastava S, et al. Should patients with challenging anatomy be offered endovascular aneurysm repair? *J Vasc Surg*. 2003; 38(5): 990–996.

19. Wanhainen A, Van Herzeele I, Bastos Goncalves F, et al. Editor's choice – European society for vascular surgery (ESVS) 2024 clinical practice guidelines on the management of abdominal aorto-iliac artery aneurysms. *Eur J Vasc Endovasc Surg*. 2024; 67(2): 192–331.

20. Yammine H, Briggs CS, Stanley GA, et al. Advanced techniques for treating juxtarenal and pararenal abdominal aortic aneurysms: Chimneys, periscopes, sandwiches and other methods. *Tech Vasc Interv Radiol*. 2018; 21(3): 165–174.

21. Patel RP, Katsargyris A, Verhoeven ELG, et al. Endovascular aortic aneurysm repair with chimney and snorkel grafts: Indications, techniques and results. *Cardiovasc Intervent Radiol*. 2013; 36(6): 1443–1451.

22. Meekel JP, van Schaik TG, Lely RJ, et al. Gutter characteristics and stent compression of self-expanding vs balloon-expandable chimney grafts in juxtarenal aneurysm models. *J Endovasc Ther*. 2020; 27(3): 452–461.

23. de Beaufort HWL, Cellitti E, de Ruiter QMB, et al. Midterm outcomes and evolution of gutter area after endovascular aneurysm repair with the chimney graft procedure. *J Vasc Surg*. 2018; 67(1): 104–112.

24. Pilz da Cunha G, Lemmens CC, Mees BME. Chimney endovascular aneurysm repair from below. *Eur J Vasc Endovasc Surg*. 2020; 60(5): 780.

25. Verlato P, Foresti L, Bloemert-Tuin T, et al. Long-term outcomes of chimney endovascular aneurysm repair procedure for complex abdominal aortic pathologies. *J Vasc Surg*. 2024; 80(3): 612–620.

26. Moulakakis KG, Mylonas SN, Avgerinos E, et al. The chimney graft technique for preserving visceral vessels during endovascular treatment of aortic pathologies. *J Vasc Surg*. 2012; 55(5): 1497–503.

27. Colvard B, George Y, Chakfe N, Swanstrom L. Current aortic endografts for the treatment of abdominal aortic aneurysms. *Expert Rev Med Devices*. 2016; 13(5): 475–486.

28. Concannon J, Moerman KM, Hynes N, Sultan S, McGarry JP. Influence of shape-memory stent grafts on local aortic compliance. *Biomech Model Mechanobiol*. 2021; 20: 2373–2392.

29. Schoretsanitis N, Georgakarakos E, Argyriou C, Ktenidis K, Geogiadis GS. A critical appraisal of endovascular stent-grafts in the management of abdominal aortic aneurysms. *Radiol Med*. 2017; 122: 309–318.

30. Dalbosco M, de Mello Roesler CR, Silveira PG, Fancello EA. Numerical study on the effect of stent shape on suture forces in stent-grafts. *J Mech Behav Biomed Mater*. 2020; 110: 1–8.

31. Hahl T, Kurumaa T, Uurto I, Protto S, Vaaramaki S, Suominen V. The effect of suprarenal graft fixation during endovascular aneurysm repair on short- and long-term renal function. *J Vasc Surg*. 2022; 76(1): 96–103.

32. Georgakarakos E, Kratimenos T, Koutsoumpelis A, Georgiadis GS. The Bolton Treo endograft for treatment of abdominal aortic aneurysms: Just another trimodular platform? *Expert Rev Med Devices*. 2018; 15(1): 5–14.

33. Marone EM, Rinaldi LF, Lovotti M, Palmieri P, Argentieri A. The Bolton Treo endograft: Single-center preliminary experience. *Ann Vasc Surg*. 2019; 56: 139–146.

34. Georgakarakos E, Karaolanis GI, Argyriou C, Papatheodorou N, Karangelis D, Georgiadis GS. Update on the TREO endograft device: Overview of its safety and efficacy. *Expert Rev Med Devices*. 2022; 19(1): 31–35.

35. Orrico M, Ronchey S, Alberti V, et al. Outcomes of endovascular repair of abdominal aortic aneurysms in narrow aortic bifurcations using the ultra-low profile "INCRAFT" device: A retrospective multicenter study. *J Vasc Surg*. 2020; 72(1): 122–128.

36. Bertoglio L, Logaldo D, Marone EM, Rinaldi E, Chiesa R. Technical features of the INCRAFT™ AAA stent graft system. *J Cardiovasc Surg*. 2014; 55(5): 705–715.

37. Ricotta JJ, Oderich GS. The Cook Zenith AAA endovascular graft. *Perspect Vasc Surg Endovasc Ther*. 2008; 20(2): 67–173.

38. Verzini F, Romano L, Parlani G, et al. Fourteen-year outcomes of abdominal aortic endovascular repair with the Zenith stent graft. *J Vasc Surg.* 2017; 65(2): 318–329.

39. Chen JF, Brahmandam A, Harris S, Fischer U, Nassiri N. Elucidating the role of the AFX2 endograft in endovascular treatment of aortic pathology. *Ann Vasc Surg.* 2022. doi: 10.1016/j.avsg.2022.04.042.

40. Tsolakis IA, Kakkos SK, Papageorgopoulou CP, et al. Improved effectiveness of the repositionable GORE EXCLUDER AAA endoprosthesis featuring the C3 delivery system compared with the original GORE EXCLUDER AAA endoprosthesis for within the instructions for use treatment of aortoiliac aneurysms. *J Vasc Surg.* 2019; 69(2): 394–404.

41. Poublon CG, Holewijn S, van Sterkenburg SMM, Tielliu IFJ, Zeebregts CJ, Reijnen MMPJ. Long-term outcome of the GORE EXCLUDER AAA endoprosthesis for treatment of infrarenal aortic aneurysms. *J Vasc Interv Radiol.* 2017; 28(5): 637–644.

42. Freyrie A, Gallitto E, Gargiulo M, et al. Results of the endovascular abdominal aortic aneurysm repair using the Anaconda aortic endograft. *J Vasc Surg.* 2014; 60(5): 1132–1139.

43. Vukovic E, Czerny M, Beyersdorf F, et al. Abdominal aortic aneurysm neck remodeling after Anaconda stent graft implantation. *J Vasc Surg.* 2018; 68(5): 1354–1359.

44. Eagleton MJ, Stoner M, Henretta J, et al. Safety and effectiveness of the TREO stent graft for the endovascular treatment of abdominal aortic aneurysms. *J Vasc Surg.* 2021; 74(1): 114–123.

45. Murray D, Szeberin Z, Benevento D, et al. A comparison of clinical outcomes of abdominal aortic aneurysm patients with favorable and hostile neck angulation treated by endovascular repair with the Treovance stent graft. *J Vasc Surg.* 2020; 71(6): 1881–1889.

46. Broos PPHL, Stokmans RA, van Sterkenburg SMM, et al. Performance of the endurant stent graft in challenging anatomy. *J Vasc Surg.* 2015; 62(2): 312–318.

47. Donas KP, Torsello G, Weiss K, et al. Performance of the endurant stent graft in patients with abdominal aortic aneurysms independent of their morphologic suitability for endovascular aneurysm repair based on instructions for use. *J Vasc Surg.* 2015; 62(4): 848–854.

48. Oliveira-Pinto J, Oliveira NFG, Bastos-Goncalves FM, et al. Long-term results after standard endovascular aneurysm repair with the Endurant and Excluder stent grafts. *J Vasc Surg.* 2020; 71(1): 64–74.

49. Pratesi G, Pratesi C, Chiesa R, et al. The innovation trial: Four-year safety and effectiveness of the inCraft® AAA stent-graft system for endovascular repair. *J Cardiovasc Surg.* 2017; 58(5): 650–657.

50. Liang NL, Ohki T, Ouriel K, et al. Five-year results of the INSPIRATION study for the INCRAFT low-profile endovascular aortic stent graft system. *J Vasc Surg.* 2021; 73(3): 867–873.

51. Mazzaccaro D, Occhiuto MT, Stegher S, Righini P, Malacrida G, Nano G. Tips about the cordis INCRAFT endograft. *Ann Vasc Surg.* 2016; 30: 205–210.

52. Broda M, Eiberg J, Vogt K, et al. Midterm outcomes of aneurysm repair with the Cook Zenith Alpha abdominal endovascular graft. *J Vasc Surg.* 2022. doi: 10.1016/j.jvs.2022.03.862.

53. Bogdanovic M, Stackelberg O, Lindstrom D, et al. Limb graft occlusion following endovascular aneurysm repair for infrarenal abdominal aortic aneurysm with the Zenith Alpha, excluder, and endurant devices: A multicentre cohort study. *Eur J Vasc Endovasc Surg.* 2021; 62(4): 532–539.

54. Mertens J, Houthoofd S, Daenens K, et al. Long-term results after endovascular abdominal aortic aneurysm repair using the Cook Zenith endograft. *J Vasc Surg.* 2011; 54(1): 48–57.

55. EunAh J, Ahn S, Min SK, Mo H, Jae HJ, Hur S. Initial experience and potential advantages of AFX2 bifurcated endograft system: Comparative case series. *Vasc Specialist Int.* 2019; 35(4): 209–216.

56. Chang RW, Rothenberg KA, Harris JE, et al. Midterm outcomes for 605 patients receiving Endologix AFX or AFX2 endovascular AAA systems in an integrated healthcare system. *J Vasc Surg.* 2021; 73(3): 856–866.

57. Vetsch R, Garrett HE, Stout CL, WladisAR, Thompson M, Lombardi JV. Midterm outcomes of 455 patients receiving the AFX2 endovascular graft for the treatment of abdominal aortic aneurysm: A retrospective multi-center analysis. *PLoS One*. 2021. doi: 10.1371/journal.pone.0261623.

58. Antoniou GA, Narlawar R. Alto Endologix integrated balloon to achieve sealing ring apposition with the aortic wall: A word of caution. *J Endovasc Ther*. 2022. doi: 10.1177/15266028221095397.

59. de Donato G, Pasqui E, Panzano C, Galzerano G, Cappelli A, Palasciano G. Early experience with the new ovation Alto stent graft in endovascular abdominal aortic aneurysm repair. *EJVES Vasc Forum*. 2021; 54: 7–12.

60. Holden A, Lyden S. Initial experience with polymer endovascular aneurysm repair using the Alto stent graft. *J Vasc Surg Cases Innov Tech*. 2020; 6(1): 6–11.

61. Pratesi C, Piffaretti G, Pratesi G, Castelli P, ITER Investigators. ITalian excluder registry and results of gore excluder endograft for the treatment of elective infrarenal abdominal aortic aneurysms. *J Vasc Surg*. 2014; 59: 52–57.

62. Midy D, Bastrot L, Belhomme D, et al. Five year results of the French EPI-ANA-01 registry of AnacondaTM endografts in the treatment of infrarenal abdominal aortic aneurysms. *Eur J Vasc Endovasc Surg*. 2020; 60(1): 16–25.

63. Tigkiropoulos K, Stavridis K, Lazaridis I, et al. Outcomes of endovascular aneurysm repair using the Anaconda stent-graft. *J Endovasc T*. 2020; 27(3): 462–467.

64. Isernia G, Simonte G, Michelagnoli S, et al. Nineteen-year outcomes with the Anaconda stent graft system from two tertiary centers. *J Vasc Surg*. 2021; 74: 105–113.

65. Deery SE, Shean KE, Pothof AB, et al. Three-year results of the endurant stent graft system post-approval study (ENGAGE PAS). *Ann Vasc Surg*. 2018; 50: 202–208.

66. Singh MJ, Fairman R, Anain P, et al. Final results of the endurant stent graft system in the United States regulatory trial. *J Vasc Surg*. 2016; 64: 55–62.

67. Bisdas T, Weiss K, Eisenack M, Austermann M, Torsello G, Donas KP. Durability of the endurant stent graft in patients undergoing endovascular abdominal aortic aneurysm repair. *J Vasc Surg*. 2014; 60: 1125–1131.

68. Troisi N, Torsello G, Donas KP, Austermann M. Endurant stent-graft: A 2-year, single-center experience with a new commercially available device for the treatment of abdominal aortic aneurysms. *J Endovasc Ther*. 2010; 17: 439–448.

69. Benveniste GL, Tjahjono R, Chen O, Verhagen HJM, Bockler D, Varcoe RL. Long-term results of 180 consecutive patients with abdominal aortic aneurysm treated with the Endurant stent graft system. *Ann Vasc Surg*. 2020; 67: 265–273.

70. Zavatta M, Squizzato F, Balestriero G, et al. Early and midterm outcomes of endovascular aneurysm repair with an ultra-low-profile endograft from the Triveneto incraft registry. *J Vasc Surg*. 2021; 73(6): 1950–1957.e2.

71. Vaaramaki S, Salenius JP, Pimenoff G, Uurto I, Suominen V. Systematic long-term follow up after endovascular abdominal aortic aneurysm repair with the Zenith stent graft. *Eur J Vasc Endovasc Surg*. 2019; 58: 182–188.

72. Iwakoshi S, Ichihashi S, Higashiura W, et al. A decade of outcomes and predictors of sac enlargement after endovascular abdominal aortic aneurysm repair using Zenith endografts in a Japanese population. *J Vasc Interv Radiol*. 2014; 25: 694–701.

73. https://endologix.com/wp-content/uploads/2019/10/MM2165-Rev-01-Endologix-2016-2019-AFX- Clinical-Update.pdf.

74. Duffy JMN, Rolph R, Clough RE, et al. Stent graft types for endovascular repair of abdominal aortic aneurysms. *Cochrane Database Syst Rev*. 2013; 3: CD008447.

75. Duffy JMN, Rolph R, Waltham M. Stent graft types for endovascular repair of abdominal aortic aneurysms. *Cochrane Database Syst Rev*. 2015; 9: CD008447.

TIPS & TRICKS IN THE MANAGEMENT OF ILIAC ANEURYSMS

Toolkit A – Isolated Aneurysms of the Iliac Arteries   **172**
- Tips 1 to 5

Toolkit B – Algorithm for the Treatment of Iliac Aneurysms   **178**
- Tips 6 to 11

Toolkit C – Tips & Tricks in the Management of Hypogastric Aneurysms   **183**
- Tips 12 to 15

DOI: 10.1201/9781003567080-5

Iliac aneurysms are relatively rare, accounting for 0.5–2% of all abdominal aneurysms. The feasibility of endovascular treatment is closely tied to anatomy, the location of the distal sealing zone, and the presence of an adequate proximal neck. Ideally, both proximal and distal necks should have a segment of healthy artery of sufficient length to ensure optimal sealing. Therefore, the choice of endovascular technique depends on a careful evaluation of this anatomical parameter.

To date, there is no unanimous consensus on the minimum length required for an iliac neck to be deemed adequate. This lack of agreement is largely due to the limited number of scientific studies on the subject, reflecting the rarity of this anatomical condition. However, most reports suggest a minimum proximal and distal neck length of **at least 20 mm.** For now, we will consider this value as a reference parameter for defining neck adequacy, pending stronger evidence to clarify this issue.

From this point forward, I will assume that identifying an adequate proximal and distal neck – where "adequate" implies at least 20 mm of healthy artery – is critically important in selecting the appropriate endovascular technique.

As a result, we will refer to a classification of isolated iliac aneurysms based on this key element, which could be described as functional. A similar classification was proposed by Melas et al. in a 2011 study. The version presented here, which includes four different anatomical types (Figure 5.1), is a simplified and, in my opinion, more straightforward interpretation.

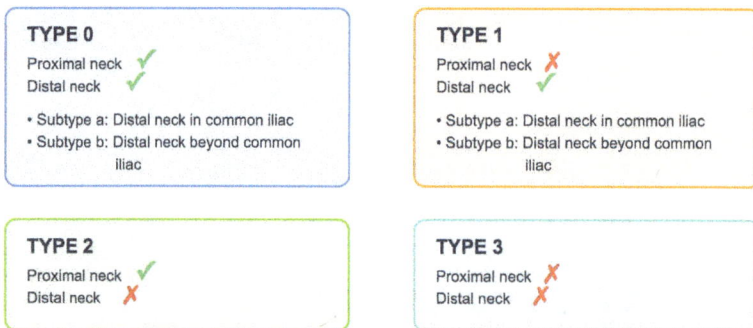

Figure 5.1 Classification of isolated iliac aneurysms.

- **Type 0:** Both a proximal and distal neck are present along the considered iliac axis (from the origin of the common iliac artery to the end of the external iliac artery) (Figures 5.2–5.2a).

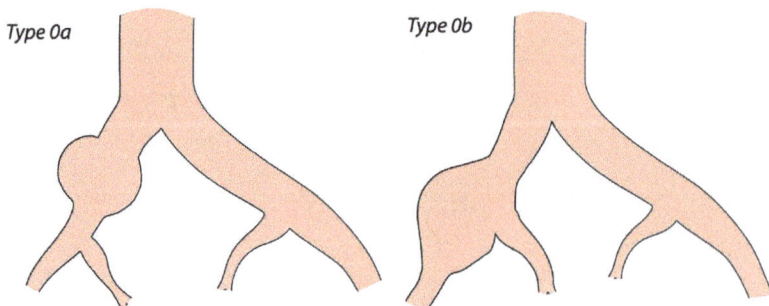

Figures 5.2–5.2a Types and subtypes of iliac aneurysms: Types 0a and 0b.

- **Type 1:** Iliac aneurysm with a distal neck but no proximal neck (Figures 5.2b–5.2c).

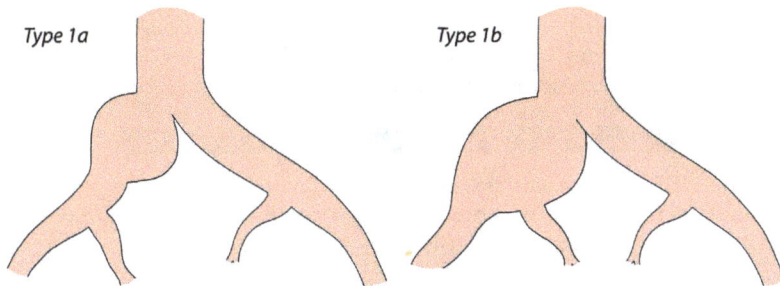

Figures 5.2b–5.2c Types and subtypes of iliac aneurysms: Types Ia and Ib.

- **Type 2:** Iliac aneurysm with a proximal neck but no distal neck (Figures 5.2d–5.2e).

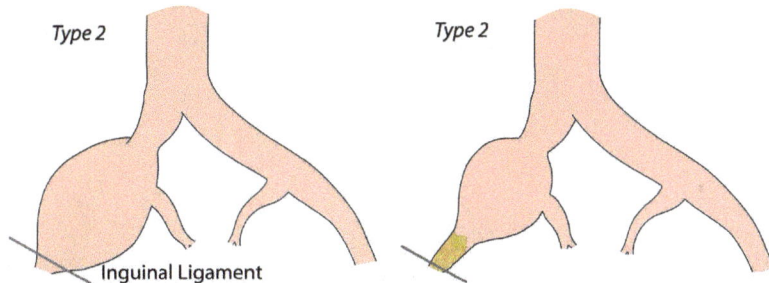

Figures 5.2d–5.2e Types and subtypes of iliac aneurysms: Type 2.

- **Type 3:** Iliac aneurysm with neither a proximal nor a distal neck (Figures 5.2f–5.2g).

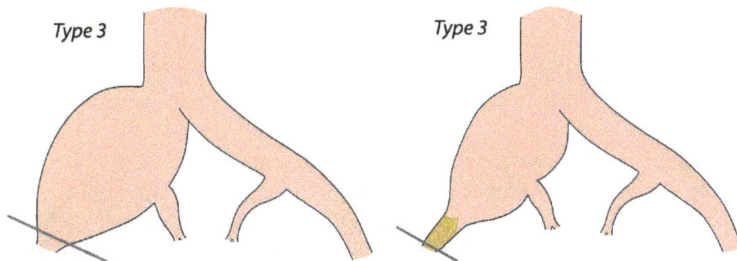

Figures 5.2f–5.2g Types and subtypes of iliac aneurysms: Type 3.

Types 0 and 1 can be further divided into two subtypes:

- **Subtype a:** The distal neck is located within the common iliac artery.
- **Subtype b:** The distal neck is located beyond the common iliac artery. In this case, it may involve the ostium of the hypogastric artery or extend into the external iliac artery.

This classification is notable for its progressive complexity: from Type 0 to Type 3, aneurysms become increasingly challenging to treat and may require procedures that are not exclusively endovascular.

One additional note: Type 0 and Type 2 iliac aneurysms, characterized by an adequate proximal neck, may also include anatomies where a bifurcated aortic endograft is already in place, and aneurysmal degeneration has occurred over time in at least one iliac axis. In such cases, the relining procedure to address the defect considers the distal portion of the iliac limb of the endograft, beyond which the disease progression has occurred, as the proximal neck.

We will now present the Tips & Tricks for treating iliac aneurysms. After clarifying the available technical and technological options, we will examine the most suitable interventional approach for each aneurysm type and subtype.

TIP #1

In hypogastric artery branching, with the current devices available on the market, the common iliac artery must be at least 40–50 mm in length and 18–20 mm in diameter. The distal landing zone in the hypogastric artery should measure at least 10 mm in length.

TIP #2

In cases of common iliac artery aneurysms (typically encountered during EVAR procedures and less commonly in isolated iliac aneurysms) when the hypogastric artery needs to be preserved, even temporarily, the **Bell Bottom Technique** can be a useful option.

This approach involves using a *flared iliac limb* that terminates at the common iliac bifurcation (Figure 5.3). These extensions typically reach diameters of up to 28 mm, allowing coverage of common iliac arteries with a distal neck diameter of up to 23–24 mm, assuming an oversizing of 15–20%.

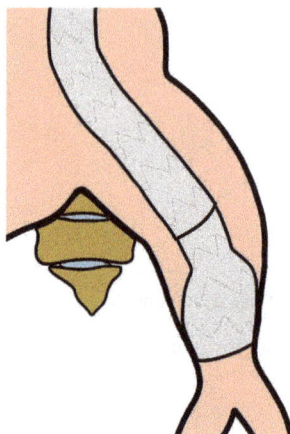

Figure 5.3 Bell Bottom Technique

If a larger diameter is required, an aortic cuff can be deployed to seal the distal neck of the common iliac artery. In case of EVAR, for approximately 50% of its length, the cuff is opened within the iliac limb extension of the bifurcated aortic endograft. Suitable cuffs for this purpose include the Cook Zenith Flex, Medtronic Endurant II, and Gore Excluder, which can accommodate diameters up to 36 mm, thereby covering a wide range of iliac diameters.

(*Note:* International reports indicate that the long-term adequacy of this technique is best for common iliac arteries with diameters up to 24–25 mm. This range is compatible with the flared iliac extensions available on the market and built for this purpose.)

TIP #3

In the case of an isolated iliac aneurysm, treatment with EVAR should be considered, as follows.

- If a concurrent abdominal aortic aneurysm is present, even if it is small. In this scenario, the procedure is primarily performed to address the iliac dilation, not the aortic aneurysm. The EVAR serves to provide the necessary proximal sealing.
- If the proximal neck in the common iliac artery is shorter than the minimum cutoff required to ensure adequate proximal sealing.

TIP #4

If treatment of the iliac bifurcation (or both bifurcations) is required while preserving the hypogastric artery, the **Sandwich Technique** offers an alternative to hypogastric artery branching. This method involves deploying two covered stents in parallel: one limb directed into the hypogastric artery and the other into the external iliac artery. The Sandwich Technique can be applied in cases of isolated iliac aneurysms (e.g., Type 0b) but is more commonly an adjunct procedure performed during an EVAR intervention.

Procedural Steps

1. Deploy the aortic endograft as usual, ensuring that the main body is inserted on the same side as the iliac axis to be treated with the Sandwich Technique. The distal end of the iliac limb should terminate approximately 10 mm above the origin of the hypogastric artery (Figure 5.4).

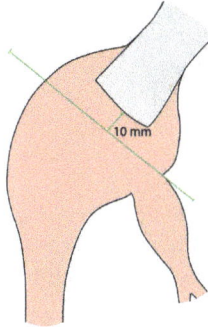

Figure 5.4 The Sandwich Technique

2. Access the hypogastric artery through left brachial (or axillary) access, advancing a 90- or 110-cm long sheath. Replace the standard guidewire with a 0.035" Teflon-coated super-stiff or extra-stiff guidewire (Figure 5.4a).

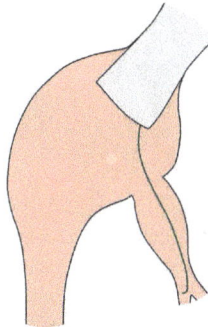

Figure 5.4a (Continued)

3. Position a self-expanding covered stent within the hypogastric artery, ensuring at least 20 mm of the hypogastric axis is covered. The stent should adequately overlap with the iliac extension stent directed toward the external iliac artery. Leave the stent in position without deploying it (Figure 5.4b).

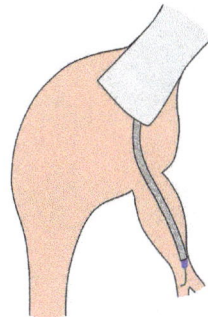

Figure 5.4b (Continued)

4. Deploy the iliac extension stent directed toward the external iliac artery following standard techniques (Figure 5.4c).

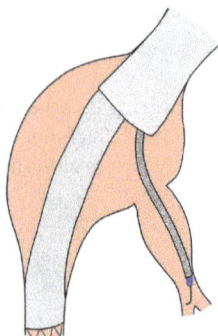

Figure 5.4c (Continued)

5. Deploy the self-expanding covered stent in the hypogastric artery, ensuring that its proximal end extends approximately 10 mm above the proximal edge of the external iliac stent. This adjustment prevents the external iliac stent from compressing the hypogastric stent against the arterial wall (Figure 5.4d).

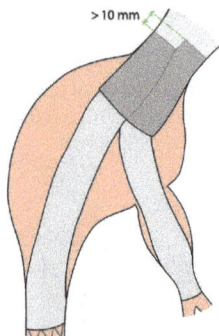

Figure 5.4d (Continued)

6. Perform molding ballooning of both the external iliac extension and the hypogastric stent. If necessary, use a Kissing Balloon Technique in the overlapped segments (Figure 5.4e).

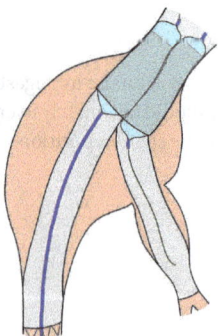

Figure 5.4e (Continued)

7. In case of EVAR, complete the procedure by deploying the contralateral iliac extension. If the contralateral iliac axis also requires hypogastric preservation, repeat all the aforementioned steps.

(*Note*: In cases of isolated Type 0b iliac aneurysms, a bifurcated aortic endograft will not be present, and the proximal landing zone will be the proximal portion of the common iliac artery. In such cases, a tubular module – either an aortic cuff or an appropriately sized covered stent – must first be deployed at this level to serve as the proximal segment for subsequent steps.)

(*Note*: The combined diameters of the stents directed toward the external iliac and hypogastric arteries should result in an oversizing of approximately 20% relative to the proximal tubular module into which they are inserted.)

The Sandwich Technique effectively excludes aneurysms involving the common iliac artery and its bifurcation. Although there is a small but present risk of gutter formation between the endograft components, this risk is generally marginal.

While largely replaced by hypogastric branching procedures using dedicated devices, the Sandwich Technique remains a viable option when anatomical criteria for safe branching cannot be met. Studies suggest that the anatomical feasibility of iliac branching is only about 50% in patients eligible for iliac aneurysm exclusion.

TIP #5

Hybrid Approach with Endovascular Iliac Bypass

In cases of abdominal aortic aneurysm with aneurysms of both common iliac arteries requiring an aorto-uniliac EVAR procedure, the **Banana Technique**, a technique sporadically reported in the literature by some authors, can be an elegant option to preserve the patency of at least one hypogastric artery. This approach is particularly useful in bailout situations, when standard treatment is anatomically unfeasible, or during endovascular management of a ruptured aneurysm.

Steps of the Banana Technique

- Deploy the aorto-uniliac endograft using standard techniques. On the side where the main body terminates in the external iliac artery, the ipsilateral hypogastric artery must be embolized beforehand.
- On the contralateral side, access the hypogastric artery via retrograde femoral access and stabilize it by replacing the standard guidewire with a 0.035" Teflon-coated super-stiff or extra-stiff guidewire.
- Deploy a self-expanding covered stent bridging the hypogastric artery to the external iliac artery. This stent revascularizes the hypogastric artery from below, via the femoral artery (Figure 5.5). Moreover, the placement of this stent eliminates the need for proximal embolization of the common iliac artery, as it will naturally be excluded by the final configuration achieved with the Banana Technique.
- Complete the procedure with the required femoro–femoral crossover bypass.

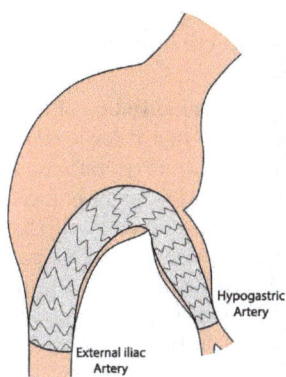

Figure 5.5 The Banana Technique

The treatment algorithm for isolated iliac aneurysms is based on the previously described morphological classification.

In this algorithm, we will consider all currently available techniques, organizing them to simplify the decision-making process while taking into account the anatomical territory where each technique performs best.

The issue of hypogastric artery preservation has long been debated, and this is a book of pure technique, which will not discuss the advisability or benefits of systematically saving the hypogastric artery. However, one consideration must be made: this algorithm refers to the unilateral treatment of iliac aneurysms.

If both the right and left iliac axes need to be treated – especially in a single surgical session – or if the treatment of aneurysms in both iliac axes is conducted during an EVAR procedure, it is essential to preserve at least one hypogastric artery using one of the techniques available and proposed herein.

TIP #6

Type 0a

This is the simplest iliac aneurysm to treat, when both the proximal and distal necks are located within the common iliac artery. In this case, the treatment will consist of the following.

- Simple exclusion by placing an iliac endograft limb or a covered stent. Both balloon-expandable and self-expanding covered stents can be effectively used, provided the deployment is precise, and the stents are adequately oversized (15–20% relative to the nominal diameter of the artery).

TIP #7

Type 0b

In this case, a proximal neck is located in the common iliac artery, but the aneurysm involves the iliac bifurcation or extends into the external iliac artery. The treatment options include the following.

- **Iliac branch device**, if anatomically feasible and preservation of the hypogastric artery is required.
- **Sandwich Technique**, if an iliac branch device is not feasible and hypogastric artery preservation is necessary. In this scenario, the procedure begins by deploying a proximal tubular module (an aortic cuff or a covered stent of appropriate diameter) in the common iliac artery, ensuring it lands at least 10 mm above the origin of the hypogastric artery. For deploying the stent in the hypogastric artery – since there is no biturcated aortic endograft – a contralateral femoral access can be used. Through this access, the hypogastric artery is cannulated, and a 0.035" Teflon-coated super-stiff or extra-stiff guidewire is positioned. A long sheath is advanced over the guidewire, with its tip landing in the hypogastric artery at a length sufficient to ensure stability. Subsequent steps are similar to those previously described.
- **Landing in the external iliac artery with embolization of the hypogastric artery**, if the hypogastric artery can be sacrificed. This raises the issue of device selection. Conical iliac endograft extensions, designed primarily for standard EVAR, are typically used. But these have a proximal diameter of approximately 16 mm, which matches the gate of the bifurcated endograft for which they are designed. Conversely, non-conical iliac endograft extensions have larger diameters, which can cause significant infolding when deployed in the external iliac artery. Some authors suggest using an **aorto-uniliac module** within the iliac axis being treated, provided that the device diameters and lengths are suitable for the anatomy. Another option involves the use of **self-expanding or balloon-expandable covered stents** (potentially two in overlapping configuration). However,

diameter mismatches can arise, as these devices often have smaller diameters that do not always align with the proximal common iliac artery. An alternative solution is to use a flared iliac endograft extension – commonly employed in the Bell Bottom Technique – in an off-label reversed fashion, deployed via contralateral, brachial, or axillary access. By inverting the proximal and distal ends of the device, it may better fit the anatomy being treated. The procedure can be completed with an additional distal iliac extension, if needed.

TIP #8

Type 1a

In this case, the anatomy is characterized by the absence of a proximal neck. The distal neck, of adequate length and caliber, is located in the distal common iliac artery. This anatomy should be addressed using a standard EVAR procedure, with landing in the distal common iliac artery.

The Bell Bottom Technique can be considered when the distal common iliac artery is dilated but still salvageable.

TIP #9

Type 1b

In this case, there is no proximal neck, and the aneurysm extends to the iliac bifurcation or into the external iliac artery.

This type of anatomy is managed with a standard EVAR procedure combined with the most appropriate iliac procedure for the specific case. The iliac gate of the bifurcated endograft transforms this anatomy into a Type 0b, making it possible to use all the previously discussed technical strategies for that anatomical scenario.

Compared to a Type 0b, this situation is even simpler to address, as the presence of the iliac gate eliminates all the proximal diameter issues previously mentioned in the related tips.

A key consideration, depending on the type of bifurcated endograft used and the lengths of the iliac axis involved in the procedure, is the preoperative decision regarding the side for introducing the main body. It is important to determine whether to proceed with the ipsilateral or contralateral gate of the bifurcated endograft to continue the iliac procedure in the most efficient and convenient way.

Finally, if preservation of the hypogastric artery is required using the Sandwich Technique, the covered stent directed to the hypogastric artery must be deployed via a brachial (or axillary) access due to the presence of the bifurcated main body in the aorta. An exception to this is when using the Endologix AFX2 endograft, which allows deployment of the stent through the contralateral femoral access.

TIP #10

Type 2

This anatomy includes iliac aneurysms with an adequate proximal neck but lacking a distal neck in the external iliac artery.

In reality, aneurysms involving the entire external iliac artery are extremely rare. However, this type also encompasses more frequently encountered anatomies, such as iliac aneurysms where a distal neck is absent due to atherosclerotic occlusion of the external iliac axis.

Technical Strategies

- **Open surgery**.
- **Hybrid Technique:** In this approach, an aorto-uniliac module is deployed and extended to the contralateral iliac axis. The procedure is completed with embolization of the hypogastric artery and

a femoro–femoral crossover bypass. If the external iliac artery is aneurysmal, the common femoral or external iliac artery should be ligated proximal to the femoral anastomosis. However, if the external iliac artery is chronically occluded, this step is unnecessary (Figures 5.6–5.6a).

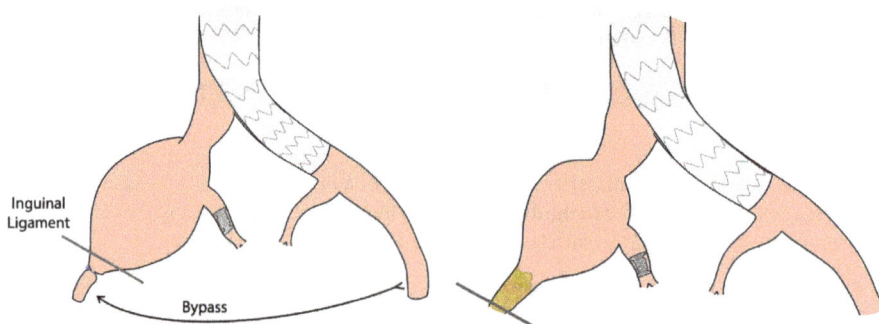

Figures 5.6–5.6a Hybrid Technique for treating Type 2 iliac aneurysms.

- **Hybrid Technique with hypogastric preservation:** If anatomical conditions permit, and an adequate landing zone is present in the hypogastric artery, some authors propose a variant of the hybrid technique, reported here for completeness of presentation. In this variation, a bifurcated main body is used to preserve hypogastric artery patency. In such cases, the iliac extension is advanced into the hypogastric artery via brachial or axillary access. The procedure is then completed with a femoro–femoral crossover bypass, with proximal ligation at the femoral anastomosis in cases of aneurysmal external iliac arteries (Figure 5.7). However, this technique is off-label, its use is anecdotal and should therefore be used with caution and sound clinical judgment.

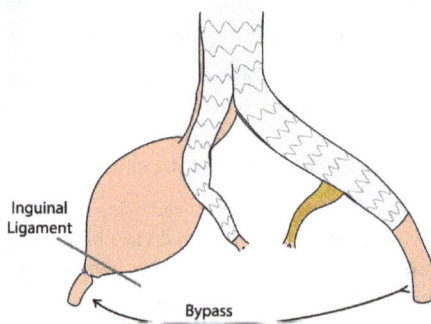

Figure 5.7 Hybrid Technique with hypogastric preservation for treating Type 2 iliac aneurysms.

- **Pure Endovascular Technique:** This approach is suitable for patients with an occluded external iliac artery who are asymptomatic or minimally symptomatic (Fontaine Stage I or Stage IIa). With an adequate proximal neck, the aneurysm can be excluded via an endovascular bypass from the common iliac artery to the hypogastric artery (Figure 5.8). The key requirement is an endovascular device compatible with the diameters and lengths of the assessed proximal and distal necks. This technique does not compromise future placement of an aorto-uniliac endograft extending into the contralateral iliac axis if required. This strategy can also be applied in cases of previous aorto-bisiliac bypass (where distal anastomoses land in the common iliac artery) or EVAR, where the distal iliac extension (prosthetic or endograft) serves as the proximal neck. A hybrid version of this technique can also address cases where the external iliac artery is aneurysmal, combining the proposed endovascular bypass with a femoro–femoral crossover bypass and ligation of the vessel proximal to the anastomosis. It is important to note that this technical approach is documented in the literature only as anecdotal cases, it is reported here for completeness of presentation and should therefore be used with caution.

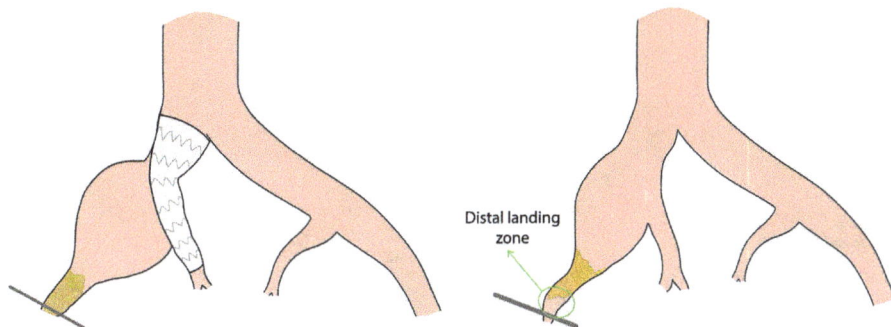

Figures 5.8–5.8a Pure endovascular technique for treating Type 2 iliac aneurysms.

- **Pure Endovascular Technique (Version 2)**: This option is also feasible for patients with a chronically occluded external iliac artery requiring revascularization. Preoperative CT angiography must confirm the presence of a patent segment of distal external iliac artery beyond the occlusion to ensure an adequate landing zone within the limits of the inguinal ligament (Figure 5.8a). In this approach, the first step is recanalization of the iliac axis using techniques described in Section 3. Once recanalization is complete, the resulting anatomy can be conceptually considered as a Type 0b, as it now has an adequate proximal and distal neck. Previously described technical strategies can then be applied. However, it is important to emphasize that recanalizing an occluded axis in aneurysmal disease requires caution. The dilated arterial wall is more fragile than in pure atherosclerotic disease. Aggressive maneuvers during the recanalization phase should be avoided to minimize the risk of arterial rupture, which is not negligible.

TIP #11

Type 3

In this type of anatomy, which is the most complex, both the proximal and distal necks are completely absent. As with Type 2, the inadequacy of the external iliac artery may be due to vessel occlusion or – less commonly – aneurysmal degeneration extending the full length of the vessel.

Therapeutic Options

- **Open surgery**.
- **Hybrid Technique:** Similar to Type 2, this approach involves deploying an aorto-uniliac endograft along the contralateral iliac axis. The procedure is completed with embolization of the hypogastric artery and a femoro–femoral crossover bypass. As with Type 2, if the external iliac artery is aneurysmal, it will be necessary to ligate the artery proximal to the femoral anastomosis.
- **EVAR with a bifurcated main body:** If preservation of the hypogastric artery is necessary and anatomical conditions allow, an EVAR procedure with a bifurcated main body can be performed. In this case, the iliac extension will be directed toward the hypogastric artery (Figures 5.9–5.9a). The procedure is completed with a femoro–femoral crossover bypass, employing the technical strategies previously described in detail, with the same considerations regarding its off-label and anecdotal use.
- **Pure Endovascular Technique:** In Type 3 anatomy, if the external iliac artery is occluded but revascularizable, recanalization can be considered, provided there is a segment of healthy, high-quality external iliac artery distal to the occlusion (Figure 5.9b). Once the external iliac axis has been revascularized, the resulting anatomy can be considered Type 1b, allowing the application of all the corresponding technical solutions.

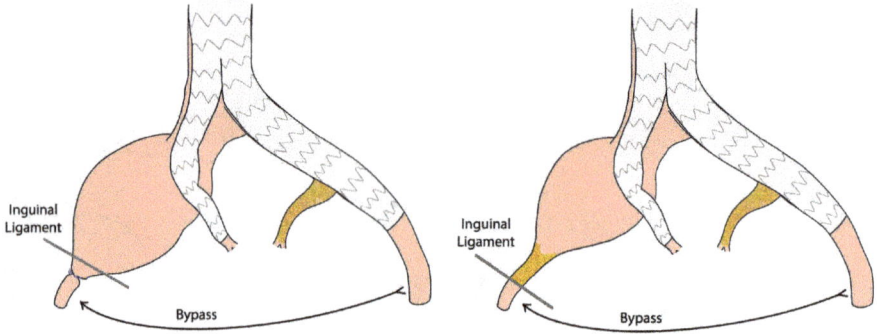

Figures 5.9–5.9a Hypogastric preservation with a bifurcated main body for treating Type 3 iliac aneurysms.

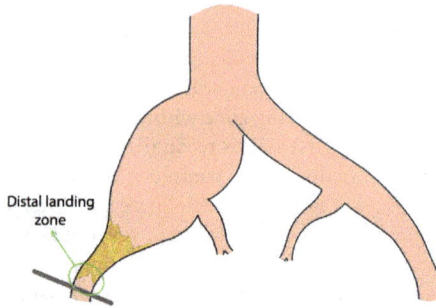

Figure 5.9b Anatomical requirements for the Pure Endovascular Technique in treating Type 3 iliac aneurysms.

These also represent a rare finding (approximately 10–30% of isolated iliac aneurysms). The previously proposed classification applies in this case as well, since hypogastric aneurysms are simply a variant of the anatomies previously discussed, sharing both anatomical and technical peculiarities. Therefore, we address them here primarily for the sake of completeness.

The treatment strategies proposed here can also be considered for managing hypogastric aneurysms associated with aortoiliac aneurysmal disease.

TIP #12

Type 0 (Figure 5.10)

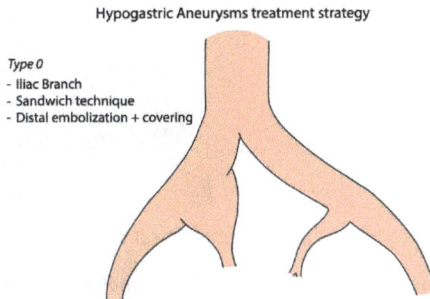

Figure 5.10 Type 0 hypogastric aneurysms and their treatment strategies.

This scenario involves the presence of an adequate proximal neck, typically located in the common iliac artery, and an adequate distal neck. The treatment strategies in this case include the following.

- **Iliac Branching**, if anatomically feasible and preservation of the hypogastric artery is necessary.
- **Sandwich Technique**, if iliac branching is not feasible.
- **Exclusion of the hypogastric aneurysm** by landing in the external iliac artery. Prior embolization of the distal neck with plugs or coils is required.

(*Note:* Hypogastric embolization techniques will be discussed in the section dedicated to the management of endoleaks.)

TIP #13

Type 1 (Figure 5.11)

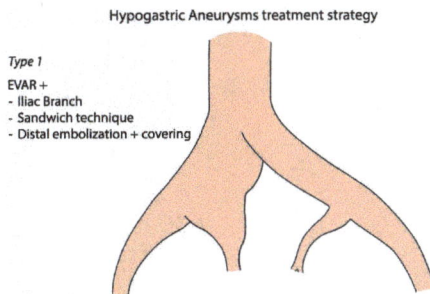

Figure 5.11 Type 1 hypogastric aneurysms and their treatment strategies.

In Type 1, the proximal neck in the common iliac artery is absent, while the distal neck is adequate, allowing for vessel preservation if necessary. The endovascular techniques applicable are the same as those for Type 0, except that in this case, a standard EVAR procedure will be required. The iliac gate of the bifurcated main body will serve as the proximal neck in this scenario.

TIP #14

Type 2 (Figure 5.12)

In this case, an adequate distal neck is absent, while the proximal neck in the common iliac artery is sufficient. The only viable endovascular option is the exclusion of the hypogastric artery through the placement of an iliac endograft extension landing in the external iliac artery. The main challenge in this scenario lies in the required embolization of the terminal branches of the hypogastric artery, which must be performed prior to its exclusion (Figure 5.12a).

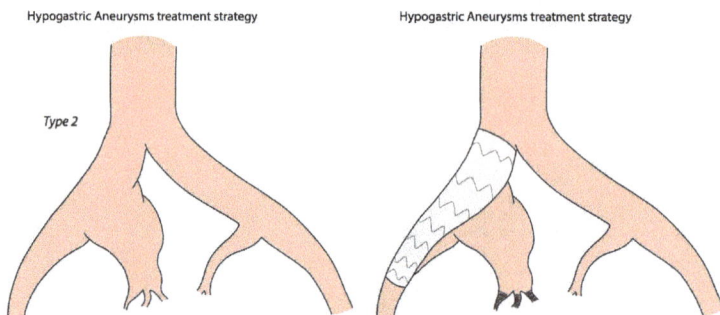

Figures 5.12–5.12a Type 2 hypogastric aneurysms and their treatment strategies.

In the context of a hypogastric aneurysm, superselective catheterization of all terminal branches can be particularly challenging but is essential to prevent retrograde backflow from the contralateral hypogastric artery, which could otherwise lead to sac growth over time. If this phase becomes overly prolonged, the following staged approach may be considered.

- **Stage 1:** Embolization of the terminal branches of the hypogastric artery.
- **Stage 2:** Treatment of the aneurysm.

Since the treatment involves only the iliac axis – requiring the deployment of an iliac module originating in the common iliac artery and landing in the external iliac artery – the same diameter matching issues between the common iliac artery and external artery apply, as discussed in *Tip #7* in this section addressing Type 0b iliac aneurysms.

TIP #15

Type 3 (Figure 5.13)

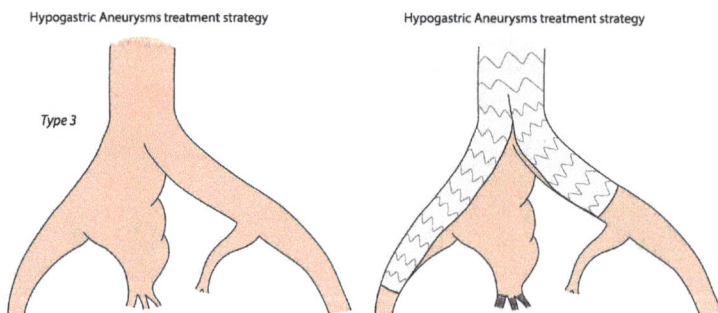

Figures 5.13–5.13a Type 3 hypogastric aneurysms and their treatment strategies.

In this case, both the proximal and distal necks are completely absent, and the only viable option is the execution of a standard EVAR with landing in the external iliac artery, preceded by embolization of the terminal branches of the hypogastric artery (Figure 5.13a). As with the previous variant, it is reasonable to consider planning the procedure in two surgical stages.

REFERENCES

1. Melas N, Saratzis A, Dixon H, et al. Isolated common iliac artery aneurysms: A revised classification to assist endovascular repair. *J Endovasc Ther*. 2011; 18(5): 697–715.

2. Wanhainen A, Van Herzeele I, Bastos Goncalves F, et al. Editor's choice – European society for vascular surgery (ESVS) 2024 clinical practice guidelines on the management of abdominal aorto-iliac artery aneurysms. *Eur J Vasc Endovasc Surg*. 2024; 67(2): 192–331.

3. Hans SS, Shepard AD, Weaver MR, et al. *Endovascular and Open Vascular Reconstruction. A Practical Approach*. London: Taylor & Francis; 2018. Vol. 12, pp. 75–85.

4. Cooper D, Odedra B, Haslam L, et al. Endovascular management of isolated iliac artery aneurysms. *J Cardiovasc Surg*. 2015; 56(4): 579–586.

5. Schneider PA. Technical aspects of treating aortic aneurysms. In: *Endovascular Skills: Guidewire and Catheter Skills for Endovascular Surgery*. 4th ed. Boca Raton, FL: CRC Press; 2020. pp. 408–435.

6. Moore WS. Aneurysms of the aorta and iliac arteries. In: *Vascular and Endovascular Surgery: A Comprehensive Review*. 8th ed. Philadelphia, PA: Elsevier Saunders; 2013. pp. 779–807.

7. Massmann A, Mosquera Arochena NJ, Shayesteh-Kheslat R, et al. Endovascular anatomic reconstruction of the iliac bifurcation with covered stentgrafts in sandwich-technique for the treatment of complex aorto-iliac aneurysms. *Int J Cardiol*. 2016; 222: 332–339.

8. Lobato AC, Camacho-Lobato L. The sandwich technique to treat complex aortoiliac or isolated iliac aneurysms: Results of midterm follow-up. *J Vasc Surg*. 2013; 57(2): 26S–34S.

9. Fossaceca R, Guzzardi G, Di Terlizzi M, et al. Long-term efficacy of endovascular treatment of isolated iliac artery aneurysms. *Radiol Med*. 2013; 118(1): 62–73.

10. Fossaceca R, Guzzardi G, Cerini P, et al. Isolated iliac artery aneurysms: A single-centre experience. *Radiol Med*. 2015; 120(5): 440–448.

11. Lobato AC. Sandwich technique for aortoiliac aneurysms extending to the internal iliac artery or isolated common/internal iliac artery aneurysms: A new endovascular approach to preserve pelvic circulation. *J Endovasc Ther*. 2011; 18(1): 106–111.

12. Oliveira-Pinto J, Martins P, Mansilha A. Endovascular treatment of iliac aneurysmal disease with internal iliac artery preservation: A review of two different approaches. *Int Angiol*. 2019; 38(6): 494–501.

13. Mazzaccaro D, Righini P, Zuccon G, et al. The reversed bell-bottom technique (ReBel-B) for the endovascular treatment of iliac artery aneurysms. *Catheter Cardiovasc Interv*. 2020; 96(4): E479–E483.

14. Rodrigues DVS, Frazao VHA, de Araujo Junior RT, et al. Endovascular repair of ruptured external iliac artery pseudoaneurysm and arteriovenous fistula using reversed bell-bottom technique. *J Vasc Surg Cases Innov Tech*. 2022; 9(1): 101087.

15. Fargion AT, Masciello F, Pratesi C, et al. Results of the multicenter pELVIS registry for isolated common iliac aneurysms treated by the iliac branch device. *J Vasc Surg*. 2018; 68(5): 1367–1373.

16. Giaquinta A, Ardita V, Ferrer C, et al. Iliac branch stent-graft Italian trial collaborators. Isolated common iliac artery aneurysms treated solely with iliac branch stent-grafts: Midterm results of a multicenter registry. *J Endovasc Ther*. 2018; 25(2): 169–177.

17. Telles GJ, Razuk Filho Á, Karakhanian WK, et al. Dilatation of common iliac arteries after endovascular infrarenal abdominal aortic repair with bell-bottom extension. *Braz J Cardiovasc Surg*. 2016; 31(2): 145–150.

18. Pagliariccio G, Gatta E, Schiavon S, et al. Bell-bottom technique in iliac branch era: Mid-term single stent graft performance. *CVIR Endovasc*. 2020; 3(1): 57.

19. Volteas P, Giannopoulos S, Koudounas G, et al. Endovascular treatment of aortoiliac aneurysms with the bell-bottom technique: A systematic review and meta-analysis. *Vasc Endovascular Surg*. 2025; 59(2): 143–152.

20. Coppi G, Tasselli S, Silingardi R, et al. Endovascular preservation of full pelvic circulation with external iliac-to-internal iliac artery "cross-stenting" in patients with aorto-iliac aneurysms. *J Vasc Interv Radiol.* 2010; 21(10): 1579–1582.

21. Zhorzel S, Busch A, Trenner M, et al. Open versus endovascular repair of isolated iliac artery aneurysms. *Vasc Endovascular Surg.* 2019; 53(1): 12–20.

22. Charisis N, Bouris V, Rakic A, et al. A systematic review on endovascular repair of isolated common iliac artery aneurysms and suggestions regarding diameter thresholds for intervention. *J Vasc Surg.* 2021; 74(5): 1752–1762.

23. Leon LR Jr, Mills JL, Psalms SB, et al. A novel hybrid approach to the treatment of common iliac aneurysms: Antegrade endovascular hypogastric stent grafting and femorofemoral bypass grafting. *J Vasc Surg.* 2007; 45(6): 1244–1248.

24. Perini P, Mariani E, Fanelli M, et al. Surgical and endovascular management of isolated internal iliac artery aneurysms: A systematic review and meta-analysis. *Vasc Endovascular Surg.* 2021; 55(3): 254–264.

25. Bekdache K, Dietzek AM, Cha A, et al. Endovascular hypogastric artery preservation during endovascular aneurysm repair: A review of current techniques and devices. *Ann Vasc Surg.* 2015; 29(2): 367–376.

26. Kouvelos GN, Katsargyris A, Antoniou GA, et al. Outcome after interruption or preservation of internal iliac artery flow during endovascular repair of abdominal aorto-iliac aneurysms. *Eur J Vasc Endovasc Surg.* 2016; 52(5): 621–634.

27. Simonte G, Parlani G, Farchioni L, et al. Lesson learned with the use of iliac branch devices: Single centre 10 year experience in 157 consecutive procedures. *Eur J Vasc Endovasc Surg.* 2017; 54(1): 95–103.

28. Yang M, Li L, Liu Y. Therapeutic management of isolated internal iliac artery aneurysms. *J Vasc Surg.* 2020; 72(6): 1968–1975.

29. Cao Z, Zhu R, Ghaffarian A, et al. A systematic review and meta-analysis of the clinical effectiveness and safety of unilateral versus bilateral iliac branch devices for aortoiliac and iliac artery aneurysms. *J Vasc Surg.* 2022; 76(4): 1089–1098.e8.

30. Wooster M, Armstrong P, Back M. Hypogastric preservation using retrograde endovascular bypass. *Ann Vasc Surg.* 2018; 51: 170–176.

ADVANCED TIPS & TRICKS IN THE MANAGEMENT OF ENDOLEAKS AND PSEUDOANEURYSMS

Toolkit A – **Tips & Tricks in Endoleak Treatment**   **188**
- Tips 1 to 8

Toolkit B – **Tips & Tricks in the Percutaneous Treatment of Iatrogenic Femoral Pseudoaneurysms**   **205**
- Tips 9 to 15

DOI: 10.1201/9781003567080-6

We are still far from having the ideal or definitive endograft in our hands, meaning a device with the characteristics described in Section 4 of this volume. This fact remains an ongoing observation (at least for me), arising from the need to systematically verify the consequences of all the inherent imperfections present in current devices.

These imperfections become even more evident when – after overcoming the perioperative phase – we compare the success rates of endovascular treatment for abdominal aortic aneurysm with those of traditional open surgery. The latter may appear more alarming in the immediate postoperative period, yet it remains reliable over the long term.

The main challenges associated with endovascular treatment primarily stem from the following critical issues.

- Endoleaks and endograft migrations.
- Life-long instrumental monitoring (a direct consequence of the previous point).
- Higher reintervention rates compared to open surgery (also a consequence of the first issue).

The endoleak issue, therefore, becomes an urgent problem that, in my opinion, should be addressed on a large scale, first on a theoretical level before a practical one. What do I mean by this, and how does it relate to the predominantly practical focus of this volume?

My observation is quite simple: endovascular treatment is perfect for atherosclerotic occlusive disease. In fact, it was originally developed for this purpose, starting with the first angioplasty ever performed in Switzerland in the 1970s by interventional radiologist Andreas Gruntzig. The results of endovascular treatment for occlusive disease are excellent and continue to improve year after year.

However, all the imperfections that have emerged in the endovascular treatment of aneurysmal disease, in my opinion, stem from an intrinsic limitation of its current conceptual paradigm. To exclude an aortic aneurysm, current endografts (with few exceptions, though these present other critical issues) merely place stents along the aortic wall. The theoretical problem I refer to arises precisely here: the radial force exerted by these stents on a potentially degenerative wall with a tendency to dilate. In this sense, the EVAR technique can almost be considered a therapeutic paradox, a kind of strange loop or recursive system. (Do you recall Escher's drawings?)

And if you think about it – in front of a patient with an aortic aneurysm – the very first step we take to prevent a Type 1 endoleak actually reinforces this technological paradox: in our preoperative planning, we primarily focus on *ensuring adequate oversizing*.

The radial force exerted by endografts on the aortic wall is not inert, and a growing number of studies have been focusing on this issue in recent years. It tends to cause what is known as Aortic Neck Dilation (AND) in a not negligible percentage of patients, the progression and real consequences of which remain unclear or possibly underestimated. Addressing this issue would require a true paradigm shift in the treatment of aneurysmal disease, but we are still far from achieving that.

However, reassured by the simplicity and high immediate postoperative success rates of this highly convenient technology, we continue to rely on it – despite the consequent Type 1 endoleaks and endograft migrations it entails.

Type 2 endoleaks, on the other hand, stem from another intrinsic imperfection, not just of endograft devices but of the EVAR procedure itself. Unlike open surgery, EVAR is incapable of achieving definitive aneurysmectomy through the opening of the aneurysmal sac and the endosaccular ligation of patent aortic collaterals. Current treatments for Type 2 endoleaks seem more like patches in comparison, and the preventive embolization of the sac, proposed by some authors to address this shortcoming, has shown mixed results and there is currently insufficient evidence to recommend its routine use.

Finally, there is the issue of endograft migration, though its incidence remains rare. Here again, the problem stems from a technological gap in current devices. Most endografts (with the exception of the AFX2 by Endologix) rely on barbs positioned along the proximal stent ring for fixation. These barbs pierce the aortic wall, anchoring the device in place. However, this anchorage is not definitive – it can be suboptimal or compromised by factors such as a heavily calcified aortic wall or an angulated neck, which may lead to imperfect apposition of the endograft. Once again, we are far from the reliability guaranteed by a surgical anastomosis.

In this section, we will describe some of the available solutions to address and mitigate these complications.

TYPE 1A ENDOLEAKS

It is first necessary to establish a distinction between primary Type 1A endoleaks – those detected during the completion angiography at the end of the index procedure – and secondary Type 1A endoleaks, which are diagnosed during follow-up. This distinction is justified by the fact that primary forms are often related to a technical failure or a failure in preoperative planning. In some cases, the possibility of a primary Type 1A endoleak is a risk that operators knowingly accept when dealing with a patient with a particularly challenging aortic neck who is unfit for procedures more complex than standard EVAR.

Secondary forms, on the other hand, are frequently the result of long-term device failure or disease progression. The treatment strategy for primary forms differs from that of secondary ones, and they will therefore be addressed separately.

TIP #1

Primary Type 1A Endoleaks

The escalation strategy initially involves – If a Type 1A endoleak is detected during the angiography performed at the end of the EVAR procedure – repeating molding ballooning of the proximal segment of the endograft, followed by another angiographic assessment. In many cases, this simple and harmless maneuver is sufficient and resolves the issue.

If this approach fails, other possible solutions include the following, sequentially.

- If an additional infrarenal landing zone is available (proximal to the endograft but not yet utilized), a proximal aortic cuff can be deployed flush with the renal arteries to maximize every millimeter of healthy aortic neck (Figure 6.1). It is important to specify that aortic cuffs are not intended to increase radial force on the segment of the aortic neck already covered by the endograft but rather to extend the sealing zone when an uncovered portion of the aortic neck remains.
- If the endograft has already been deployed flush with the renal arteries, adding an additional aortic cuff will not improve sealing (Figure 6.1a). In this scenario, the use of EndoAnchors may be beneficial, as they firmly secure the device to the aortic neck. It should be noted that EndoAnchors can be planned proactively for patients with short aortic necks (according to the manufacturer's data, as described in Section 4, the combined use of the Endurant II endograft and EndoAnchors allows for infrarenal treatment in necks as short as 4 mm) or reverse-tapered necks, when the patient is deemed unfit for more complex procedures.
- Alternatively, in the absence of an additional usable aortic neck for sealing, some authors have anecdotally proposed over the years the use of a large Palmaz stent deployed at the level of the infrarenal neck, with the rationale of providing additional radial force. The impact on the renal arteries is minimal, but the efficacy of this tool has never been conclusively demonstrated. Furthermore, reintervention rates are not negligible. For these reasons, this maneuver should be reserved only for bailout situations or emergency settings.
- If none of the previous techniques are feasible, or if it is deemed that a better treatment strategy exists but is not available during the index procedure, then terminating the intervention and planning a short-term elective reintervention may represent an option.

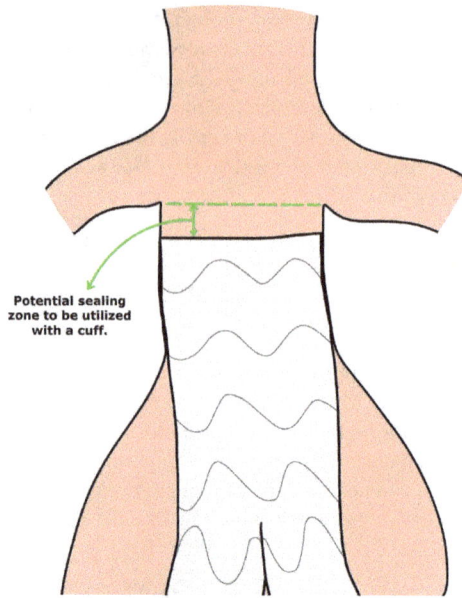

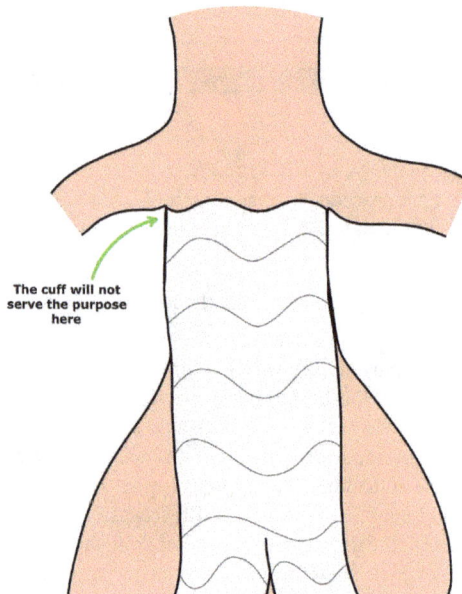

Figures 6.1–6.1a Primary Type 1A endoleak management.

TIP #2

The Use of the Heli-FX EndoAnchor System

The Heli-FX EndoAnchor system by Medtronic consists of the following.

1. A guide catheter that is steerable, with its maneuverability enabled by a rotating knob on the handle. It has a 16 French diameter and a 62 cm length, and is available in two versions: 22 mm and 28 mm, compatible with aortic necks measuring 18–28 mm and 28–32 mm, respectively.

2. An applicator catheter, which measures 12 Fr in diameter and 86 cm in length.

3. A cassette preloaded with ten EndoAnchors, each measuring 4.5 mm in length and 3 mm in diameter.

According to the manufacturer's indications, the Heli-FX system has been tested and evaluated in terms of safety and efficacy with these commercially available endografts: Medtronic Endurant, Cook Zenith, and Gore Excluder. Therefore, its use is recommended exclusively with these devices.

- After initial flushing maneuvers and a preparation phase, the device will be ready for use. (A green light on the introducer system handle will illuminate once preparation is complete.)

- At this point, the first EndoAnchor can be loaded into the applicator catheter. Once loaded, its correct positioning must be visually verified: the EndoAnchor should be fully seated within its catheter without protruding beyond its tip (Figure 6.2). Even minimal protrusion of the EndoAnchor beyond the catheter tip indicates mispositioning (Figure 6.2a), requiring optimization or complete reloading.

- The implantation process can now begin. Under fluoroscopic guidance, the guiding catheter is advanced over a 0.035" extra-stiff guidewire until it reaches the desired position, specifically the proximal segment of the endograft, where the EndoAnchors will be deployed (Figure 6.2b). If the Heli-FX system is being used during the index EVAR procedure, the aortic endograft deployment must already be completed. At this stage, it is advisable to verify the proper navigation of the guiding catheter along the iliac arteries and within the endograft. In the presence of severely tortuous or calcified iliac arteries, its advancement may be challenging; if this occurs, placing a long sheath may facilitate the advancement of the system.

**Endoanchor
correctly loaded**

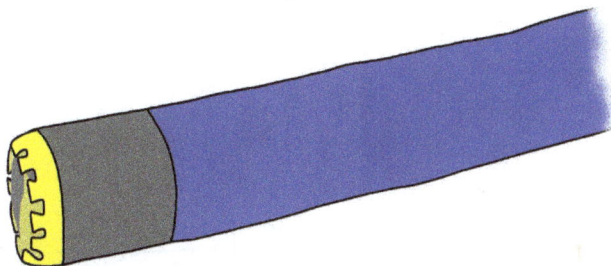

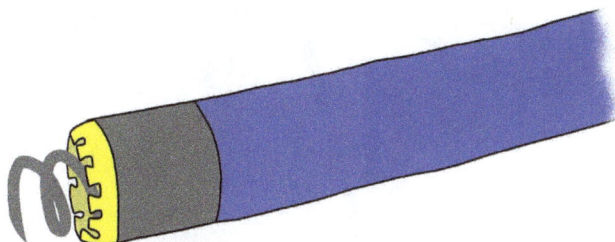

**Endoanchor
improperly loaded**

Figures 6.2–6.2a EndoAnchor implantation: Before proceeding with the implantation, check whether the EndoAnchor has been correctly loaded into its applicator.

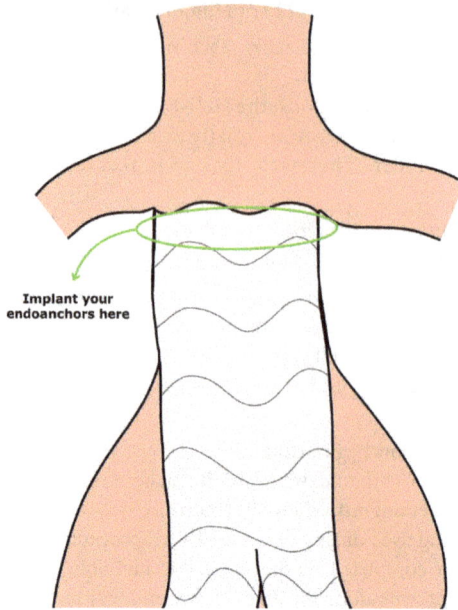

Figure 6.2b EndoAnchor implantation: The proximal segment of the endograft is the target site for implantation.

- Once the guiding catheter has been positioned at the target site, its obturator must be removed, and the tip steered to align it with the specific site on the endograft where the first EndoAnchor will be implanted (Figure 6.2c).

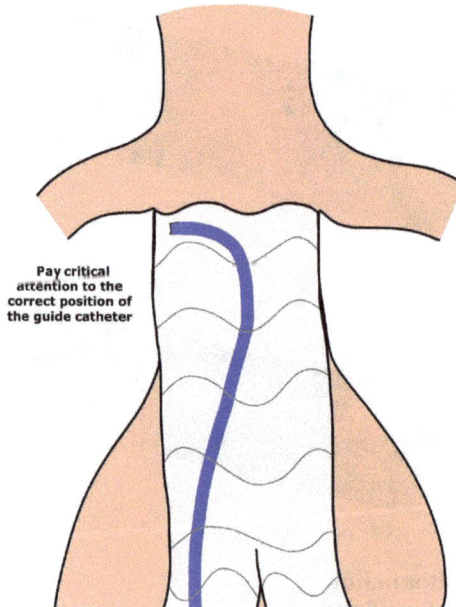

Figure 6.2c (Continued)

- The tip of the guiding catheter features a radiopaque marker, whose position should be carefully verified to ensure optimal placement on the endograft wall. This phase is critical, as effective and precise EndoAnchor deployment requires that the guiding catheter tip be oriented perpendicularly to the endograft (Figure 6.2d).

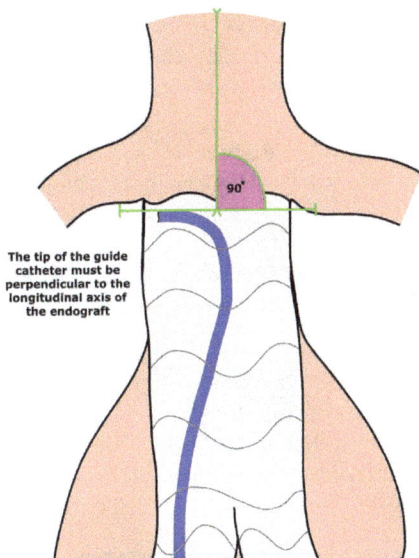

The tip of the guide catheter must be perpendicular to the longitudinal axis of the endograft

Figure 6.2d (Continued)

- At this point, the applicator catheter is advanced through the guiding catheter until it emerges from the tip of the latter. When resistance is encountered during its advancement, this indicates that the tip of the applicator is correctly positioned against the endograft wall.
- Before proceeding with EndoAnchor deployment, the positioning of both the guide catheter and applicator catheter must be reverified (both distal portions should be perpendicular to the longitudinal axis of the endograft; Figures 6.2e–6.2f). If not perfectly perpendicular, the system will

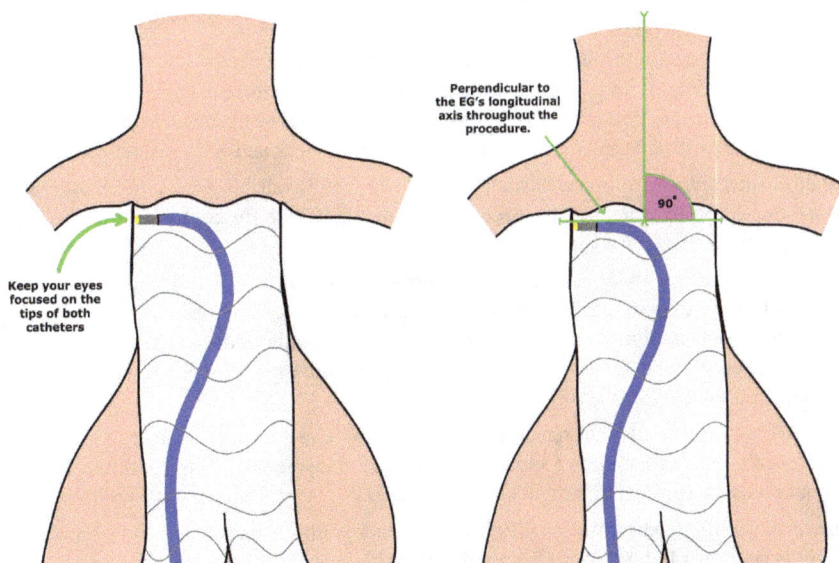

Keep your eyes focused on the tips of both catheters

Perpendicular to the EG's longitudinal axis throughout the procedure.

Figures 6.2e–6.2f (Continued) The tips of the guiding catheter and the applicator catheter must be oriented perpendicular to the longitudinal axis of the endograft.

be misaligned, increasing the risk of an ineffective, incorrect, or incomplete implantation.

- The EndoAnchor deployment sequence begins laterally on the endograft while maintaining the fluoroscope in an anteroposterior view. Subsequently, by rotating the fluoroscope to a lateral position, the anterior and posterior segments of the endograft are treated.

- Each EndoAnchor implantation is automatic and consists of two stages. Stage 1 provides partial deployment, while Stage 2, once the correct EndoAnchor position has been confirmed at the end of Stage 1, completes the implantation. Throughout the procedure, the guiding and applicator catheters must remain firmly stabilized.

(*Note*: At the end of Stage 1, if there is any doubt about the correct positioning of the EndoAnchor, it can be retracted using the retrieval button on the handle and repositioned before final deployment.)

***

According to the manufacturer's recommendations, for aortic diameters up to 29 mm, a minimum of four EndoAnchors should be deployed, whereas for diameters between 30 mm and 32 mm, at least six EndoAnchors are required.

At the end of the implantation, the following steps should be performed in sequence.

- Remove the applicator from the guiding catheter.
- Straighten the guiding catheter by deflecting its steerability control, using the rotating knob.
- Reinsert the obturator into the guiding catheter, and within it, advance a 0.035" extra-stiff guidewire. The catheter is then removed from the circulation, leaving the guidewire in place.

TIP #3

Secondary Type 1A Endoleaks

- It is not uncommon to encounter secondary Type 1A endoleaks in which – at least on angio-CT assessment – despite confirming the presence of sac refilling, the sealing between the aortic neck (which appears to be of good quality) and the endograft seems adequate in terms of length and device apposition. In these cases – when the issue may be related to an *undersized* oversizing during the index procedure or early degenerative changes of the aortic neck not yet clinically evident – it is possible to attempt sealing optimization by performing molding ballooning of the proximal segment of the endograft using a suitably sized aortic balloon. If this maneuver is unsuccessful, the use of EndoAnchors in this anatomical scenario may effectively secure the device to the aortic wall.

- An alternative reported in the literature is the use of a Palmaz stent deployed along the entire length of the proximal endograft neck, in order to apply additional radial force to enhance sealing. However, as already mentioned in *Tip #1*, its use remains anecdotal and has been associated with a non-negligible risk of dilative degeneration, both at the infrarenal neck and at the level of visceral aorta.

- If a high-quality, unused infrarenal aortic neck segment is still available, we can take advantage of this anatomical feature by proximally extending the endograft with the deployment of an aortic cuff of appropriate length and diameter.

- If the infrarenal aortic neck is insufficient to ensure optimal sealing with these techniques, it may be advisable – before proceeding with more extensive proximal extensions – to assess the feasibility of EndoAnchors implantation. As a reminder, EndoAnchors are indicated when at least 4 mm of usable infrarenal neck is present. This procedure does not compromise subsequent proximal extension strategies and is effective in a lot of cases.

- In the absence of any usable infrarenal neck – or in complex anatomies whereby previous maneuvers are not feasible – the transition to a suprarenal endograft implantation using FEVAR or BEVAR techniques must be considered, provided that the patient's anatomy and clinical conditions allow it.

- In emergency settings, when off-the-shelf branched endografts are unavailable (or the anatomy does not permit their implantation), combining the Chimney Technique with the deployment of an aortic cuff or tube graft can be considered, if technically feasible and in the presence of a suitable suprarenal neck.

- Sac embolization, performed via a transealing approach through the proximal aortic neck, should be reserved for bailout situations when previous techniques have failed or proved ineffective, and when the patient's clinical condition precludes more invasive procedures. It should be noted that this technique is not standardized and has been anecdotally reported in the literature. The transealing maneuver, performed between the aortic wall and the endograft, must allow for the passage of a guiding catheter (typically introduced via a brachial access; however, thanks to modern steerable catheters, femoral access is also feasible). Within this catheter, a microcatheter is advanced, which must securely reach the refilled aortic chamber (Figure 6.3). A sacculography is then performed to confirm the diagnosis, assess the dimensions and extent of the cavity, and identify the presence of other types of endoleaks. Embolization is then carried out using glues, embolic agents, or coils. At the end of the procedure, the proximal neck sealing should be reassured via molding ballooning (Figure 6.3a).

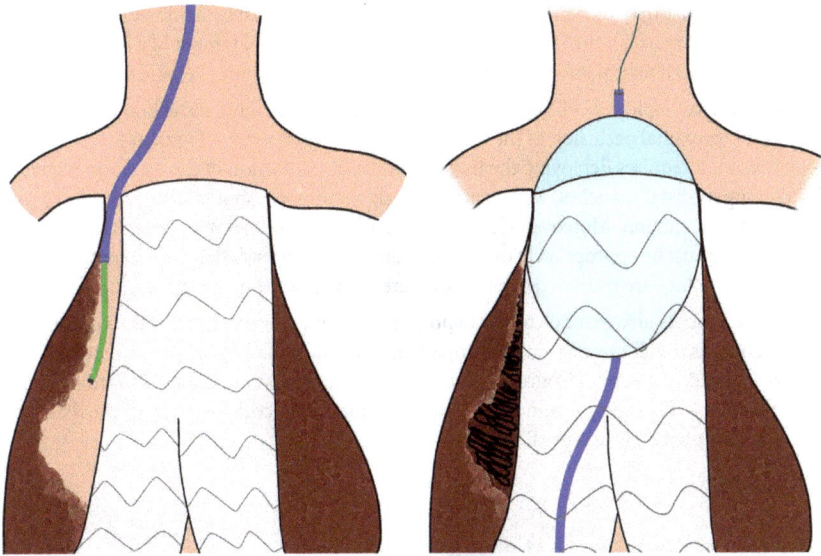

Figures 6.3–6.3a Bailout treatment of secondary Type 1A endoleak using embolization through the proximal transealing technique.

- In cases of persistent Type 1A endoleak, when therapeutic failure has occurred or endovascular techniques are deemed unfeasible, conversion to open surgery remains the only option. However, this procedure should be entrusted to high-volume centers specializing in complex aortic surgery. For an in-depth study of open surgical techniques in post-EVAR conversion surgery, I recommend reading an excellent volume authored by Chiesa R. et al. titled *Tips & Tricks in Open Vascular Surgery* (2016; Minerva Medica – Torino).

TIP #4

Type 1b Endoleaks: This tip will be very brief. The key point to remember is that the strategy for resolving this type of endoleak must focus on ensuring an adequate distal sealing zone along the affected iliac arteries.

For further details, please refer to the relevant Tips in Section 5.

TYPE 2 ENDOLEAKS

Hypogastric Artery Embolization

It is always advisable to perform preventive embolization of the hypogastric artery that will be covered by an endograft if the distal landing zone is located in the external iliac artery. The embolization technique will vary depending on the anatomical situation and the diameter of the hypogastric artery to be treated, as follows.

- Embolization of the common trunk of the hypogastric artery – shortly after its ostium – should be performed if the vessel is healthy and not involved in aneurysmal degeneration. In this case, its distal branches must be preserved, as they will ensure regular perfusion of the pelvic viscera through collateral circulation from the contralateral side (Figures 6.4–6.4a). The embolization of the common trunk of the hypogastric artery must be performed precisely and meticulously, avoiding the risk – especially when using coils – that they may migrate distally. Two approaches can be adopted for this purpose (see A. Sarcina in the References): the first method involves the distal deployment of a large-caliber coil, onto which smaller-caliber coils are then packed (Scaffolding Technique – Figure 6.4b).

- Alternatively, the first deployed coil can be anchored to the first emerging distal branch before proceeding with proximal occlusion of the trunk (Anchoring Technique – Figure 6.4c). While this technique is valid, it requires deploying the first coil in the distal portion of the common trunk, with the risk of occluding its distal branches, which, as previously mentioned, should be preserved. Therefore, it should be used with caution. Moreover, if embolization of the common trunk is performed using a plug instead of coils, it must be appropriately oversized relative to the artery's diameter to ensure effective wall fixation; generally, plugs are oversized by 50% compared to the target diameter.

- If the dilatative process also extends to the hypogastric artery, embolization of the common trunk is disadvantageous, as it will not guarantee complete exclusion of the hypogastric aneurysm, which, in this scenario, would be fed by retrograde circulations. In such cases, the appropriate – albeit more complex and time-consuming – solution is embolization using coils for each of the distal branches of the diseased hypogastric artery (Figure 6.4d).

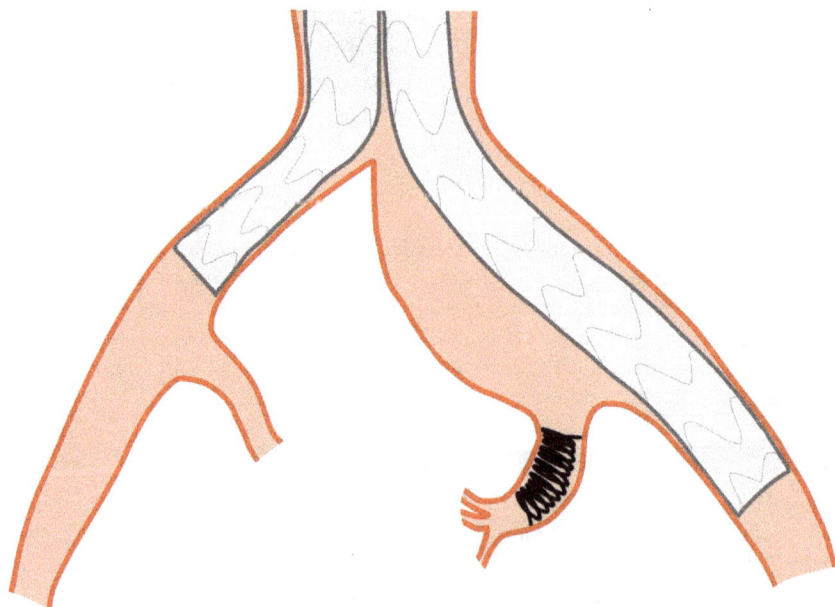

Figure 6.4 Hypogastric artery embolization techniques.

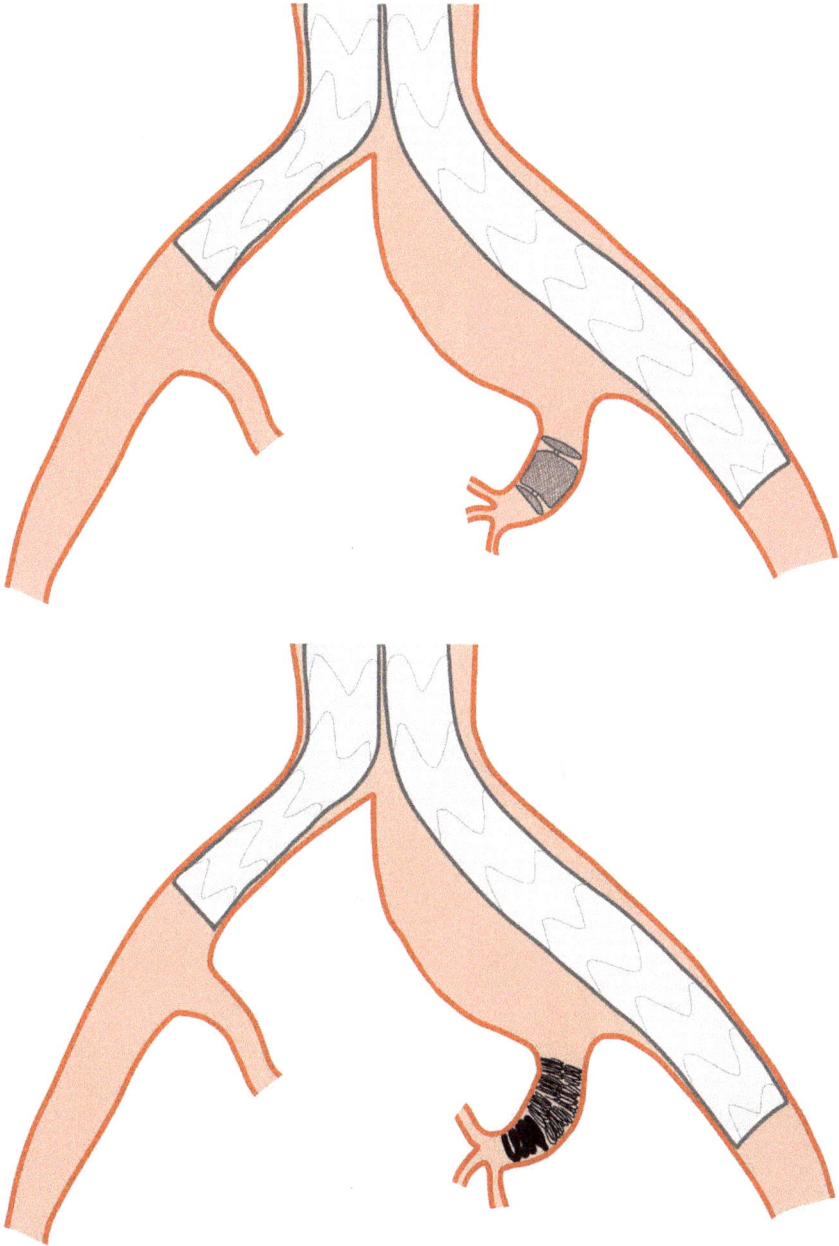

Figures 6.4a–6.4b (Continued)

It should be noted that a two-stage surgical approach can be considered if the patient is treated electively, and prolonged embolization times are expected. In Stage 1, only hypogastric embolization is performed, while in Stage 2, the EVAR procedure is carried out.

For further details regarding the management of iliac arteries involving the hypogastric arteries, refer to Section 5.

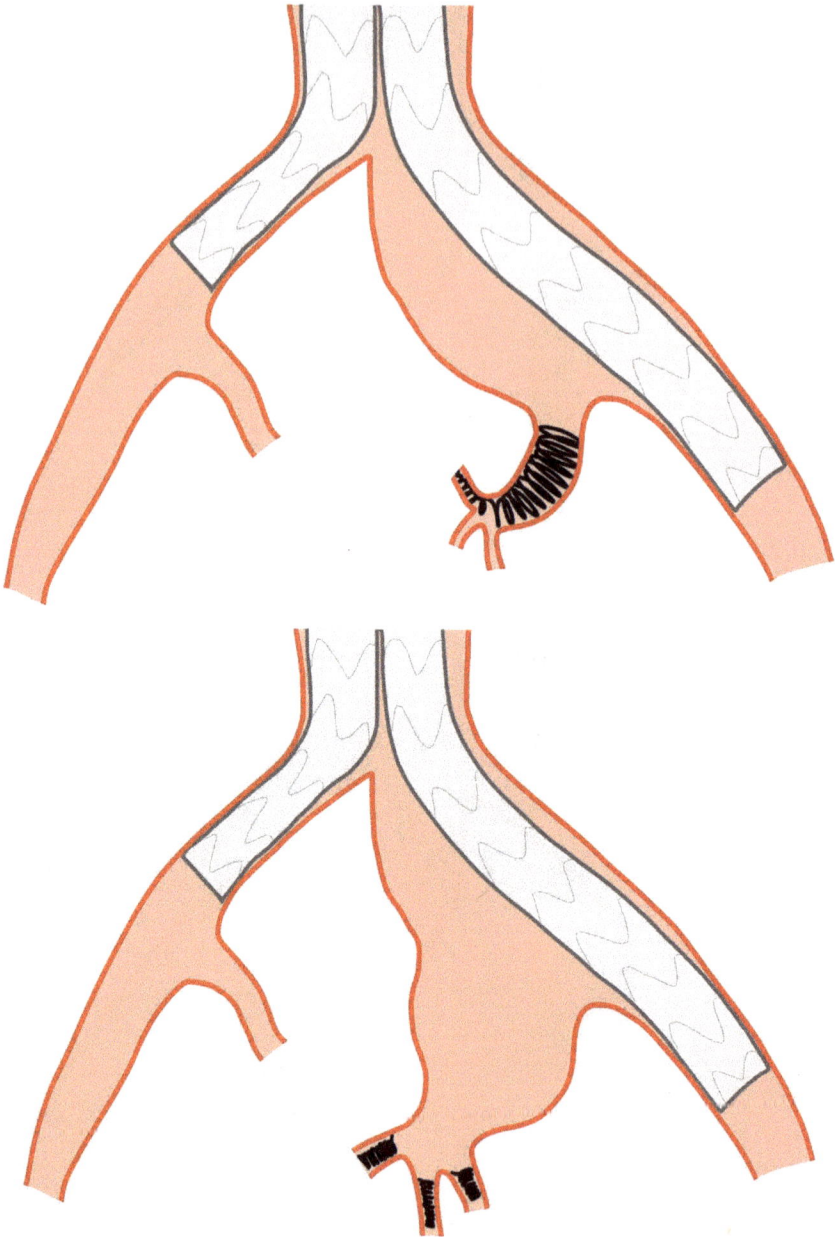

Figures 6.4c–6.4d (Continued)

TIP #6

Type 2 Endoleak Treatment

A detailed arteriography must be performed. For this purpose, in addition to an angiogram acquired from the aorta – if the preoperative CTA has not identified the branch supplying the endoleak – angiograms should also be obtained from the superior mesenteric artery and each hypogastric artery.

Angiographic acquisitions should be prolonged to allow contrast medium to reach the afferent branches of the leak and the nidus. Additionally, multiple projections, including steep oblique views, are recommended.

Angiography will often help us understand the behavior of the endoleak. It is now well established that Type 2 endoleaks – particularly those with multiple afferent and efferent branches – behave similarly to arteriovenous malformations, and their management should conceptually follow similar principles. In these cases, there will be one or more afferent branches feeding the nidus, followed by one or more efferent branches exiting from the aneurysm sac.

Ideally, the efferent branches should be embolized first, followed by the nidus, and finally the afferent branches.

Once embolization is complete, prolonged angiographic acquisitions should be repeated to rule out additional endoleaks that may have become evident after treating the most significant one. This is not an uncommon occurrence and underscores the need for continuous long-term follow-up after the procedure.

Techniques

If the Endoleak Originates from the Inferior Mesenteric Artery

- Gain a femoral access and cannulate the superior mesenteric artery using a catheter with an appropriate curve. The choice of catheter will depend on the angle at which the vessel originates from the aorta; the most commonly used catheters are the Cobra, SIM, IM, and RIM.
- If the aorto-mesenteric angle is excessively acute, a left brachial access may be considered, as it allows for direct anterograde navigation and provides greater support in such cases compared to the femoral approach.
- Once the superior mesenteric artery has been securely engaged, a guiding catheter is positioned within it to ensure adequate system stability.
- Using a coaxial system consisting of a 150 cm microcatheter and a 0.021" guidewire, the middle colic artery is catheterized, and the Riolan's arcade is traversed until reaching the inferior mesenteric artery. Alternatively, if the Riolan's arcade is not identifiable, of poor quality, or incomplete, the more peripheral marginal arcade of Drummond can be navigated – if feasible.

If the Endoleak Originates from Lumbar the Branches

- Preoperative CTA or angiography should be used to determine from which femoral artery and which hypogastric artery access should be obtained (Figure 6.5). The hypogastric artery that gives rise to the ilio-lumbar artery – supplying or connecting with the lumbar arteries responsible for the endoleak – should be selected as the access point to the sac.
- Once the hypogastric artery has been cannulated and adequate stability of the guiding system is achieved, a coaxial system consisting of a microcatheter and a 0.021" guidewire (preferably 150 cm in length in this case as well) is introduced to navigate through the ilio-lumbar artery and reach the sac via the lumbar branches targeted for embolization (Figure 6.5a).

(*Note*: The middle colic artery, Riolan's arcade, and the ilio-lumbar artery are small-caliber branches prone to spasm or arterial thrombosis. To prevent this, all necessary technical and pharmacological precautions – already described in *Tip #13* of Section 2 – should be taken.)

***

THE TRANSEALING TECHNIQUE

Through this technical expedient, it is possible – when the necessary conditions are met – to access the aneurysm sac by using the distal sealing zone of one of the two iliac modules as a *forced* entry point.

First, it is crucial to determine whether a suitable iliac artery is present. This evaluation is critical and should be conducted preoperatively, focusing – in order of importance – on the following anatomical and radiological findings:

- **Areas where the iliac endograft margin is not perfectly apposed to the arterial wall:** It is not uncommon – due to the aneurysm remodeling that occurs over weeks, months, or years after endograft implantation – for infolding or bird-beaking (or simply an imprecise apposition of the iliac module

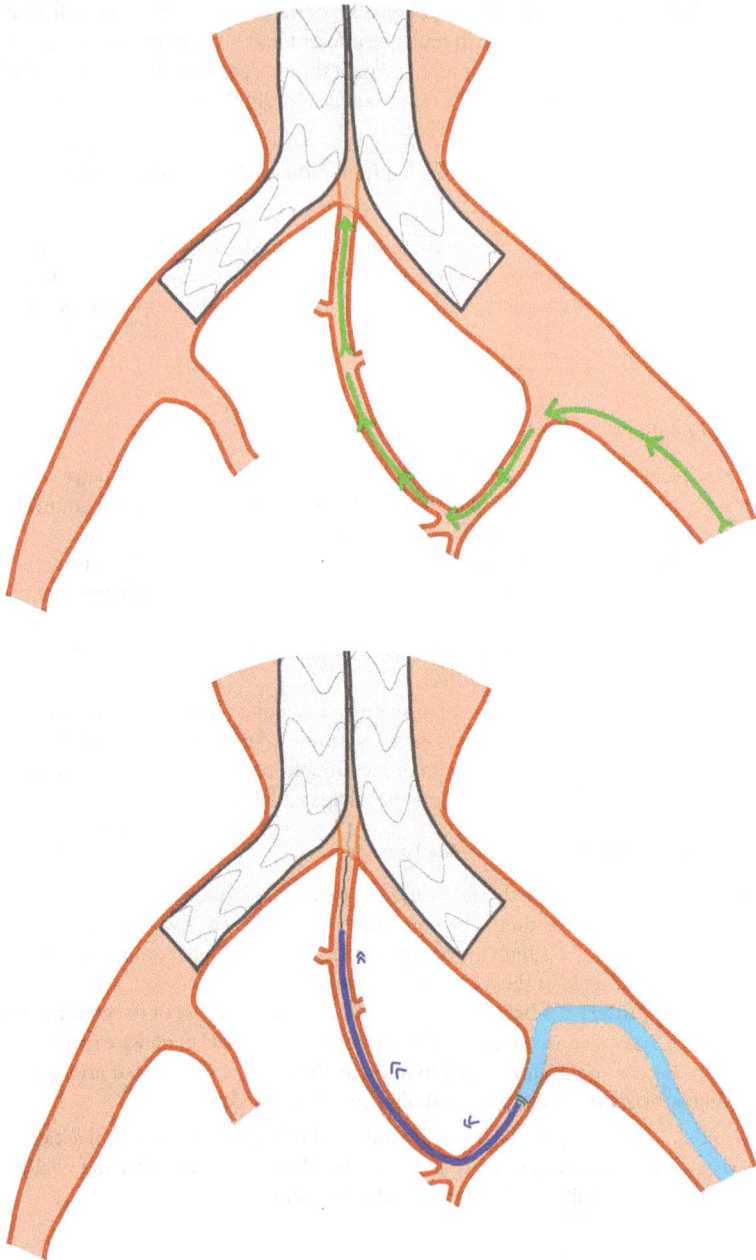

Figures 6.5–6.5a Type 2 endoleak treatment using the translumbar approach.

to the arterial wall) to develop along the iliac sealing zone. These areas can be leveraged as an actual gate to access the sac (Figure 6.6).

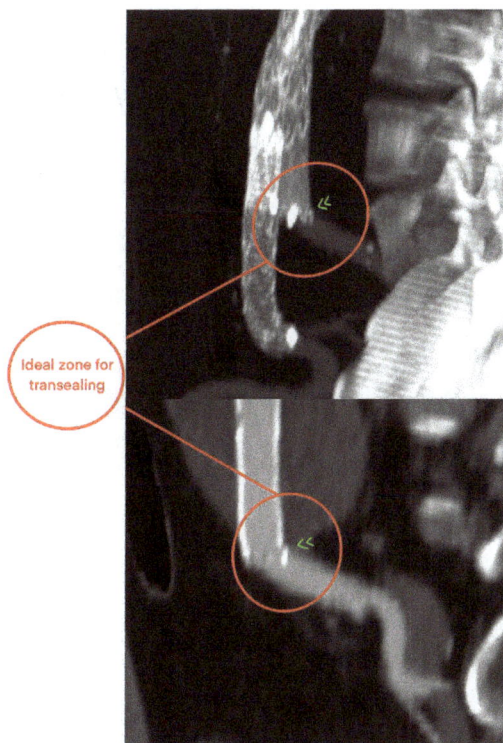

Figure 6.6 Treatment of Type II endoleak using the Transealing Technique.

- **Iliac modules landing in the common iliac artery**, as the Transealing Technique performed on the external iliac artery – often diseased or of small caliber – may lead to vessel wall complications.
- **The iliac axis converging toward the sac** from the side closest to the nidus.

Technical Steps of the Transealing Technique

1. The procedure begins with femoral arterial access on the side corresponding to the iliac artery to be navigated. An extra-stiff guidewire is positioned in the descending thoracic aorta to provide stable support. Over the extra-stiff guidewire, a 9 Fr long sheath is advanced. A second 0.035" hydrophilic guidewire is inserted into the sheath, parallel to the extra-stiff one.

2. A Bern catheter is loaded onto the hydrophilic guidewire. To support the catheter, the femoral sheath is positioned so that only the distal, angled portion of the Bern catheter emerges. The extra-stiff guidewire remains firmly in place in the descending thoracic aorta.

3. Instead of the Bern catheter, if available, a Piton GC catheter can be used. This catheter has two distal exit ports – one central and one lateral – and should be loaded onto both guidewires (hydrophilic and extra-stiff). The extra-stiff guidewire emerges from the lateral port of the Piton catheter, maintaining its position in the descending thoracic aorta, while the hydrophilic guidewire is used for navigation and exits from the catheter's central port.

4. Regardless of whether a Piton or Bern catheter is used, it must be directed toward the area where an apposition defect between the endograft and the arterial wall is identified. At this point, using the hydrophilic guidewire (acting like a Socratic gadfly!), access is forced into the plane between the endograft and the arterial wall, creating an entry passage (Figure 6.6a). This maneuver is similar to the subintimal technique commonly used for CTO recanalization. The goal is to advance the guidewire through this space until it reaches the aneurysm sac (Figure 6.6b).

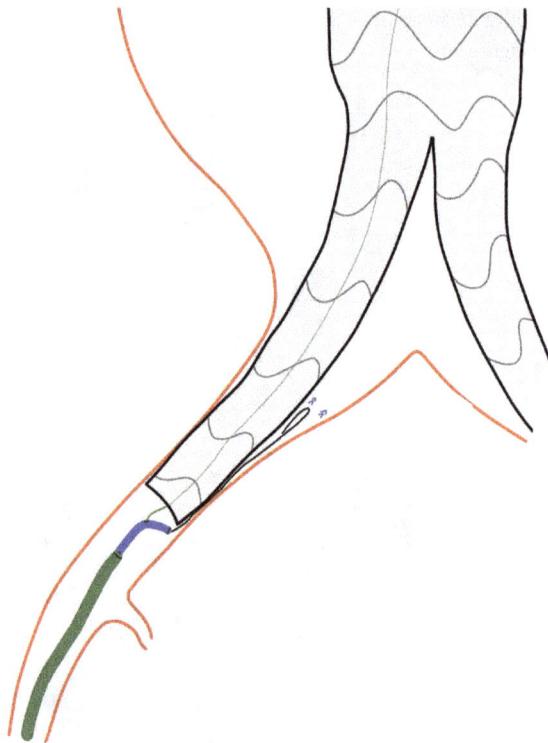

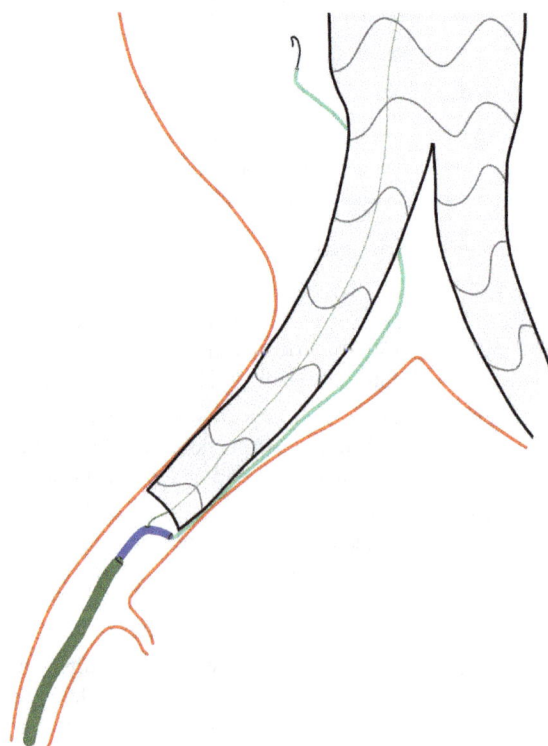

Figures 6.6a–6.6b (Continued)

5. Once the sac is reached, a 5 Fr long sheath is advanced into the nidus. In many cases, it will advance directly into it, while in other cases, additional guidewire and catheter maneuvers will be required. Correct positioning can be verified by observing backflow from the sheath's side port or by performing a sac angiography.

6. Once inside the sac, a sac angiography is performed to define the endoleak's characteristics, confirm its type (excluding other types of endoleaks), and plan the treatment. It is worth noting that sac angiography should not be performed using a power injector but rather with a syringe (personally, I prefer 10 cc syringes), using a controlled and steady push without excessive force. The embolization is carried out using glue, coils, or liquid embolic agents. (There is no definitive evidence favoring one material over the others.)

7. After embolization, and once the guidewire/catheter system has been removed from the sac, an aortic balloon is advanced over the extra-stiff guidewire and used to perform a molding ballooning of the entire iliac sealing zone affected by the procedure. This step is crucial for restoring the integrity of the apposition between the endograft and the arterial wall (Figure 6.6c).

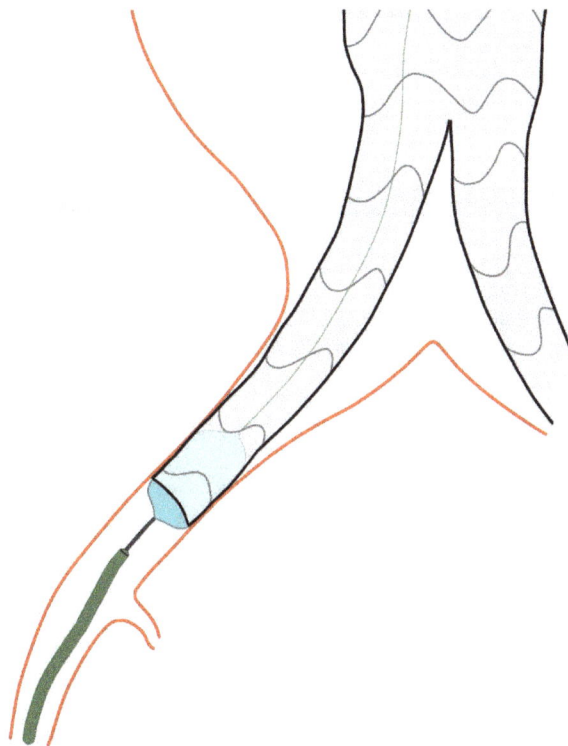

Figure 6.6c (Continued)

8. At the end of the procedure, an aortography is performed to rule out additional endoleaks. Particular attention should be given to identifying potential Type 1b endoleaks at the level of the iliac endograft module used as the access point.

(*Note:* The Transealing Technique is particularly useful in cases when preoperative CTA or initial aorto-arteriography does not reveal navigable lumbar or mesenteric collaterals for microcatheter access. In these cases, it allows for both diagnosing the endoleak via sac angiography and performing embolization in a single procedure.)

TYPE 3 ENDOLEAKS

TIP #7

Type 3a Endoleaks

The treatment of this type of endoleak usually involves relining the implant by interposing a bridging endograft, as previously described – both textually and iconographically – in *Tip #1* of Section 4.

The only two scenarios in which relining is not feasible are as follows.

- The iliac module disconnection is complete, and its proximal migration has occurred beyond the emergence of the gate of the main body (Figure 6.2b, Section 4). In this case, the therapeutic options include the following.
    1. Open surgery.
    2. Hybrid surgery involving the occlusion of the disconnected iliac module with a plug positioned in its proximal portion, followed by definitive exclusion of the sac through the placement of an aorto-uni-iliac endograft deployed via the contralateral iliac axis, combined with a crossover femoro–femoral bypass.

- A Type 3A endoleak occurs in Endologix AFX2 endografts, when, due to the specific design of this device, an endovascular resolution is not feasible, necessitating open surgery. For a detailed description, refer to the dedicated section in Section 4.

TIP #8

Type 3b Endoleaks

This type of endoleak, caused by a tear in the endograft fabric at the level of the aortic body or one of the iliac modules, should be treated by relining the main body or the iliac module responsible for the issue. This may sometimes require deploying a new bifurcated endograft within the existing one.

The treatment of this type of endoleak is imperative; therefore, if endovascular solutions are not feasible, an open or hybrid surgical approach must be planned.

Iatrogenic pseudoaneurysms of the femoral artery represent one of the most common complications of percutaneous procedures performed to treat peripheral arterial and cardiac diseases (following coronary, valvular, or – more rarely – electrophysiological interventions, the latter due to accidental puncture of the femoral artery).

Their management requires a thorough understanding of anatomical variations and the available therapeutic options, which must be tailored to the specific characteristics of the lesion that needs to be addressed.

MORPHOLOGICAL CLASSIFICATION

To simplify the therapeutic approach, I propose a classification derived from my clinical experience over many years and numerous treated cases, intended to provide practical and reproducible criteria. This classification identifies the following two main anatomical categories.

1. **Sessile Pseudoaneurysms (Type 1):** These are located adjacent to the femoral artery and are characterized by a broad implantation base on the artery, without a well-defined neck. The following two subtypes can be distinguished.
   a) **Type 1A (Figure 6.7):** The tract is of small caliber, its diameter usually measuring 1–2 mm.

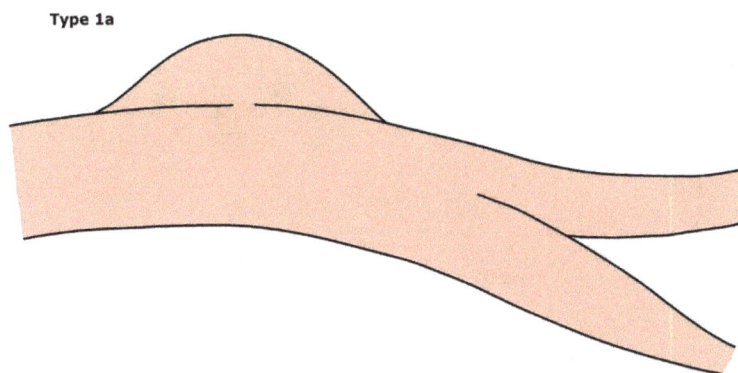

Figure 6.7 Type 1A pseudoaneurysm

   b) **Type 1B (Figure 6.7a):** The tract is larger than Type 1A, resembling an actual tear in the arterial wall.

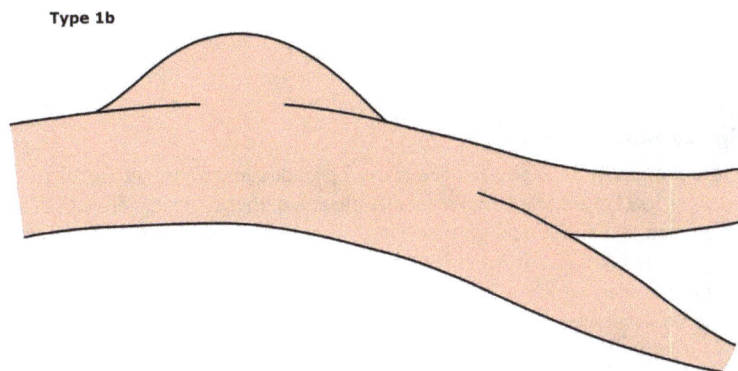

Figures 6.7a Type 1B pseudoaneurysm.

2. **Pedunculated Pseudoaneurysms (Type 2):** These are separated from the artery by a well-defined neck, whose length varies depending on the subtype.

    a)   **Type 2A** (Figure 6.8): Characterized by a short neck, less than 10 mm in length.

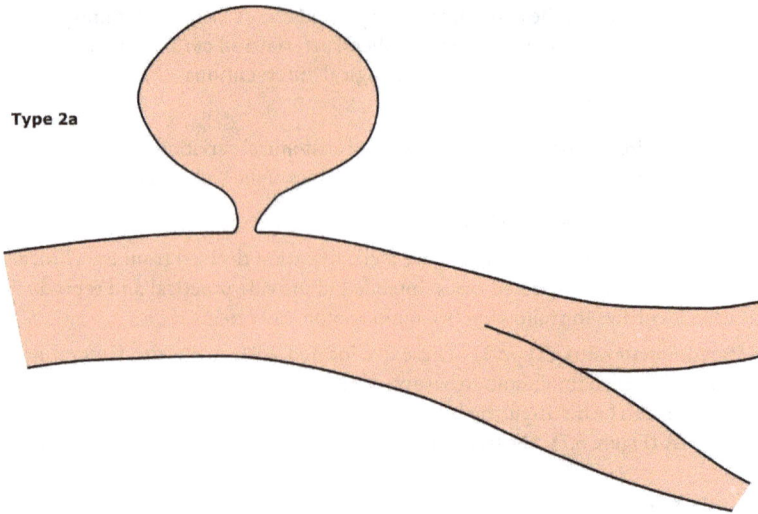

Type 2a

Figure 6.8 Type 2A pseudoaneurysm.

    b)   **Type 2B** (Figure 6.8a): Characterized by a longer neck than Type 2A

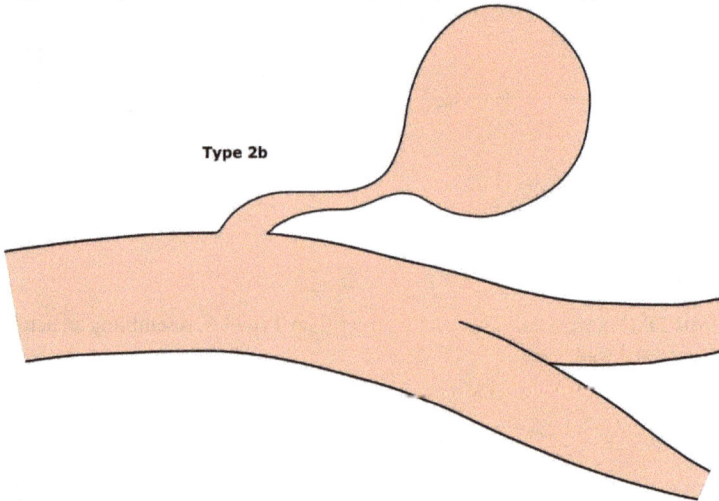

Type 2b

Figure 6.8a Type 2B pseudoaneurysm.

It is important to note that although multichambered pseudoaneurysms – characterized by multiple interconnected cavities (Figure 6.9) – are frequently observed, these variants do not affect the classification or the therapeutic management proposed here. From a treatment perspective, attention should be focused solely on the main sac, which is directly connected to the femoral artery via the neck. Treating this primary chamber, which is responsible for the high-pressure supply to the entire lesion, generally leads to spontaneous thrombosis of the other compartments.

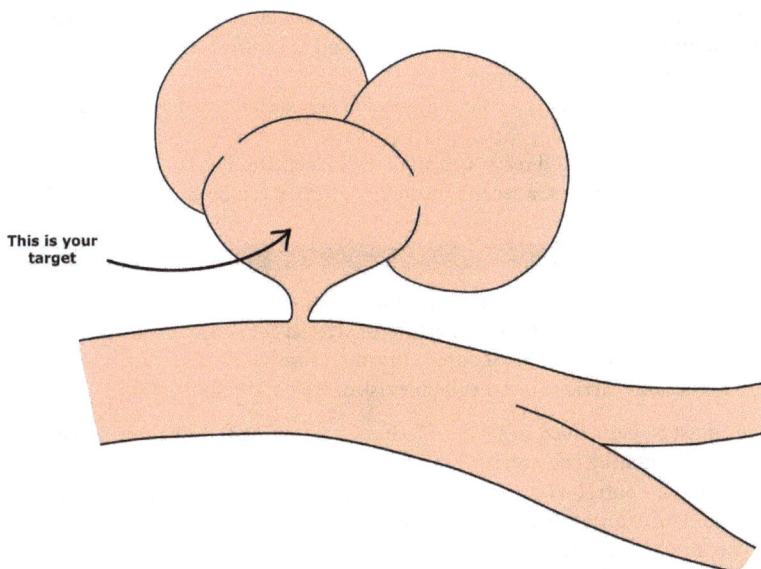

This is your target

Figure 6.9 In multichambered pseudoaneurysms, the target of treatment must be the chamber that communicates with the neck.

***

In text that follows, we will discuss several tips related to the treatment techniques for this type of lesions. Subsequently, I will propose a therapeutic approach, which in the author's experience has been associated with an exceptionally low rate of major complications.

TIP #9

Embolization of Pseudoaneurysms Using Thrombin Injection

This method should be used only for pseudoaneurysms with a pedunculated implantation base on the artery – thus, for Type 2, according to the classification just proposed. In the case of a sessile pseudoaneurysm, as we will see shortly, the risk of thrombin embolization into the arterial circulation is not negligible.

The necessary steps for a successful thrombin embolization are the following.

- Prepare a 1 ml syringe with 400 IU of thrombin (depending on the thrombin concentration in the vial used, draw 400 IU of thrombin and, if necessary, add sodium chloride to reach a total volume of 1 ml).
- This amount is generally sufficient to embolize a sac measuring up to 3–4 cm in diameter. Larger lesions may require a higher volume, while smaller ones may only need half the dose. Given the average size of the pseudoaneurysms encountered in practice, it is advisable to start with 400 IU of thrombin.
- The pseudoaneurysm sac should be punctured under ultrasound guidance using a 22G echogenic needle. It is crucial to pay close attention to the needle selection, as not all are perfectly echogenic. The risk is that the needle tip may not be clearly visible, which is essential to ensure it is not positioned inside the artery or adjacent to it. In the absence of specific alternatives, high-quality needles commonly used for distal retrograde arterial punctures are a good option. Alternatively, a butterfly needle can be used; in this case, the operator manages both the butterfly needle and the ultrasound probe, while a second operator handles the syringe and the injection of the thrombin mixture.
- If the pseudoaneurysm sac is multichambered, it is sufficient to embolize only the sac communicating with the neck. It is rarely necessary to embolize the others.
- Under continuous ultrasound monitoring, inject the thrombin mixture very slowly, 0.1–0.2 cc at a time (approximately 0.1 cc every 15 seconds), pausing for a few seconds between injections and using color Doppler to assess the progressive degree of thrombosis achieved.

- Only the strictly necessary amount should be injected, stopping as soon as thrombosis is complete. After a few minutes, re-evaluate the area with ultrasound to confirm complete sac obliteration or determine if an additional dose is required.
- At the end of the procedure, apply gentle compression and keep the patient on bed rest for at least 6 hours.
- The following day, an ultrasound reassessment of the treated area is recommended. If the pseudoaneurysm remains partially patent, a second thrombin injection can be attempted.

TIP #10

An elegant approach to pseudoaneurysm occlusion involves the use of percutaneous closure devices normally employed for post-procedural hemostasis of arterial access sites. This endovascular solution is particularly well suited for Type 1A pseudoaneurysms, as we have already discussed, since thrombin injection in sessile lesions carries a non-negligible risk of systemic embolization.

This technique must be performed in a hybrid fashion, combining fluoroscopic and ultrasound guidance, the latter facilitating percutaneous pseudoaneurysm cannulation and management; if needed, angiographic control via crossover access from the contralateral femoral artery can be obtained. This guidance can confirm the diagnosis and precisely define the lesion's location; it can also assist in completing the procedure once the guidewire has gained access to the arterial circulation, if other maneuvers are needed.

PROCEDURE STEPS

- The pseudoaneurysm sac is punctured with an angiographic needle under ultrasound guidance.
- With the needle held in a fixed position inside the pseudoaneurysm sac, the guidewire of a sheath is advanced into the sac (alternatively, a standard 0.035" Teflon-coated guidewire, such as the Emerald, can be used). Under ultrasound visualization, the guidewire is carefully maneuvered to cross the tract of the pseudoaneurysm, allowing access to the artery.
- A key technical tip is to orient the beveled edge of the needle downward, and similarly, the J-tip of the guidewire should also face downward. The maneuver consists of advancing the guidewire beyond the pseudoaneurysm tract and then retracting it while keeping its tip in contact with the lower wall of the sac (Figure 6.10). Once the guidewire engages the tract, it will "hook" onto it, allowing forward advancement into the arterial lumen (Figure 6.10a). The correct placement of the guidewire within the iliac–femoral axis is confirmed fluoroscopically.

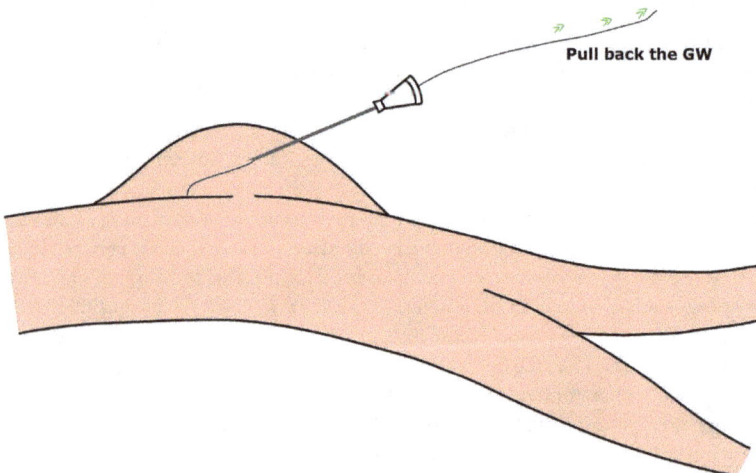

Pull back the GW

Figure 6.10 How to engage the tract with a ultrasound-guided guidewire for the treatment of pseudoaneurysms using a closure device.

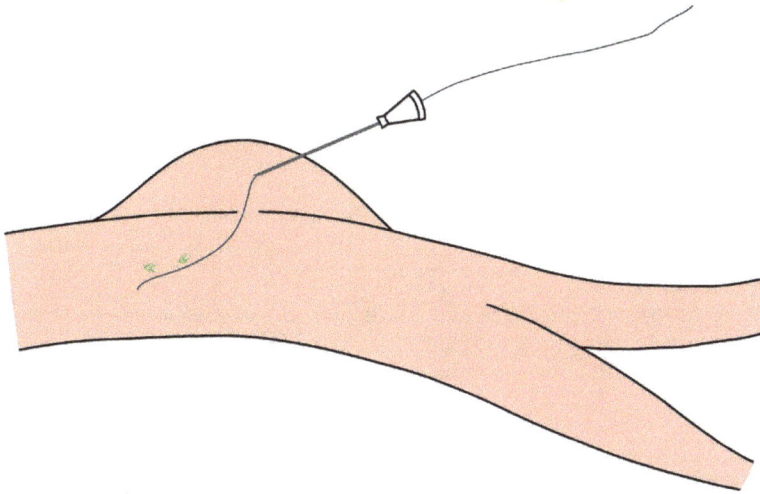

Figure 6.10a (Continued)

- At this point, a standard 6 Fr or 7 Fr sheath is advanced over the guidewire into the artery. Its position is confirmed by angiographic control.
- The procedure is completed by deploying the vascular closure device according to standard technique. By sealing the tract, the closure system achieves hemostasis and obliteration of the pseudoaneurysm. The most commonly used percutaneous closure system is ProGlide, but Angioseal and Femoseal have also been reported in the literature for this application.

It should be noted that the use of closure devices in this technique is off-label and has only been described in a limited number of reports. Therefore, it should be employed with caution and sound clinical judgment, exclusively by experienced operators and under strict ultrasound guidance.

TREATMENT STRATEGIES

The therapeutic approach proposed here varies according to the subtype of pseudoaneurysm and has been developed based on clinical experience accumulated over several years and multiple cases. The success rate is extremely high, with minimal complications.

TIP #11

Type 1A Pseudoaneurysms

1. At present, I consider open surgery the first-choice treatment for this type of lesion. As we will soon discuss, ultrasound-guided compression is not well suited for this variant, while thrombin injection poses a significant risk of reflux into the arterial circulation due to the broad implantation base and direct contact with the femoral artery, potentially leading to distal embolization.

2. Although technically challenging, an alternative could be percutaneous obliteration using closure devices such as ProGlide, FemoSeal, or AngioSeal, as previously described, following the recommendations already provided regarding the use of an off-label technique.

TIP #12

Type 1B Pseudoaneurysms

In this anatomical configuration, the best therapeutic option is surgery. The presence of a large tract prevents the use of closure devices, as they will not anchor properly to the tract walls. Thrombin injection is highly risky for the same reasons described for Subtype 1A. Ultrasound-guided compression is usually ineffective.

TIP #13

Type 2A Pseudoaneurysms

This configuration represents one of the most favorable anatomical scenarios for ultrasound-guided thrombin injection. The presence of the neck effectively isolates the sac from the artery, minimizing the risk of arterial embolization.

Percutaneous obliteration using closure devices, as previously described and with the same recommendations, can also be considered; however, the presence of the neck, even if short, may make cannulation of the femoral artery more challenging.

If the percutaneous approach proves ineffective or impractical, surgical intervention remains a valid alternative. In selected cases, ultrasound-guided manual compression can also be attempted, but the short neck may make it difficult to apply the necessary pressure to exclude the sac from the arterial circulation.

TIP #14

Type 2B Pseudoaneurysms

1. I consider ultrasound-guided manual compression the first-line treatment in this configuration. The length of the neck allows optimal positioning of the ultrasound probe, enabling compression of the neck and interruption of arterial flow to the sac. In fact, ultrasound-guided manual compression requires a key anatomical condition: the presence of a neck that can be effectively compressed externally. The neck should be the primary ultrasound target (Figure 6.11), as compressing only the sac is ineffective and does not stop the arterial flow feeding the pseudoaneurysm. This is the main reason for the high failure rate of this technique, which is often misapplied, resulting in considerable effort for the operator and discomfort for the patient. Compression with the probe should be maintained for the time required to achieve effective thrombosis of the sac, typically no less than 20–40 minutes. A rotation of multiple operators is advisable, with shifts every 5–7 minutes, ensuring that compressive force is not reduced and the probe position remains unchanged. If sealing of the lesion is not achieved within 60 minutes, the method should be abandoned.

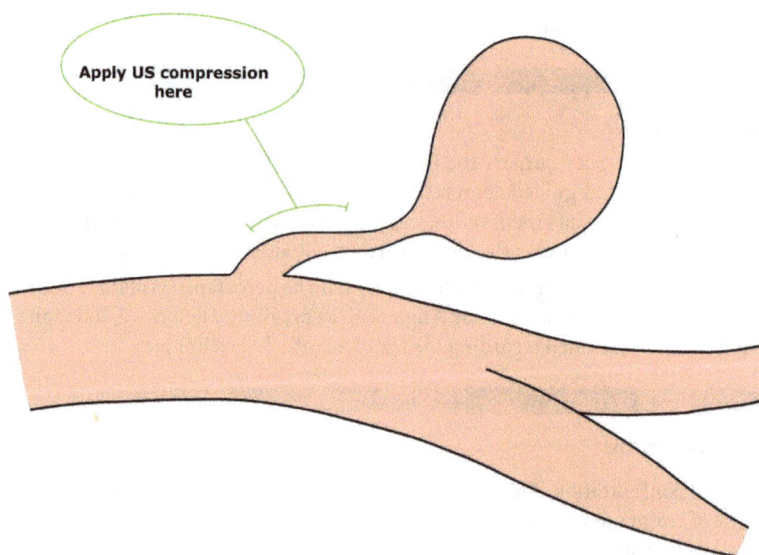

Apply US compression here

Figure 6.11 The correct location of ultrasound-guided compression for effective pseudoaneurysm treatment.

2. An alternative technique proposed by some authors involves hydrocompression of the subcutaneous tissue above the neck using a tumescent anesthetic solution (composed of 45 ml of sodium chloride and 15 mL of 1% lidocaine). The procedure then continues with standard ultrasound-guided compression. This approach offers the following two advantages.

   a) The tumescent solution assists and reinforces ultrasound-guided compression, leading to faster occlusion.

   b) The operator can apply less pressure on the skin, making the technique easier and less physically demanding. Additionally, the anesthesia improves patient comfort and pain tolerance.

3. If manual compression fails, ultrasound-guided thrombin injection remains a viable alternative, as this anatomical configuration provides a favorable safety profile.

4. As a last resort, surgical intervention is always an option, though the effectiveness of the described techniques makes it rarely necessary in this subtype.

TIP #15

In the case of a symptomatic pseudoaneurysm (pain, neurological symptoms due to femoral nerve compression) or rupture, the proposed subtypes become irrelevant, and the only feasible option is surgery. In these cases, the goal is not simply to resolve the issue by occluding the sac but rather to perform direct arterial repair through suture closure of the arterial breach, combined with sac evacuation and pseudoaneurysmectomy. Only in this way can the affected area be adequately decompressed, effectively resolving the neurological symptoms.

REFERENCES

1. Barton M, Grüntzig J, Husmann M, et al. Balloon angioplasty – the legacy of Andreas Grüntzig, M.D. (1939–1985). *Front Cardiovasc Med.* 2014; 1: 15.

2. Oliveira NFG, Oliveira-Pinto J, van Rijn MJ, et al. Risk factors, dynamics, and clinical consequences of aortic neck dilatation after standard endovascular aneurysm repair. *Eur J Vasc Endovasc Surg.* 2021; 62(1): 26–35.

3. Ahmad W, Weidler P, Salem O, et al. Implications of aortic neck dilation following thoracic endovascular aortic repair. *J Vasc Surg.* 2023; 78(6): 1402–1408.

4. Filis KA, Galyfos G, Sigala F, et al. Proximal aortic neck progression: Before and after abdominal aortic aneurysm treatment. *Front Surg.* 2017; 4: 23.

5. Chatzelas DA, Loutradis CN, Pitoulias AG, et al. A systematic review and meta-analysis of proximal aortic neck dilatation after endovascular abdominal aortic aneurysm repair. *J Vasc Surg.* 2023; 77(3): 941–956.

6. Mascoli C, Faggioli G, Gallitto, et al E. Tailored sac embolization during EVAR for preventing persistent type II endoleak. *Ann Vasc Surg.* 2021; 76: 293–301.

7. Chen Q, Zhang Y, Lei K, et al. Efficacy and safety of prophylactic intraoperative sac embolization in EVAR for abdominal aortic aneurysm: A meta-analysis. *Front Surg.* 2023; 9: 1027231.

8. Mathlouthi A, Yei K, Guajardo I, et al. Prophylactic perigraft arterial sac embolization during EVAR: Minimizing type II endoleaks and improving sac regression. *Ann Vasc Surg.* 2023; 93: 103–108.

9. Chun JY, de Haan M, Maleux G, et al. CIRSE standards of practice on management of endoleaks following endovascular aneurysm repair. *Cardiovasc Intervent Radiol.* 2024; 47(2): 161–176.

10. Abdulrasak M, Resch T, Sonesson B, et al. The long-term durability of intra-operatively placed palmaz stents for the treatment of type Ia endoleaks after EVAR of abdominal aortic aneurysm. *Eur J Vasc Endovasc Surg.* 2017; 53(1): 69–76.

11. Arthurs ZM, Lyden SP, Rajani RR, et al. Long-term outcomes of Palmaz stent placement for intraoperative type Ia endoleak during endovascular aneurysm repair. *Ann Vasc Surg.* 2011; 25(1): 120–126.

12. Qamhawi Z, Barge TF, Makris GC, et al. Editor's choice – systematic review of the use of endoanchors in endovascular aortic aneurysm repair. *Eur J Vasc Endovasc Surg.* 2020; 59(5): 748–756.

13. Arko FR 3rd, Stanley GA, Pearce BJ, et al. Endosuture aneurysm repair in patients treated with endurant II/IIs in conjunction with Heli-FX EndoAnchor implants for short-neck abdominal aortic aneurysm. *J Vasc Surg.* 2019; 70(3): 732–740.

14. Jordan WD Jr, Mehta M, Ouriel K, et al. One-year results of the ANCHOR trial of EndoAnchors for the prevention and treatment of aortic neck complications after endovascular aneurysm repair. *Vascular.* 2016; 24(2): 177–186.

15. de Vries JP, Ouriel K, Mehta M, et al. Analysis of EndoAnchors for endovascular aneurysm repair by indications for use. *J Vasc Surg.* 2014; 60(6): 1460–1467.

16. de Vries JP, Ouriel K, Mehta M, et al. Analysis of EndoAnchors for endovascular aneurysm repair by indications for use. *J Vasc Surg.* 2014; 60(6): 1460–1467.

17. Masoomi R, Lancaster E, Robinson A, et al. Safety of EndoAnchors in real-world use: A report from the manufacturer and user facility device experience database. *Vascular.* 2019; 27(5): 495–499.

18. Giudice R, Borghese O, Sbenaglia G, et al. The use of EndoAnchors in endovascular repair of abdominal aortic aneurysms with challenging proximal neck: Single-centre experience. *JRSM Cardiovasc Dis.* 2019; 8. doi: 10.1177/2048004019845508.

19. van Schaik TG, Meekel JP, Hoksbergen AWJ, et al. Systematic review of embolization of type I endoleaks using liquid embolic agents. *J Vasc Surg.* 2021; 74(3): 1024–1032.

20. Chaikof EL, Dalman RL, Eskandari MK, et al. The society for vascular surgery practice guidelines on the care of patients with an abdominal aortic aneurysm. *J Vasc Surg.* 2018; 67(1): 2–77.

21. Mangialardi N, Orrico M, Ronchey S, et al. Open conversion after EVAR. In: Chiesa R, Setacci C, editors. *Tips and Tricks in Open Vascular Surgery.* Torino: Edizioni Minerva Medica; 2017. pp. 42–45.

22. Ultee KHJ, Büttner S, Huurman R, et al. Editor's choice – systematic review and meta-analysis of the outcome of treatment for type II endoleak following endovascular aneurysm repair. *Eur J Vasc Endovasc Surg.* 2018; 56(6): 794–807.

23. Akmal MM, Pabittei DR, Prapassaro T, et al. A systematic review of the current status of interventions for type II endoleak after EVAR for abdominal aortic aneurysms. *Int J Surg.* 2021; 95: 106138.

24. Bryce Y, Lam CK, Ganguli S, et al. Step-by-step approach to management of type II endoleaks. *Tech Vasc Interv Radiol.* 2018; 21(3): 188–195.

25. Rampoldi A, Barbosa F. Embolizzazione preventiva delle arterie ipogastriche. In: Sarcina A, editors. *Endoleak di II Tipo Post-EVAR.* Torino: Edizioni Minerva Medica; 2015. pp. 32–36.

26. Görich J, Rilinger N, Sokiranski R, et al. Embolization of type II endoleaks fed by the inferior mesenteric artery: Using the superior mesenteric artery approach. *J Endovasc Ther.* 2000; 7(4): 297–301.

27. Coppi G, Saitta G, Coppi G, et al. Transealing: A novel and simple technique for embolization of type 2 endoleaks through direct sac access from the distal stent-graft landing zone. *Eur J Vasc Endovasc Surg.* 2014; 47(4): 394–401.

28. Webber GW, Jang J, Gustavson S, et al. Contemporary management of postcatheterization pseudoaneurysms. *Circulation.* 2007; 115(20): 2666–2674.

29. Jiaxin L, Yan L, Sheng Z, et al. Case report: Successful and effective percutaneous closure of a deep femoral artery pseudoaneurysm using proglide device. *Front Surg.* 2023; 10: 1109243.

30. Kodama T, Yamaguchi T, Fujiwara H, et al. Successful endovascular repair of complicated pseudoaneurysm using Perclose ProGlide: A novel concept. *Clin Case Rep.* 2022; 10(11): e6655.

31. Gong X, Zhang W, Sang L, et al. Successful treatment of a femoral pseudoaneurysm by ultrasonographically-guided application of a suture-mediated closure device. *J Clin Ultrasound.* 2021; 49(3): 286–289.

32. Coley BD, Roberts AC, Fellmeth BD, et al. Postangiographic femoral artery pseudoaneurysms: Further experience with US-guided compression repair. *Radiology.* 1995; 194(2): 307–311.

33. Algin O, Mustafayev A, Ozmen E. Iatrogenic superficial external pudendal artery pseudoaneurysm: Treatment with Doppler US-guided compression. *Iran J Radiol.* 2014; 11(2): e7228.

34. Fellmeth BD, Roberts AC, Bookstein JJ, et al. Postangiographic femoral artery injuries: Nonsurgical repair with US-guided compression. *Radiology.* 1991; 178(3): 671–675.

35. Kim KW, Lee C, Im G, et al. Optimal thrombin injection method for the treatment of femoral artery pseudoaneurysm. *J Thromb Haemost.* 2024; 22(5): 1389–1398.

36. Ergun O, Çeltikçi P, Güneş Tatar İ, et al. Percutaneous thrombin injection treatment of a femoral artery pseudoaneurysm with simultaneous arterial balloon occlusion: Case report and review of the literature. *Turk Kardiyol Dern Ars.* 2016; 44(8): 684–689.

37. Yoo T, Starr JE, Go MR, et al. Ultrasound-guided thrombin injection is a safe and effective treatment for femoral artery pseudoaneurysm in the morbidly obese. *Vasc Endovascular Surg.* 2017; 51(6): 368–372.

38. Kurzawski J, Janion-Sadowska A, Zandecki L, et al. Comparison of the efficacy and safety of two dosing protocols for ultrasound guided thrombin injection in patients with iatrogenic femoral pseudoaneurysms. *Eur J Vasc Endovasc Surg.* 2020; 59(6): 1019–1025.

39. Kuma S, Morisaki K, Kodama A, et al. Ultrasound-guided percutaneous thrombin injection for post-catheterization pseudoaneurysm. *Circ J.* 2015; 79(6): 1277–1281.

40. Jargiełło T, Sobstyl J, Światłowski Ł, et al. Ultrasound-guided thrombin injection in the management of pseudoaneurysm after percutaneous arterial access. *J Ultrason.* 2018; 18(73): 85–89.

INDEX

Note: Page numbers in *italics* indicate a figure on the corresponding page.

abdominal aortic aneurysms (AAAs), 129
  for challenging necks in, *see* necks, challenging, in AAAs
  endografts with infrarenal fixation, *see* infrarenal endograft
  endografts with suprarenal fixation, *see* suprarenal fixation, endografts with
  infrarenal, *see* infrarenal AAAs
acute arterial lesions
  completion angiography, 84, *84*
  femoral trifurcation, 82–85, *83*
  fresh lesion and chronic lesion, distinguishing, 81
  hybrid surgical techniques, 82
  mechanical thromboaspiration, 85
  primary stenting, 81, 82, *82*
  Rendezvous Technique, 84–85, *85*
  for stenting, 81, *82*
  thromboembolectomy, 83, *83*
ActiveSeal, 160
Anaconda endograft, 140, 155
anastomotic stenosis, PTA of, 79–81, *79*
Anchoring Technique, 196
AngioSeal, 17, 38, 209
aortic endoclamping, 134, *135*, 136
aortic endograft, 38, 109–113, 151
Aortic Neck Dilation (AND), 188
aortoiliac pathology
  brachial access
    advantages, 95
    disadvantages, 96
  in CTOs for iliac recanalization procedures, 92, 92–93
  dual access during iliac recanalization, 93, *93–95*, 95
  management of percutaneous access in, 92
  stenting of both iliac arteries via single femoral access, 95, *96*
aortoiliac stenoses
  balloon-expandable stent deployment, 97, *97*
  critical stenosis or CTO, 99, 99–100
  Crush Stent Technique, 105, *105–107*
  for eccentric and calcified lesions, 100
  during iliac catheterization, 100
  kissing stent approach, 100, *102*
  occlusion of common iliac artery, 103, *104*, 105
  during PTA, 103
  self-expanding stents, 103
  stenting of contralateral common iliac artery, 102–103, *102–103*
  V-stenting approach, 100, *101*

arterial lesions, *see* acute arterial lesions
arteriovenous fistula (AVF), 16, 58, 71, 136
atherectomy devices
  directional (excisional) atherectomy, 73
  laser atherectomy, 74
  orbital atherectomy, 73–74
  rotational atherectomy, 73
atraumatic balloons, 72–73, *72*

"ballerina" deployment, 138
Banana Technique, *177*, 177–178
Bell Bottom Technique, 174, *174*, 179
Bern catheter, 28, 31, 138, 201
BEVAR technique, 141, 162, 194
bird-beaking, 199
Bolton Treo, 127, 157, *157*
Buddy Wire Technique, 24–25, *25*, 70, 133

Cap Morphology, 42, *43*
catheters
  Bern-type catheter, 28, 31
  guiding catheters and long sheaths, 30
  with heparinized saline solution, 29
  homemade snare, 31–34, *31–34*
  during infrainguinal POBA, 36
  Mother and Child Technique, 30, *30*
  Pigtail or UF catheter, 29
  stenting of pre-occlusive stenoses/chronic occlusions, 35
  using a twisting maneuver, 28, *28*
CERAB (Covered Endovascular Reconstruction of the Aortic Bifurcation) Technique, 160
  aortic balloon to proximal portion of endograft, 109, *109*
  in aortic thrombosis, 112, *112*
  balloon-expandable covered stents, 113
  Chimney Technique, 112
  evaluating visceral circulation, 112
  in patients with Leriche syndrome, 112
  procedural technique, 108–111, *108–111*
  to reduce hemodynamic alterations, 108, 113
  use of Endologix AFX2 endograft, 112
challenging necks, in AAAs, *see* necks, challenging, in AAAs
Chimney Technique (ChEVAR), 150, *150–153*, 162
  Acute Aortic Syndromes, 153
  access strategy, 151
  aortic dissection, 153
  contraindications, 153

pararenal aortic PAU, 153
preoperative planning, 151
risk of complications, 150
stenting, 153
technical procedure, 151
stent types, 153
Chocolate balloon, 72–73
chronic limb-threatening ischemia (CLTI), 42, 81
chronic total occlusion (CTO), 21
  critical stenosis, 99, 99–100
  crossing algorithm, see CTO crossing algorithm
  guidewires, see CTO guidewires
  for iliac recanalization procedures, 92, 92–93
  proximal cap of, 21–23, 21–23
  recanalization, see CTO recanalization, CTO
    recanalization, complex
  types, 42–43
common femoral artery (CFA), 8, 17
  for antegrade access, 6, 66, 67
  hydrophilic guidewire into, 12
  post-TEA restenosis of, 72
  quality of ipsilateral, 4
  vessel preparation of, 73
contralateral gate cannulation
  Anaconda endograft implantation, 140
  "ballerina" deployment, 138
  cannulation of, 136, 138, 138, 139, 140
  catheter use, 137–138
  extended procedural times, 137
  preoperative CT angiography, 137, 137–138
  snare use, 141
Cook Zenith, 127, 158, 174, 191
Cordis Incraft, 158
Crush Balloon Technique, 52, 52
Crush Stent Technique, 105, 105–107
CTO crossing algorithm, 65, 65
  management techniques, 65
  with PTA catheter, 66–68, 67, 68
CTO guidewires
  characteristics of
    lubricity, 44
    penetrability, 44
    pushability, 43
    steerability, 44
    torquability, 44
    trackability, 43
  escalation, 44
    drilling, 46, 46
    perforating, 47, 47
    sliding, 45, 45
  for high tip-load guidewires, 51, 51
  re-entry, 50–52
  subintimal technique, 48–50, 49
CTO recanalization
  angiography, 42
  clinical practice, 42
  crossing algorithm, 42–43
  CTOP classification, 42–44, 43
  guidewires, see CTO guidewires

subintimal technique, 48, 50
supportive catheter use, 44
CTO recanalization, complex
  0.014" guidewires, 64
  access, 64
  advanced subintimal techniques, 52–55
    Crush Balloon Technique, 52, 52
    Double Balloon Technique, 54–55, 55
    Parallel Wire Technique, 53, 53
    SAFARI Technique, 53–55, 53
  imaging
    angiography, 63
    anteroposterior projection, 63, 64
    lateral projection, 61, 63
  nitrates, 64
  pedal plantar loop, 61, 62–63
  retrograde recanalization techniques, 55–58
    access, 64
    accessing SFA, 58
    advancing guidewire, 58
    anteroposterior projection, 63, 63–64
    arterial spasm prevention, 56
    choice of needle, 58
    flossing wire technique, 58
    fluoroscopic puncture, 56
    hemostasis, 58
    nitroglycerin solution, 56–58
    popliteal artery access, 58
    recanalization tips, 63
    retrograde puncture of tibial, peroneal, or dorsalis
      pedis arteries, 56
    sheathless technique, 58
    ultrasound-guided puncture, 56
  transcollateral technique, 58, 59–61, 60–61
Custom Seal, 161, 161
cutting balloons, 71, 71–72

de novo lesions, 78
Diamondback 360, 73
directional (excisional) atherectomy, 73
distal embolization, 81
"dogbone effect," 69, 69
Double Balloon Technique, 52, 55, 55
Drilling Technique, 46, 46, 65
drug-coated balloons (DCBs), 68, 70, 73
  deployment, 78–79, 78
  long sheaths or guiding catheters use, 79
  use of,, 78–80
  and vessel diameter, 79, 79
"Dumbbell Aorta," 149, 149

Emboshield NAV6 (Abbott), 75
EndoAnchors, 189, 191, 193
Endoconduit Technique, 130, 131, 132, 133
endoleak treatment, 188–189
  Type IA endoleaks, 189–195
    Heli-FX EndoAnchor system, 190–194, 191–193
    primary Type IA endoleaks, 189, 190
    secondary Type IA endoleaks, 194–195, 195

Type Ib endoleaks, 195
Type II endoleaks, 197–203
    hypogastric artery embolization, 196–197, *196–198*
    Transealing Technique, 199, 201, *202*, 203, *203*
    treatment, 198–199, *200*
Endologix AFX2,158, *159*
Endologix ALTO, 160–161, *161*
Endologix Nellix, 162, *163*
Endowedge Technique, 145–146, *146*, 155

FemoSeal, 17, 37, 209
FEVAR technique, 38, 141, 162, 194
Flossing Wire Technique, 55, 58, 67, 93, 133
Fogarty catheter, 82, 83

Gore Excluder, *154*, 154–155
guidewires
    Bern or Straight catheter, 26, *26*
    Buddy Wire Technique, 24–25, *25*
    guidewire bending, 23–24, *24*
        Boston V18, 23
        double bend, *23*, 24
        J-curve, *23*, 24
        single bend, *23*, 24
    high tip-load guidewires, 21
    hydrophilic guidewires, *20*, 20–21
    from interventional cardiology, 26
    nitrile gloves, 21
    proximal cap of CTO, 21–23, *21–23*
    reverse-curved bend, 26, *26*
    Reverse Wire Technique, 26, *26,*

Hawk systems, 73
Heli-FX EndoAnchor system, 190–194, *191–193*
hemorrhage, 80, 134
hemostasis for percutaneous access
    adhesive bandage, 37
    for antegrade accesses, 38
    closure devices, 38
    for large arterial accesses, 38
    manual compression, 37
hockey stick probe, 56
homemade snare, 31–34, *31–34*
    alternative method, 33–35, *33–35*
hypogastric aneurysms
    Type 0, *183*, 183
    Type 1, *183*, 183
    Type 2, *184*, 184
    Type 3, 184, *184*

iatrogenic femoral pseudoaneurysms, percutaneous treatment of
    embolization with thrombin injection, 208
    morphological classification, 205–208
        pedunculated pseudoaneurysms (Type II), *206*, 206–208
        sessile pseudoaneurysms (Type I), 205–208, *208*

pseudoaneurysm occlusion, 208–211, *210*
symptomatic pseudoaneurysm, 211
treatment strategies, 209
Type IA pseudoaneurysms, 209
Type IB pseudoaneurysms, 209
Type IIA pseudoaneurysms, 210
Type IIB pseudoaneurysms, *210*, 210–211
iliac aneurysms, management of
    algorithm for, 178
        Type 0a, 178
        Type 0b, 178–179
        Type 1a, 179
        Type 1b, 179
        Type 2, 179–181, *180*, *181*
        Type 3, 184, *184*
    of hypogastric aneurysms, *see* hypogastric aneurysms
    isolated aneurysms of the iliac arteries, *see* isolated iliac aneurysms
iliac arteries, management of
    calcifications, 133
    iliac stenosis, 130, *131–132*, 133
    occlusions, 133–134, *134*
    tortuosities, 133
iliac–femoral recanalizations, 114
    5 Fr sheath placement, 114
    arms away from radiation, 114
    CTO recanalization, 114–115
    during endarterectomy, 115, *115–118*
    endovascular phase targets, 118–120
    femoropopliteal axis, 118
    hemostasis of surgical site, 120, *120*
    hybrid revascularization procedures, 114
    into proximal segment, 120, *120*
    puncture techniques, 119, *120*
    service access, 120, *120*
iliac stenosis, 130, *131–132*, 133
    Endoconduit Technique, 130, *131*, *132*, 133
    endografts, low-profile, 130
    Open Conduit Technique, 130, *131*, *132*
    Paving & Cracking Technique, 130
    progressive dilation, 130
    PTA, 130
inferior mesenteric artery (IMA), 112, 129, 199
infrarenal AAAs
    accessory renal arteries, 129
    aortic endoclamping, 134, *135*, 136, *136*
    contralateral gate cannulation, 136–143
    during EVAR procedure, 127
    Flossing Technique with brachial access, 128–129, *128*
    iliac extension within aneurysmal sac, 124, *124–126*
    during intraoperative phase, 127, *127*
    iliac artery management, 129–134
    in residual stenosis, 127, *128*
    of superior mesenteric artery (SMA), 129
    in trimodular endograft, 126, *126*
infrarenal endografts
    algorithm for selecting, 162, 164–166, *166*
    complications, 153

Gore Excluder, *154*, 154–155
Terumo Anaconda, 155, *155*
intravascular lithotripsy, *see* Shockwave system
isolated iliac aneurysms
    Banana Technique, *177*, 177–178
    Bell Bottom Technique, 174, *174*
    classification of, 172, *172*
    in iliac artery aneurysms, 174
    in hypogastric artery branching, 174
    in isolated iliac aneurysm, 174
    Sandwich Technique, 174–177, *175–176*
    types and subtypes of, 172–173, *172–173*

Jetstream, 73
Jotec E-Tegra, 162

Kilt Technique, 147–150, *148–150*
Kissing Balloon Technique, 70, 108, 151, 176
kissing stent approach, 100, *102*

laser atherectomy, 74

Manta system, 38
Medtronic Endurant II, 157
micrometric-release stents, 81
Mother and Child Technique, 30, *30*
MynxGrip and MynxControl, 37

necks, challenging, in AAAs
    aortic cuff, 147,
    aneurysm curvature of, *143*
    Chimney Technique, *see* Chimney Technique
    with contemporary endograft molding ballooning
      and releasing, 144, *144*
    defined, 141
    "Dumbbell Aorta," 149, *149*
    endograft deployment, 142
    Endowedge Technique, 145–146, *146*
    establishment of EVAR, 141
    extra-stiff guidewire, *144–145*
    with FEVAR/BEVAR techniques, 141
    Gore Excluder, 145
    highly angulated aorta, 147, *147–148*
    Kilt Technique, 147–148, *148*
    microscalloping, 145–147
    neck angle calculation, 141, *141*
    Type IA endoleak, risk of developing, 141

Open Conduit Technique, 130, *131, 132*
orbital atherectomy, 73–74

Palmaz stent, 189, 194
Parallel Wire Technique, 53, *53*
Pararenal aortic ulcers (PAUs), 160
Paving & Cracking Technique, 130
pedal plantar loop, 61, *62–63*
percutaneous access
    antegrade access
      under fluoroscopy, *7*, 7–10

guidewire into profunda femoral artery, 7, 8, *8*
guidewire into superficial femoral artery, 9, *9, 10*
for infrainguinal pathology, 4
injecting contrast, 10
at origin of SFA, 4–5
removing catheter, 10
aortic bifurcation, 4, 12, 38
in aortoiliac pathology, *see* aortoiliac pathology
axillary access
    contraindications for, 16
    under ultrasound guidance, 16, *16*
brachial access
    indications for, 14
    steps, 14–15, *14–15*
calcification of arterial wall, 18
femoral puncture, anatomy of, 17, *17*
fully fluoroscopic femoral access, 16–17
fully ultrasound-guided technique, 16–17
hybrid approach
    initial fluoroscopic guidance, 17
    pre-procedural ultrasound mapping, 17
    reverse hybrid approach, 18
    with ultrasound guidance, 18
introducer into artery resistance, 18–19, *18–19*
planning access, 4
retrograde femoral access, 4
    crossover access, 10–12
    under fluoroscopy, 10
    navigating difficult bifurcation crossings,
      12–13, *13*
ultrasound-guided arterial puncture, 5–7
percutaneous transluminal angioplasty (PTA)
of anastomotic stenosis, 80, *80*
aortoiliac stenoses and occlusions during, 103
catheter, CTO crossing algorithm, 66–67, *67*
iliac stenosis, 130
wall injury from, 68, *68*
Perforating Technique, 47, *47*
Pigtail catheter, 11, 29, 114, 138
popliteal aneurysms
    endovascular feasibility, 86
    using endovascular technique, 86
popliteal CTOs, 73
Preclose Technique, 38
ProGlide, 38, 209
pseudoaneurysm formation, 80

radiation protection principles
    bed position, 2, *2*
    digital zoom, 3
    fluoroscopic imaging, 3
    image field using collimation, 2, *2*
    intervention plan, 4
    positioning protective devices, 2
    pulsed fluoroscopy, 3
    radiation-protective shields, 3, *3*
    ultrasound-guided arterial puncture, 3
Railroad Technique, 14
Rendezvous Technique, 84, *85*

restenoses, 78

Reverse Wire Technique, 26, *26,*

Rotarex (BD), 73

rotational atherectomy, 73

ruptured abdominal aortic aneurysms (rAAA), 136

sacculography, 195

SAFARI (Subintimal Arterial Flossing with Antegrade–
    Retrograde Intervention) Technique, 52–55, *53,*
    58, 95

Sandwich Technique, 174–179, *175–176,* 183

Scaffolding Technique, 196, *196*

self-expanding, closed-cell stents, 81

self-expanding covered stents, 82

Shockwave system, 74

Sirolimus, 78

Sliding Technique, 45, *45,* 65

snare, 139, *see also* homemade snare

SpiderFx (Medtronic), 75

Supera Stent, 70

superficial femoral artery (SFA)

    for antegrade access, 6

    antegrade puncture, *10, 10*

    de novo lesions in, 74

    femoral trifurcation, 75–76

    origin of, 5, 7, 72

    patency of, 4

    proximal, 66

    thrombosis of, 81

superior mesenteric artery (SMA), 112, 129, 198, 199

suprarenal fixation, endografts with

    Cook Zenith, 158

    Cordis Incraft, 158

    Endologix AFX2, 158–161, *159*

    Endologix ALTO, 160–162, *161*

    Endologix Nellix, 161, *163*

    Jotec E-Tegra, 162

    Medtronic Endurant II, 157

    Terumo Bolton Treo, 157, *157*

Teleflex, 38

Tensoplast, 37

Terumo Anaconda, 155, *155*

Terumo Bolton Treo, 157, *157*

thromboembolectomy, 83, *83*

thrombosis or embolization, 81

Transcollateral Technique, 58, *59–61,* 60–61

Transealing Technique, 199, 201, *202,* 203, *203*

    tortuosities, 133

UF catheter, 29

ultrasound-guided arterial puncture, 5

    guidewire into superficial femoral artery, 6

    needle, advancement 6

    needle control, 6

    positioning the probe, 5–6, *5–6*

    pre-puncture scanning, 5

vessel preparation

    atherectomy devices

        directional (excisional) atherectomy, 73

        laser atherectomy, 74

        orbital atherectomy, 73–74

        rotational atherectomy, 73

    atraumatic balloons, 72–73, *72*

    cutting balloons, *71,* 71–72

    and infrainguinal pathology, 74–78

        endovascular treatment of popliteal aneurysms,
            77, *77*

        femoral trifurcation endarterectomy, 76, *76*

        occlusions characterized by fresh thrombosis,
            76, 76

        placement in the deep femoral artery, 75, *75*

        use of distal filters, 74, *75–77*

    objectives of, 68

    rationale for, 68–70

        in highly calcified lesions, 70

        pressure distribution and "dogbone effect," 69, *69*

        restenosis and recoil risks, 70

        wall injury from traditional PTA, 68, *68*

    Shockwave system, 74

    scoring balloons, 72, *72*

    Ten Commandments for, 70–71, *71*

V-stenting approach, 100, *101*

W-shaped stent configuration, 156, 162

Z-shaped stent designs, 156

For Product Safety Concerns and Information please contact our EU
representative GPSR@taylorandfrancis.com
Taylor & Francis Verlag GmbH, Kaufingerstraße 24, 80331 München, Germany